The Role of Cholesterol in Atherosclerosis: New Therapeutic Opportunities

Merck Sharp & Dohme International
Medical Advisory Council
New Milton, Hampshire, England

July 13–14, 1987

Editors

Scott M. Grundy, M.D.
Alexander G. Bearn, M.D.

Hanley & Belfus, Inc.   Philadelphia

Library of Congress Cataloging-in-Publication Data
Main entry under title:

The role of cholesterol in atherosclerosis.

    "Merck Sharp & Dohme International Medical Advisory Council, New Milton, Hampshire, England, July 13-14, 1987.
    Includes bibliographies and index.
    1. Atherosclerosis—Congresses.   2. Cholesterol—Physiological effects—Congresses.   3. Anticholesteremic agents—Congresses.   4. Blood lipoproteins—Congresses.
    I. Grundy, Scott M.   II. Bearn, Alexander G., 1923–
III. Medical Advisory Council (Merck, Sharp & Dohme International)
RC692.R65   1988   616.1'36071   87-33542
ISBN 0-932883-13-3

Published by Hanley & Belfus, Inc., 210 South 13th Street, Philadelphia, Pennsylvania 19107, USA

Contents

v

Contributors and Participants

ALFRED W. ALBERTS, B.S.
Distinguished Senior Scientist
Biochemical Regulation Department
Merck Sharp & Dohme
Research Laboratories
Rahway, New Jersey, U.S.A.

A. WILLIAM ASSCHER, M.D.,
  F.R.C.P.
Professor
Department of Renal Medicine
University of Wales College of Medicine
Royal Infirmary
Cardiff, Wales, U.K.

SIR RICHARD BAYLISS, K.C.V.O.,
  M.D., F.R.C.P.
Honorary Consultant Physician and
  Endocrinologist
Westminster Hospital
London, England, U.K.

ALEXANDER G. BEARN, M.D.,
  F.R.C.P.
Senior Vice President
Medical & Scientific Affairs
Merck Sharp & Dohme International
Rahway, New Jersey, U.S.A.

KONRAD E. BLOCH, Ph.D.
Higgins Professor of Biochemistry
Conant Laboratories
Department of Chemistry
Harvard University
Cambridge, Massachusetts, U.S.A.

C. BOYD CLARKE
Senior Director, Cardiovascular Products
Corporate Human Health Marketing
Merck & Co., Inc.
Rahway, New Jersey, U.S.A.

JAMES I. CLEEMAN, M.D.
Coordinator
National Cholesterol Education Program
National Heart, Lung, and Blood
  Institute
National Institutes of Health
Bethesda, Maryland, U.S.A.

PIERRE CORVOL, M.D.
Director
Vascular Pathology and Renal
  Endocrinology Unit
Institut National de la Santé et de la
  Récherche Médicale
Paris, France

RAMZI S. COTRAN, M.D.
Chairman, Department of Pathology
Brigham and Women's Hospital
F.B. Mallory Professor of Pathology
Harvard Medical School
Boston, Massachusetts, U.S.A.

PROF. SIR COLIN T. DOLLERY,
  M.B., Ch.B., F.R.C.P.
Professor of Clinical Pharmacology
Department of Clinical Pharmacology
Royal Postgraduate Medical School
Hammersmith Hospital
London, England, U.K.

DETLEV GANTEN, M.D., Ph.D.
Professor, Department of Pharmacology
University of Heidelberg
Scientific Director, German Institute for
  High Blood Pressure Research
Heidelberg, West Germany

SCOTT M. GRUNDY, M.D., Ph.D.
Director, Center for Human Nutrition
Chairman, Department of Clinical
  Nutrition
University of Texas Health Science
  Center at Dallas
Dallas, Texas, U.S.A.

vii

JOEL W. HAY, Ph.D.
Senior Research Fellow
The Hoover Institution
Stanford University
Stanford, California, U.S.A.

HIROO IMURA, M.D.
Professor and Chairman
Second Division
Department of Medicine
Kyoto University
School of Medicine
Kyoto, Japan

COLIN I. JOHNSTON, M.B., B.S.,
   F.R.A.C.P.
Professor of Medicine
University of Melbourne
Austin Hospital
Heidelberg, Victoria, Australia

DESMOND G. JULIAN, M.D.,
   F.R.C.P.
Consultant Medical Director
British Heart Foundation
London, England, U.K.

MICHAEL J. S. LANGMAN, M.D.,
   F.R.C.P.
Professor of Internal Medicine
University of Birmingham
Queen Elizabeth Medical Centre
Birmingham, England, U.K.

LOUIS LASAGNA, M.D.
Dean, Sackler School of Graduate
   Biomedical Sciences
Director, Center for the Study of Drug
   Development
Tufts University
Boston, Massachusetts, U.S.A.

JOHN G. G. LEDINGHAM, M.D.,
   F.R.C.P.
May Reader in Medicine
University of Oxford
Honorary Consultant Physician
Oxford Area Health Authority
Oxford, England, U.K.

CLAUDE LENFANT, M.D.
Director, Department of Health and
   Human Services
National Institutes of Health
National Heart, Lung and Blood Institute
Bethesda, Maryland, U.S.A.

BARRY LEWIS, M.D., Ph.D., F.R.C.P.
Professor
Department of Clinical Pathology and
   Metabolic Disorders
St. Thomas's Hospital
London, England, U.K.

RUEDI P. LÜTHY, M.D.
Professor of Medicine
Chief, Division of Infectious Diseases
Department of Medicine
University Hospital
Zürich, Switzerland

ROBERT W. MAHLEY, M.D., Ph.D.
Director
Gladstone Foundation Laboratories for
   Cardiovascular Disease
Professor of Pathology and Medicine
University of California, San Francisco
San Francisco, California, U.S.A.

KALMAN C. MEZEY, M.D.
Clinical Professor of Medicine
University of Medicine & Dentistry of
   New Jersey
Newark, New Jersey, U.S.A.

J. MICHAEL MUNRO, M.B.B.S.
Research Fellow
Department of Pathology
Brigham and Women's Hospital
Harvard Medical School
Boston, Massachusetts, U.S.A

FEDERICO MONCLOA, M.D.
Group Director, Clinical Research
Merck Sharp & Dohme Research
   Laboratories
Woodbridge, New Jersey, U.S.A.

S. RAGNAR NORRBY, M.D., Ph.D.
Professor and Chairman
Department of Infectious Diseases
University of Umeå
Umeå University Hospital
Umeå, Sweden

DEREK K. NORTH, M.D., F.R.C.P.
Professor of Medicine
University of Auckland
Auckland, New Zealand

D. KEITH PETERS, M.B., F.R.C.P.
Regius Professor of Physic
University of Cambridge
Cambridge, U.K.

PHILIP A. POOLE-WILSON, M.D.,
   F.R.C.P.
Professor of Cardiology
The Cardiothoracic Institute and National
   Heart Hospital
London, England, U.K.

KALEVI PYÖRÄLÄ, M.D.
Professor
Internal Medicine
Clinical Medicine Department
University of Kuopio
Kuopio, Finland

JOHAN H. C. REIBER, Ph.D.
Director, Laboratory for Clinical and
   Experimental Image Processing
Thoraxcenter
Erasmus University Rotterdam
Rotterdam, The Netherlands

HEONIR ROCHA, M.D.
Head, Nephrology Department
Medical School of the Federal University
   of Bahia
Bahia, Brazil

FRANK M. SACKS, M.D.
Assistant Professor of Medicine
Brigham and Women's Hospital
Harvard Medical School
Boston, Massachusetts, U.S.A.

EVE E. SLATER, M.D.
Executive Director
Biochemistry & Molecular Biology
Merck Sharp & Dohme Research
   Laboratories
Rahway, New Jersey, U.S.A.
Associate Clinical Professor of Medicine
Columbia University College of
   Physicians and Surgeons
New York, New York, U.S.A.

ROBERT L. SMITH, Ph.D.
Senior Director of Medicinal Chemistry
Merck Sharp & Dohme
Research Laboratories
West Point, Pennsylvania, U.S.A.

THOMAS W. SMITH, M.D.
Chief, Cardiovascular Division
Brigham and Women's Hospital
Professor of Medicine
Harvard Medical School
Boston, Massachusetts, U.S.A.

PETER H. STONE, Ph.D
Associate Director,
Samuel A. Levine Cardiac Unit
Brigham and Women's Hospital
Assistant Professor of Medicine
Harvard Medical School
Boston, Massachusetts, U.S.A

KINSUKE TSUDA, M.D.
Department of Medicine
Kyoto University Faculty of Medicine
Kyoto, Japan

RICARDO VERONESI, M.D.
Professor of Infectious Diseases
Faculty of Medicine
University of São Paulo
São Paulo, Brazil

YAWARA YOSHITOSHI, M.D.
Director
The Japanese Red Cross Medical Center
Tokyo, Japan

Foreword

The ceaseless battle against disease is not confined to the boundaries of nations, nor is it likely that the outcome will be determined by the efforts of solitary genius. Medical science is cumulative, its revelations the end products of shared intellect and creative energy, which, when laced with serendipitous discovery, ultimately lead humankind nearer to solving the biological mysteries of life.

Throughout the world there have been ample rewards from this highly productive interaction as inquiring minds acting on new information from every corner have uncovered the root causes and pathological mechanisms of many elusive diseases and, in some cases, have developed new and dramatic medicines for their prevention or cure. Human beings, a bustling social species armed with the facility of language, cannot resist the expression of an idea; it is an idea codified in language and resilient to refutation that provokes and propels us onward.

But while the core of science is universal, medical practice and health needs vary greatly from country to country and from culture to culture. Thus, the Medical Advisory Council (MEDAC) was founded in 1973 as a forum for the discussion and evaluation of advances in medical science, changing trends in medical thinking, approaches to drug therapy, and the major issues confronting medicine throughout the world. The collective insights of MEDAC members, coupled with those of invited speakers, all chosen for their distinguished achievements in the fields of medicine and science, should provide a better understanding of the health needs of our times.

In these meetings we continue to exchange, "tossing into the center the products of our separate imaginations," to use the words of Dr. Lewis Thomas, Chancellor of Memorial Sloan-Kettering Cancer Center in New York. This is an ineluctable and satisfying process because it works. Dr. Thomas perhaps has said it best:

> It is in the abrupt, unaccountable aggregation of random notions, intuitions, known in science as good ideas, that the high points are made . . . an active field of science is like an immense anthill; the individual almost vanishes into the mass of minds tumbling over each other, carrying information from place to place, passing it around at the speed of light . . . (until) there suddenly emerges, with the purity of a slow phrase of music, a single new piece of truth about nature.

In this spirit, members of MEDAC convene annually, and in the exchange of facts, ideas, random notions, and intuitions, such as those that are presented in this volume, lies the exhilarating possibility that new truths about nature may emerge that in turn will help us as physicians to prevent disease and improve the health and welfare of our patients.

1

Opening Statement

When the program for this year's MEDAC meeting was planned, it was decided that a major part of the symposium would be devoted to roundtable discussions. This would provide the opportunity for a number of topics to be discussed as fully and constructively as possible. There were four roundtable discussions in all, each with a chairman and five or six panelists. The discussions were directed by the chairmen and questions from the delegates were addressed by the panelists.

It was felt that verbatim transcripts of the roundtable discussions would become unmanageable. Therefore, the material has been arranged under topic headings; this provides a more structured presentation while retaining the flavor and thrust of each discussion.

We are deeply indebted to Ms. Elaine Gill and Dr. William Whimster and their staffs for their superb editorial efforts at the MEDAC symposia over the years. Their congeniality has made the meetings more enjoyable for everyone, and their competence has helped to create an interesting and impressive library of symposia proceedings.

Opening Remarks

The 1986 MEDAC Meeting included as part of its program a number of roundtable discussions. These proved a most effective means of enabling particularly important or contentious topics to be discussed as fully as possible. A similar format was adopted for the 1987 MEDAC Meeting.

This year, there were four roundtable discussions. The subjects covered ranged from the prevalence of atherosclerosis and attitudes towards cholesterol reduction, to the medical and economic implications of the effective reduction of serum cholesterol, the effective use of lipid-lowering drugs, and areas of future opportunity in clinical and scientific research.

In preparing the roundtable discussions for publication, the intention has not been to produce a consensus opinion. Consensus reports on this subject, from such authoritative bodies as the National Institutes of Health, have been produced in the past and referred to during the Meeting. Professor Lasagna, during one of the roundtable discussions, commented that consensus reports were usually achieved by sequestering everyone in a room in the evening. By about 2 a.m., agreements, which would not normally have been reached, tend to fall into place. We should, he said, simply admit that there is controversy in many important areas, and that there just is no firm consensus.

While no consensus may have been reached, or even attempted, it became very clear during the course of these discussions that there were a number of areas that were of great concern to almost all the participants. For example, just how serious is a raised serum cholesterol? What effect does it have on the incidence of coronary heart disease? How important are other risk factors, or the presence of multiple risk factors? Who should be treated—the young, the elderly, the moderate- or the high-risk individuals? When should diet and when should lipid-lowering drugs be used? There were also more contentious issues such as can we actually demonstrate benefit from reducing serum cholesterol in terms of reduced mortality from CHD, and have the necessary trials been conducted to demonstrate the efficacy and safety of lipid-lowering drugs? All of these subjects recurred in more than one of the roundtable discussions. Although the material presented appears as recorded speech and is arranged under headings to improve readability, the basic content of each roundtable has not been altered. In this way, the topics of greatest general concern are highlighted; cross-referencing of these topics between roundtables has also been introduced.

The discussions which have taken place, both in the roundtables and following the individual presentations, produced some very lively and fruitful debate. And despite Professor Lasagna's abhorrence of consensus, it is clear that some clear patterns of agreement on the important role of cholesterol in atherosclerosis have begun to emerge.

Alexander G. Bearn
July 1987

The Role of Cholesterol in Atherosclerosis:
New Therapeutic Opportunities, edited by S. M. Grundy
and A. G. Bearn, Hanley & Belfus, Inc., Philadelphia.

Pathogenesis of Atherosclerosis: Recent Concepts

Ramzi S. Cotran and J. Michael Munro

Atherosclerosis-related diseases, such as myocardial infarction, strokes, and gangrene, account for about half of the deaths in the United States and Western Europe, and for a great deal of morbidity. Although the precise pathogenesis of such a widespread disorder is still far from established, two major series of advances in the past 15 years have greatly increased our knowledge of the mechanisms of atherosclerosis: first are the advances in cell and molecular biological techniques which have been applied to the study of the cells that make up the vascular wall — smooth muscle and endothelium; and second, the spectacular advances in our understanding of the abnormalities of lipid metabolism in this disorder. This chapter reviews briefly a few selected aspects of the pathogenesis of atherosclerosis that relate to the possible role of lipids in the development of the lesions.

Any concept or concepts of atherogenesis must account for (1) the role of the major risk factors, particularly hyperlipidemia, hypertension and smoking in the development of atheromatous plaques, (2) the mechanisms of smooth muscle proliferation, which is a fundamental process in atherogenesis, (3) the presence of lipid in most lesions, and (4) the focal nature of the lesions and their localization to the intima.

The fundamental lesion of atherosclerosis is the *atheromatous or fibro-fatty plaque*. This is the lesion that causes narrowing of the artery, predisposes to thrombosis, calcifies, and causes weakening of the muscle and aneurysmal dilatation. There are other lesions that may be precursors of the atheromatous plaque (as examples, the fatty streak, the intimal cushion, diffuse intimal thickening, and the gelatinous lesion) but those cause no narrowing of the lumen. Although the appearance of plaques may vary, virtually all plaques have combinations of the following components: (1) connective tissue cells, which have been identified as proliferating smooth muscle cells; (2) a great deal of extracellular connective tissue composed of collagen, elastic tissue and proteoglycans; (3) lipid, mostly in the form of cholesterol and cholesteryl esters, present both extracellularly and within lipid-laden cells called foam cells; (4) inflammatory cells, principally macrophages; and (5) a variable amount of necrotic debris. The more complicated plaque will also show calcification, ulceration, superimposed thrombosis, hemorrhage and aneurysmal dilatation.

5

The distribution of these plaques is important. The most common site is the lower descending aorta, predominantly around the ostia of the major branches, followed by the coronary arteries, usually within the first 6 cm, the arteries of the lower extremities, the descending thoracic aorta, the internal carotids, and the circle of Willis. Some of this localization can be explained by hemodynamic factors, such as sheer stress or turbulent flow, but certainly not all of it. Why, for example, do some patients have disease only in the coronary arteries and not in the brain, and vice versa, and why do some have severe aortic atherosclerosis with clear coronary vessels?

Fatty streaks are grossly visible, intimal, slightly raised, yellow areas which are narrow and longitudinally-oriented. Microscopically, they consist of subendothelial aggregates of foam cells, which are cells whose cytoplasm is filled with lipid droplets—mostly cholesterol and cholesterol esters. Recent studies in which monoclonal antibodies were used as cell markers have shown that a majority of the foam cells in fatty streaks are macrophages, with the rest being of smooth muscle derivation. Little extracellular lipid is present in fatty streaks.

Fatty streaks appear in the aortas of all children over one year, regardless of geography, sex, race or environment, and by the third decade of life they cover about 30% of the aortic intimal surface. They subsequently decrease in number as plaques begin to predominate. They are most common in the thoracic aorta. Are fatty streaks the early or precursor forms of the important fibro-fatty plaque? The issue is controversial and will not be reviewed here. On balance, it appears that fatty streaks are of universal occurrence and distribution, and most, especially those in the aorta, either disappear or remain harmless. In certain locations (e.g., in coronary arteries) and especially in the predisposed individual, these streaks may conceivably evolve into fibrous plaques.

CONCEPTS OF ATHEROGENESIS

Although there are investigators who still argue for the primacy of one etiological agent or pathogenetic mechanism, or one necessary sequence of events in atherogenesis, the current trend is to consider atherosclerosis as a response of the vascular wall to a variety of initiating agents and to admit that multiple pathogenetic mechanisms contribute to the formation of plaques.[1,2] To simplify this chapter, the concept of atherosclerosis as a response to injury is discussed first, and then the possible role of lipids in this response is examined. Finally alternative concepts that consider the lesions of atherosclerosis as neoplastic proliferations of smooth muscle are briefly mentioned.

Atherosclerosis as a Response to Injury

The response-to-injury hypothesis, based on the early proposals made by Virchow, was formulated by Ross and his colleagues in the mid-seventies[3] and modified in the mid-eighties.[1] It postulates that mechanical, chemical, toxic, viral, or immunological stimuli cause endothelial "injury," followed by elaboration of factor(s) that lead to migration and proliferation of smooth muscle cells into the intima and secretion of connective tissue components, including collagen, proteoglycans, and elastic tissue. With repeated or chronic insults, typical atheromatous plaques form. Hypercholesterolemia markedly accentuates the lesions by causing increased lipid infiltration or by contributing to endothelial injury or both. Let us review the various components of the response to injury hypothesis as they are currently understood.

Endothelial Injury

Smooth muscle proliferation and lesions resembling atheromatous plaques can be most readily produced in experimental animals by endothelial denudation, such as by a balloon catheter, and, indeed, the 1976 version of the "reaction to injury" hypothesis postulated that denudation, followed by platelet aggregation and release of platelet-derived growth factor, were necessary if not important components of the response.[3] It soon became apparent, however, that actual denudation was not a feature of hypercholesterolemia-induced atherosclerosis[4,5] and that platelets are neither necessary nor sufficient to cause the lesions.[6] It has also become clear that the endothelium may respond to stimuli by alterations in any one of its many functional properties (endothelial dysfunction),[7,8] or by induction of new properties often associated with the elaboration of new surface proteins.[9] For example, hemodynamic changes such as altered shear stress or turbulent flow induce shape changes, increased fluid pinocytosis and increased endothelial replication without causing endothelial necrosis.[10,11] Platelets can adhere to intact endothelium treated with chemicals or transformed by SV40 virus in cultures.[7] Interleukin-1 (IL 1) induces increased procoagulant activity of endothelium,[12,13] increased adhesion of leukocytes to endothelium,[14] and the synthesis of a new surface protein molecule.[15] Hypercholesterolemia or hypercholesterolemic serum lipoproteins promote monocyte adhesion to endothelium in vivo[16] and in vitro.[17] Hypertension and hyperlipidemia appear to increase focally endothelial replication,[6,18] possibly resulting from transient foci of denudation. Reidy and Schwartz[19] have shown that detachment of single endothelial cells is quickly followed by replacement from adjacent cells— a form of non-denuding injury. These transient foci of injury might not cause significant platelet adhesion but can be associated with foci of increased permeability. Heparin-like proteoglycan molecules, derived from endothelium, cause smooth muscle growth inhibition, and their loss may promote proliferation.[20,21] All of these are examples in which a response to injury can occur in the vascular wall without overt endothelial denudation and which could theoretically initiate a sequence of events that may lead to the development of an atheromatous lesion.

Smooth Muscle Proliferation

Smooth muscle proliferation is a critical event in the development of an atheromatous plaque. Smooth muscle cells are the main cellular components of the fibrous cap, and it is the smooth muscle cells that synthesize the considerable amounts of connective tissue matrix, including collagen, elastic tissue, and proteoglycans, which characterize the lesions of atherosclerosis. They can also accumulate lipid and become foam cells.

What then are the chemical stimuli underlying smooth muscle proliferation? *Platelet-derived growth factor (PDGF)*, the first postulated growth factor in atherogenesis, remains one of the most likely candidates, as it is produced by four cell types involved in the lesion—platelets, macrophages, endothelium, and smooth muscle.[1,22] It can induce both smooth muscle migration and proliferation. PDGF is present in the alpha granules of platelets and megakaryocytes and is released in the platelet-release reaction. It is a highly cationic protein composed of two chains (A and B) with molecular weights of approximately 30,000 daltons. PDGF binds to smooth muscle cells by way of high-affinity receptors, resulting in a multitude of biological events (in addition to the induction of migration and proliferation), including increased endocytosis, cholesterol synthesis, and expression of LDL receptors. It is also a potent vasoconstrictive agent.[23]

PDGF, or PDGF-like molecules, are secreted by a number of different cell types, including platelets,[22] macrophages,[24] endothelial cells,[25] and smooth muscle cells.[26,27] Production of macrophage-derived PDGF is enhanced by activation of macrophages with lipopolysaccharide, immune complexes, and other agents. Endothelial cells in culture also produce a PDGF-like molecule, whose release is stimulated by endotoxin and phorbol esters. Although *in vivo* intact arteries have very low levels of mRNA for PDGF, it is possible that synthesis and release can be induced *in vivo* by certain stimuli; for example, some component of hypercholesterolemic serum. Smooth muscle cells also secrete a growth factor that is PDGF-like.[26,27] Whereas aortic smooth muscle from adult rats has receptors for PDGF, it does not secrete it; however, similar smooth muscle cells from newborn rats secrete a PDGF-like molecule but lack PDGF receptors. Atherosclerotic lesions of rats have the same characteristics as smooth muscle from newborn rats, that is, they secrete PDGF, and have decreased numbers of receptors compared to uninjured smooth muscle. Such findings suggest that regulation of PDGF expression by the smooth muscle cells themselves may be an important determinant of their proliferative state.

There are other potential smooth muscle growth factors, apparently distinct from PDGF, that are produced by endothelium, smooth muscle and macrophages, but these have not been well-characterized.[28] TGF-beta is present in platelets—it causes inhibition of subconfluent smooth muscle cell and proliferation of such cells in agar.[29] Hyperlipidemic serum has also been reported to cause smooth muscle proliferation in culture.

Smooth muscle proliferation can also theoretically be ascribed to the loss of inhibitory molecules present in the vascular wall. Several such molecules have been described, including heparin-like molecules secreted by endothelial cells,[20,21] and proteoglycans from the media, presumably formed by smooth muscle.[30]

There is, therefore, no scarcity of growth factors or mechanisms that can account for smooth muscle proliferation within the plaque. It must be admitted, however, that it is difficult to be certain of precise mechanisms that are relevant *in vivo*. Pharmacological agents and antibodies that inhibit platelet adhesion or platelet function, and anti-platelet antibodies have been shown to inhibit the acute smooth muscle proliferation that occurs after endothelial denudation,[31,32] but these agents have other confounding effects. To date it has not been possible to suppress proliferation consistently with anti-PDGF antisera. Clowes *et al.* have been able to suppress with heparin, including non-anticoagulant heparin, the acute proliferative response after air-induced endothelial injury, suggesting that loss of the inhibiting effect of endothelial heparin-like molecules may play a role *in vivo* in this model.[33]

Monocytes and Macrophages

The participation of monocytes and macrophages in atherosclerosis was indicated by the early ultrastructural studies of Still and O'Neal in 1962[34] (and by others subsequently), who showed electron micrographs of monocytes adhering to and penetrating the endothelium in rats fed a hypercholesterolemic diet. These studies, however, were largely forgotten because of the preoccupation in the 1970s with the smooth muscle cell as the central cell type of atherosclerosis.

The careful studies of Gerrity and his associates in which scanning and transmission electron microscopy were used to examine the earliest stages of lesion formation in experimental hyperlipidemia in swine[16,35,36] put to rest any doubts that monocytes are involved.[16] These authors found that the earliest change, which occurred within 2 weeks on a hypercholesterolemic diet in pigs (and fully 10 weeks before the first subintimal lesions occurred), consisted of increased adhesion of blood monocytes to the endothelial lining. They showed images of monocytes penetrating between endothelial cells into the subintima, where they appeared to convert to intimal lipid-laden foamy cells. Since at these early stages, smooth muscle proliferation is scant, there was little doubt, even without the use of specific markers for macrophages, that the vast majority of the cells in the early lesions are indeed monocyte-derived. The increased monocyte adhesion early in hypercholesterolemia and the essential subsequent series of events have now been confirmed in subhuman primates,[37,38] rats[39] and atherosclerosis-prone pigeons.[40]

Recent work indicates that fatty-streak foam cells in humans are also predominantly macrophages. Using immunohistochemical techniques and cell markers, it has been shown that up to 90% of the cells are leukocyte-derived, depending on the precise area within the lesion.[41] In fibro-fatty lesions, the predominant cell type was also the macrophage.[42,43] In fibrous plaques, smooth muscle cells predominated, though variable numbers of macrophages were also present.[43] Advanced plaques were most heterogeneous but still contained macrophages. It should be stressed that cell-marker studies also demonstrate the presence of lymphocytes, mostly T lymphocytes, in both fatty streaks[41] and fibro-fatty plaques.[42]

The possible mechanisms of increased monocyte adhesion to endothelium in hypercholesterolemia are just beginning to be examined. Rogers *et al.* found that peritoneal macrophages from hypercholesterolemic rats showed increased adhesion to cultured endothelial cells.[44] Preincubation of endothelial cells in culture using beta-VLDL from cholesterol-fed rabbits leads to an increase in the adherence of human mononuclear cells.[17] The increased adhesion in these studies was modest and the mechanisms involved were not examined. Recent studies have also shown that a variety of factors can induce increased adhesion of leukocytes to endothelium *in vitro* by acting primarily on leukocytes (e.g., complement components),[45] primarily on endothelial cells (interleukin-1),[14] or on both cell types (e.g., tumor necrosis factor).[46] Adhesion molecules on leukocytes (e.g., the CDW 18 complex) and endothelium (ELAM-1)[47] are involved in these interactions. Whether they play a role in the monocyte adhesion in hypercholesterolemia deserves to be investigated.

Factors that favor monocyte emigration into the arterial wall in atherosclerosis have also been examined. Several authors have described factors derived from arterial tissue extracts[48] or cultured smooth muscle cells[49] that are capable of increasing monocyte emigration *in vitro*. These molecules have not been characterized in any detail. Once monocyte emigration into the intima has occurred, a variety of macrophage- and/or endothelial-derived factors, including PDGF, complement fragment C5a, and leukotriene B4, may be involved in the recruitment of additional monocytes into the lesions, as these substances all have been shown to have chemotactic activity for monocytes.

The mechanism by which macrophages in the intima become foam cells has been studied by several investigators. In early studies, Goldstein, Brown and their associates incubated peritoneal mouse macrophages with high concentrations of LDL but were not able to convert them into foam cells.[50] However, beta-VLDL from animals fed cholesterol and VLDL from hypertriglyceridemic humans bind to the beta-VLDL receptor (genetically distinct from the LDL receptor), resulting in internalization and hydrolysis, reesterification of cholesterol, and its storage in lipid droplets, producing a foam cell.[51] In addition, if the LDL is modified chemically by acetylation, acetoacetylation, or conjugation with malondialdehyde, it is taken up rapidly and actively by macrophages, and foam cells readily form in culture (see ref. 50 for review). These chemically-modified forms are taken up because of the presence on the surface of macrophages of a specific receptor, termed the acetyl-LDL, or scavenger receptor, which is not susceptible to feed-back inhibition as is characteristic of the LDL receptor.[52] It must be said, however, that despite the ease by which foam cells can be induced with these modified LDL's *in vitro*, there is no evidence that such modified LDL's are present *in vivo*; it is *theoretically* possible that sufficient malondialdehyde is produced during platelet aggregation to achieve appreciable local concentration of malondialydehyde-modified LDL.[53] Another modification of LDL that leads to its uptake by macrophages is oxidation.[2] Oxidized LDL uptake occurs also by way of the acetyl LDL receptor, and is saturable as is the case for any receptor-mediated uptake. The effect is due to peroxidation of the LDL and is dependent on the presence of metal ions in the culture. Endothelial cells,[54] smooth muscle cells,[55] and macrophages[56] markedly enhance LDL oxidation, which can also occur in the presence of high metal concentrations, without cells. Although it is theoretically possible that such oxidatively-modified LDL's may be the determinants of foam cell formation *in vivo*, firm evidence is lacking. Oxidatively-modified LDL has some other potentially atherogenic influences to be detailed later.

In view of the large number of biological activities and secretory products elaborated by macrophages, a great number of adverse actions can be ascribed to the macrophage within the atheromatous plaque.[57] It must be stressed here that by immunocytochemical evidence many of the macrophages in the plaques appear to bear activation markers.[42,57a] Of particular importance to atherosclerosis are the following points:

1. Interleukin 1 (IL 1) and tumor necrosis factor (TNF), both produced by activated macrophages, are capable of inducing increased monocyte adhesion, as described earlier.[14] Likewise, LTB_4 and C5a are macrophage products that are chemotactic for leukocytes. These two activities, increased adhesion and increased chemotaxis, may form an amplification mechanism for the recruitment of further leukocytes into the atheromatous plaque.

2. Macrophages may produce toxic substances such as oxygen metabolites and proteases that may injure neighboring cells and may be responsible for the central necrosis which occurs regularly in large atheromatous plaques. Oxygen metabolites may cause endothelial injury and, indeed, in the studies of Faggiotto *et al.*[37,38] endothelial denudation did occur in the vicinity of large foam-laden macrophages about 5 months after the induction of hypercholesterolemia. These oxidation products may also potentially oxidize LDL, which has cytotoxic effects on cultured smooth muscle cells, fibroblasts, and endothelial cells.[58,59]

3. Along with platelets, macrophages can produce 12 HETE, which is chemokinetic for smooth muscle cells. The formation of this compound is increased when macrophages are incubated with acetyl LDL. This has been postulated to play a role in the migration of smooth muscle cells into the intima.

4. Macrophages may have a role in the apparent regression that occurs in experimental animals fed high levels of cholesterol and then switched to low-lipid diets.[60]

5. Finally, and perhaps most importantly, macrophages secrete factors that induce the proliferation of fibroblasts, smooth muscle cells, and endothelium.[61,62] As stated, smooth muscle cell growth activity in macrophages is PDGF-like.[24] Macrophages also secrete IL 1, which is a mitogen for fibroblasts, fibroblast growth factor, and angiogenesis factors,[62] perhaps accounting for the neovascularization characteristic of advanced plaques.

Lipids and Atherosclerosis

The evidence linking hyperlipidemia to atherogenesis is overwhelming[2] and is discussed elsewhere in this publication. Unfortunately, the precise mechanisms by which the increased levels of cholesterol induce the lesions are still unclear. Several mechanisms, however, have been postulated on theoretical grounds and from experimental studies. Most of these link low-density lipoprotein (LDL) and beta-very low density lipoprotein (β-VLDL) to atherogenesis. LDL is the major carrier of cholesterol in plasma and is the molecule which is most strongly linked to the risk of coronary heart disease in epidemiological studies; β-VLDL is a beta fraction derived from chylomicrons and from VLDL but is richer in cholesterol and has a beta rather than a pre-beta mobility in electrophoresis.

Increases in plasma levels of LDL may *increase the rate of its penetration* into the artery wall and its subsequent uptake and degradation by vascular smooth muscle cells and infiltrating macrophages. As shall be discussed, the local conditions in the intima exposed to increased LDL concentrations may cause the cellular accumulation of cholesterol esters and the formation of foam cells. For example, LDL complexes to intimal proteoglycans (PG), resulting in at least two consequences: extracellular deposition of LDL-cholesterol and uptake of LDL-PG complexes by macrophages, and formation of foam cells.[63] As mentioned earlier, modified LDL and oxidatively altered LDL also promote foam cell formation.

Lipoproteins may affect *endothelial cells directly*. Foci of increased permeability,[64] increased replication,[18] altered anionic sites,[40] and increased monocyte adhesion (see above) have been shown in experimental hypercholesterolemia. *In vitro*, increased monocyte adhesion appears to be, at least in part, an endothelial-dependent effect. LDL and particularly oxidized LDL cause endothelial injury *in vitro*. It has also been postulated that chronically elevated levels of LDL may increase the number of cholesterol molecules in the plasma membranes of cells, including endothelial cells, affecting endothelial cell malleability and causing endothelial cell retraction.[65]

Lipoproteins may have *direct effects on smooth muscle*. There is some *in vitro*, but unconfirmed, evidence that smooth muscle cell proliferation is stimulated by components of hyperlipidemic serum.[66] Platelet aggregation with subsequent release of platelet-derived growth factor and smooth muscle replication is favored by higher LDL levels.[67]

As described earlier, lipoproteins or oxidatively altered lipoproteins affect monocytes and macrophages by increasing monocyte adhesion to endothelium, causing monocyte recruitment by chemotactic mechanisms,[68] inhibition of macrophage motility,[69] and the formation of foam cells.

The Monoclonal Hypothesis

Although the concept of the response to injury coupled with the effects of hyperlipidemia are attractive mechanisms of atherogenesis, *the development of the atheromatous plaque could also be explained if smooth muscle proliferation were in fact the initial event*. Endothelial injury may then be a secondary phenomenon, or may indeed accentuate the lesion, but would be neither the first nor a necessary event. It is possible, for example, that amounts of lipid (or some lipid component) that would normally reach the smooth muscle layer in hypercholesterolemic individuals may somehow alter smooth muscle cells and trigger their proliferation. Or it may be that genetic or acquired defects cause autonomous smooth muscle proliferation. One theory that accounts for such a primary effect on smooth muscle has been proposed by Benditt and Benditt[70] and termed the monoclonal hypothesis.

Benditt and Benditt studied the distribution of A- or B-isoenzyme of X-linked glucose-6-phosphate dehydrogenase (G6PD) in atheromatous plaques of black women heterozygous for this enzyme. As expected, it was found that segments of uninvolved aortic intima and media contained both A- and B-isoenzymes. *However, fibrous plaques contained either A or B, and only seldom contained both.* This monotypic nature of the smooth muscle cells in the plaque was interpreted as evidence that plaques may, therefore, be equivalent to benign monoclonal neoplastic growths (such as leiomyomas) and are initiated by a mutation. The mutagenic effect may be exogenous (e.g., hydrocarbons, viruses), or via an endogenous metabolite (e.g., cholesterol or some of its oxidants). The monoclonality or oligoclonality of human plaques has been confirmed by some investigators (e.g., ref. 71), although the possibility exists that the oligoclonality could develop as a consequence of selection of a subpopulation of cells during the course of lesion formation.

Several pieces of evidence, however, are consistent with Benditt's concepts. Benditt's group has shown herpes virus mRNA by *in situ* hybridization in cells of human atheromatous lesions.[72] Focal fibromuscular plaques have been induced in the abdominal aorta of cockerels by repeated injections of the carcinogen dimethylbenz[a]-anthracene (DBA) and benzo[a]pyrene. DBA and methoxamine administered to cockerels in an initiation-promotion protocol also induce small focal mounds of cells in the thoracic aorta.[73] Repeated injections of the oncogenic Marek's disease virus in cockerels result in microscopic plaques in the thoracic aorta not found in controls.[74] Finally, transforming genes have been extracted from DNA samples of human coronary artery plaques.[75] While all of these findings do not make a case for Benditt's original hypothesis, they do open the question of autonomous smooth muscle proliferation as an important event in some forms of atherosclerosis.

CONCLUSIONS

Figure 1 summarizes some of the mechanisms discussed in this chapter. There is little doubt that overt endothelial injury leads to smooth muscle proliferation, and PDGF (derived from platelets, macrophages, endothelial cells and smooth muscle cells) and other growth factors can cause smooth muscle proliferation. It is clear, however, that endothelial injury need not be denuding and in fact may be subtle. Adhesion of monocytes and increased permeability of endothelium, and disturbances in growth-control properties, can occur without overt endothelial injury. Hyperlipidemia, hypertension, smoking, immune injury, and other risk factors may contribute to this endothelial dysfunction in different ways and sometimes in combination.

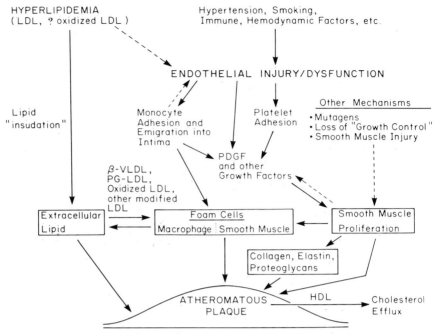

FIG. 1.   Schematic representation of possible sequence of events in atherogenesis.

Smooth muscle cells produce the collagen, elastin, and proteoglycans that form part of the atheromatous plaque. Hyperlipidemia contributes in a number of ways (as discussed earlier), and indeed, in the severely hypercholesterolemic patient, such as one with familial hypercholesterolemia, is alone sufficient to cause atherosclerosis. Foam cells of the atheromatous plaques are derived both from macrophages and from smooth muscle cells; from macrophages via the β-VLDL receptor and also possibly by way of LDL modifications, such as oxidation recognized by the acetyl-LDL receptor; and from smooth muscle cells by uncertain mechanisms. Cholesterol accumulation in the plaque should be viewed as the balance between influx and efflux, and it is possible that HDL is the molecule that helps clear the cholesterol from these accumulations. Figure 1 also depicts the possibility that smooth muscle proliferation may occur without endothelial injury at all. There are several postulated mechanisms for such an occurrence: loss of inhibitors, direct smooth muscle injury (such as by oxidized LDL), and autonomous mutagenic proliferations by the mechanisms suggested by Benditt. Clearly the scheme is full of question marks, is based largely on *in vitro* studies not yet substantiated by *in vivo* experiments, and fails to explain many of the data pertaining to atherosclerosis. It does, however, provide a framework for further studies of the relationship between cholesterol and atherosclerosis, which forms the focus of this publication.

ACKNOWLEDGMENTS

This work was supported by Grant #HL 22602 from the National Heart, Lung, and Blood Institute and NIH Training Grant #5T32 HL07627-03.

REFERENCES

1. Ross R. The pathogenesis of atherosclerosis: An update. *N Engl J Med* 1986; **314**:488–500.
2. Steinberg P. Current theories of the pathogenesis of atherosclerosis. *In:* Steinberg D, Olefsky JM, eds. *Hypercholesterolemia and Atherosclerosis. Pathogenesis and Prevention.* New York: Churchill Livingstone, 1987; 5–25.
3. Ross R, Glomset JA. The pathogenesis of atherosclerosis. *N Engl J Med* 1976; **295**:369–77.
4. Davies PF, Reidy MA, Goode TB, Bowyer DE. Scanning electron microscopy in the evaluation of endothelial integrity of the fatty lesion in atherosclerosis. *Atherosclerosis* 1976; **25**:125.
5. Goode T, Davies PF, Reidy MA, Bowyer DE. Aortic endothelial cell morphology observed *in situ* by scanning electron microscopy during atherogenesis in the rabbit. *Atherosclerosis* 1977; **27**:235.
6. Schwartz SM, Reidy MA. Common mechanisms of proliferation of smooth muscle in atherosclerosis and hypertension. *Human Pathol* 1987; **18**:240–7.
7. Gimbrone MA Jr. Endothelial dysfunction and the pathogenesis of atherosclerosis. *In:* Gotto A, ed. *Atherosclerosis V*, Proceedings of the Fifth International Symposium on Atherosclerosis. New York: Springer-Verlag, 1980; 415–25.
8. DiCorleto PE, Chisolm GM III. Participation of the endothelium in the development of the atherosclerotic plaque. *Prog Lipid Res* 1986; **25**:365–74.
9. Cotran RS, Pober JS. Endothelial activation: Its role in inflammatory and immune reaction. *In:* Simionescu N, Simionescu M, eds. *Endothelial Cell Biology.* New York: Plenum Press (1988, in press).
10. Davies PF, Dewey CF Jr, Bussolari SR, Gordon EJ, Gimbrone MA Jr. Influence of hemodynamic forces on vascular endothelial function. *J Clin Invest* 1984; **73**:1121–9.
11. Davies PF, Remuzzi A, Gordon EJ, Dewey CF Jr, Gimbrone MA Jr. Turbulent fluid shear stress induces vascular endothelial cell turnover *in vitro. Proc Natl Acad Sci USA* 1986; **83**:2114–7.
12. Bevilacqua MP, Pober JS, Majeau GR, Cotran RS, Gimbrone MA Jr. Interleukin 1 (IL-1) induces biosynthesis and cell surface expression of procoagulant activity in human vascular endothelial cells. *J Exp Med* 1984; **160**:618–23.
13. Bevilacqua MP, Pober JS, Majeau GR, Fiers W, Cotran RS, Gimbrone MA Jr. Recombinant tumor necrosis factor induces procoagulant activity in cultured human vascular endothelium: Characterization and comparison with the actions of interleukin 1. *Proc Natl Acad Sci USA* 1986; **83**:4533–7.
14. Bevilacqua MP, Pober JS, Wheeler ME, Cotran RS, Gimbrone MA Jr. Interleukin 1 acts on cultured human vascular endothelium to increase the adhesion of polymorphonuclear leukocytes, monocytes, and related leukocyte cell lines. *J Clin Invest* 1985; **76**:2003–11.
15. Pober JS, Bevilaqua MP, Mendrick DL, Lapierre LA, Fiers W, Gimbrone MA Jr. Two distinct monokines, interleukin 1 and tumor necrosis factor, each independently induce biosynthesis and transient expression of the same antigen on the surface of cultured human vascular endothelial cells. *J Immunol* 1986; **136**:1680–7.
16. Gerrity RG, Bauti HK, Richardson M, Schwartz CJ. Dietary induced atherogenesis in swine: Morphology of the intima in prelesion stages. *Am J Pathol* 1979; **95**:775–92.
17. Endemann G, Pronzcuk A, Friedman G, Lindsey S, Alderson L, Hayes KC. Monocyte adherence to endothelial cells *in vitro* is increased by β-VLDL. *Am J Pathol* 1987; **126**:1–35.
18. Florentin RA, Nam SC, Daoud AS, *et al.* Dietary-induced atherosclerosis in miniature swine, I–V. *Exp Mol Pathol* 1968; **8**:263–301.
19. Reidy MA, Schwartz SM. Recent advances in molecular pathology: Arterial endothelium—assessment of *in vivo* injury. *Exp Mol Pathol* 1984; **41**:419–34.
20. Castellot JJ Jr, Addonizio ML, Rosenberg R, Karnovsky MJ. Cultured endothelial cells produce a heparin-like inhibitor of smooth muscle cell growth. *J Cell Biol* 1981; **90**:372–84.

21. Castellot JJ Jr, Rosenberg RD, Karnovsky MJ. Endothelium, heparin and the regulation of vascular smooth muscle cell growth. *In:* Jaffe E, ed. *Biology of Endothelial Cells.* Boston: Martinus Nijhoff Publishers, 1974; 118–28.

22. Ross R, Raines EW, Bowen-Pope D. The biology of the platelet-derived growth factor. *Cell* 1986; **46**:155–169.

23. Berk BC, Alexander RW, Brock T, Gimbrone MA Jr, Webb CR. Vasoconstriction: A new activity for platelet-derived growth factor. *Science* 1986; **232**:87–90.

24. Shimokado K, Raines EW, Madtes DK, Barrett TB, Benditt EP, Ross R. A significant part of macrophage-derived growth factor consists of at least two forms of PDGF. *Cell* 1985; **43**:277.

25. DiCorleto PE, Bowen-Pope DF. Cultured endothelial cells produce a platelet-derived growth factor-like protein. *Proc Natl Acad Sci USA* 1983; **80**:1919–23.

26. Seifert RA, Schwartz SM, Bowen-Pope DF. Developmentally regulated production of platelet-derived growth factor-like molecules. *Nature* 1984; **311**:669–71.

27. Walker LN, Bowen-Pope DF, Ross R, Reidy MA. Intimal vascular smooth muscle cells secrete PDGF-like activity. *Fed Proc* 1985; **44**:737a.

28. Davies PF. Biology of disease: Vascular cell interactions with special reference to the pathogenesis of atherosclerosis. *Lab Invest* 1986; **55**:5–24.

29. Assoian RK, Sporn MB. Transforming growth factor-beta acts on aortic smooth muscle cells. *In:* Fidge NH, Nestel PJ, eds. *Atherosclerosis VII.* Amsterdam: Excerpta Medica, 1986; 459.

30. Fritze LM, Reilly CF, Rosenberg RD. An antiproliferative heparin sulfate species produced by post-confluent smooth muscle. *J Cell Biol* 1985; **100**:1041–50.

31. Friedman RJ, Stemerman MB, Wenz B, *et al.* The effect of thrombocytopenia on experimental arteriosclerotic lesion formation in rabbits: Smooth muscle cell proliferation and re-endothelialization. *J Clin Invest* 1977; **60**:1191–201.

32. Harker LA, Harlan JM, Ross R. Effect of sulfinpyrazone on homocystein-induced endothelial injury and arteriosclerosis. *Circ Res* 1983; **53**:731–9.

33. Clowes AW, Karnovsky MJ. Suppression by heparin of smooth muscle cell proliferation in injured arteries. *Nature* 1977; **265**:625.

34. Still W, O'Neal RM. Experimental studies of early atherosclerosis in the rat. *Am J Pathol* 1962; **40**:21–35.

35. Gerrity RG. The role of the monocyte in atherogenesis. I. Transition of blood-borne monocytes into foam cells in fatty lesions. *Am J Pathol* 1981; **103**:181–90.

36. Gerrity RG. The role of the monocyte in atherogenesis. II. Migration of foam cells from atherosclerotic lesions. *Am J Pathol* 1981; **103**:191–200.

37. Faggiotto A, Ross R, Harker L. Studies of hypercholesterolemia in the nonhuman primate. I. Changes that lead to fatty streak formation. *Arteriosclerosis* 1984; **4**:323–40.

38. Faggiotto A, Ross R. Studies of hypercholesterolemia in the nonhuman primate. II. Fatty streak conversion to fibrous plaque. *Arteriosclerosis* 1984; **4**:341–56.

39. Joris I, Zand T, Nunnari JJ, Krolikowski FJ, Majno G. Studies on the pathogenesis of atherosclerosis. I. Adhesion and emigration of mononuclear cells in the aorta of hypercholesterolemic rats. *Am J Pathol* 1983; **113**:341–58.

40. Lewis JC, Taylor RG, Jones ND, St. Clair RW, Cornhill JF. Endothelial surface characteristics in pigeon coronary artery atherosclerosis. I. Cellular alterations during the initial stages of dietary cholesterol challenge. *Lab Invest* 1982; **46**:123–38.

41. Munro JM, van der Walt JD, Munro CS, Chalmers JAC, Cox EL. An immunohistochemical analysis of human aortic fatty streaks. *Human Pathol* 1987; **18**:375–80.

42. Jonasson L, Holm J, Bondjers G, Hansson GK. Regional accumulations of T cells, macrophages, and smooth muscle cells in the human atherosclerotic plaque. *Arteriosclerosis* 1986; **6**:131–8.

43. Gown AM, Tsukada T, Ross R. Human atherosclerosis. II. Immunocytochemical analysis of the cellular composition of human atherosclerotic lesions. *Am J Pathol* 1986; **125**:191–207.

44. Rogers KA, Hoover RL, Castellot JJ Jr, Robinson JM, Karnovsky MJ. Dietary cholesterol-induced changes in macrophage characteristics. *Am J Pathol* 1986; **125**:284–91.

45. Harlan JM. Leukocyte-endothelial interactions. *Blood* 1985; **65**:513–525.

46. Gamble JR, Harlan JM, Klebanoff SJ, Vadas MA. Stimulation of the adherence of neutrophils to umbilical vein endothelium by recombinant tumor necrosis factor. *Proc Natl Acad Soc USA* 1985; **82**:8667–8671.

47. Bevilacqua MP, Pober JS, Mendrick DL, Cotran RS, Gimbrone MA Jr. Identification of an inducible endothelial-leukocyte adhesion molecule, E-LAM 1. *Proc Natl Acad Sci USA* (in press).

48. Gerrity RG, Goss JA, Soby L. Control of monocyte recruitment by chemotactic factors in lesion-prone areas of swine aorta. *Arteriosclerosis* 1985; **5**:55.
49. Valente AJ, Fowler SR, Sprague EA, Kelley JL, Suenram CA, Schwartz CJ. Initial characterization of a peripheral blood mononuclear cell chemoattractant derived from cultured arterial smooth muscle cells. *Am J Pathol* 1984; **117**:409–17.
50. Goldstein JL, Brown MS. Lipoprotein metabolism in the macrophage: Implications for cholesterol deposition in atherosclerosis. *Ann Rev Biochem* 1983; **52**:223.
51. Gianturco SH, Bradley WH. The β-VLDL receptor pathway of macrophages. *In:* Fidge NH, Nestel PG, eds. *Atherosclerosis VII.* Amsterdam: Elsevier Science Publishers, 1986; 495–9.
52. Goldstein JL, Ho YK, Basu SK, Brown MS. Binding site on macrophages that mediates uptake and degradation of acetylated LDL, producing massive cholesterol deposition. *Proc Natl Acad Sci USA* 1979; **79**:333.
53. Fogelman AM, Shechter I, Seager J, Hokom N, Child JS, Edwards PA. Malondialdehyde alteration of LDL leads to cholesterol ester accumulation in human monocyte-macrophages. *Proc Natl Acad Sci* 1980; **77**:221.
54. Henriksen T, Mahoney EM, Steinberg D. Enhanced macrophage degradation of LDL previously incubated with cultured endothelial cells: Recognition by receptors for acetylated LDL. *Proc Natl Acad Sci USA* 1981; **78**:6499.
55. Henriksen T, Mahoney EM, Steinberg D. Enhanced macrophage degradation of biologically modified LDL. *Arteriosclerosis* 1983; **3**:149.
56. Parthasarathy S, Printz DJ, Boyd D, Joy L, Steinberg D. Macrophage oxidation of low density lipoprotein generates a modified form recognized by the scavenger receptor. *Arteriosclerosis* 1986; **6**:505–510.
57. Nathan CF. Secretory products of macrophages. *J Clin Invest* 1987; **79**:319–326.
57a. Munro JM, Pober JS, Cotran RS. (unpublished observations)
58. Hessler JR, Robertson AL, Chisolm GM. LDL-induced cytotoxicity and its inhibition by HDL in human vascular smooth muscle cells and endothelial cells in culture. *Atherosclerosis* 1979; **32**:213.
59. Cathcart MK, Morel DW, Chisolm GM III. Monocytes and neutrophils oxidize low density lipoprotein making it cytotoxic. *J Leuko Biol* 1985; **38**:341–50.
60. Daoud AS, Fritz KE, Jarmolych J, Frank AS. Role of macrophages in regression of atherosclerosis. *Ann NY Acad Sci* 1985; **454**:101–14.
61. Martin BM, Gimbrone MA Jr, Unanue ER, Cotran RS. Stimulation of non-lymphoid mesenchymal cell proliferation by a macrophage-derived growth factor. *J Immunol* 1981; **126**:1510–15.
62. Polverini PJ, Cotran RS, Gimbrone MA Jr, Unanue ER. Activated macrophages induces vascular proliferation. *Nature* 1977; **269**:804–6.
63. Berenson G, Radhakrishnamurthy B, Srinivasan SR, Vijayagopal P, Dalferes ER. Proteoglycans and potential mechanisms related to atherosclerosis. *Ann NY Acad Sci* 1985; **454**:69–78.
64. Stemerman MB. Effects of moderate hypercholesterolemia on rabbit endothelium. *Arteriosclerosis* 1981; **1**:25.
65. Jackson RL, Gotto AM Jr. Hypothesis concerning membrane structure, cholesterol, and atherosclerosis. *In:* Paoletti R, Gotto AM Jr, eds. *Atherosclerosis Reviews.* Vol. 1. New York: Raven Press, 1976; 1–21.
66. Fisher-Dzoga K, Frazer RA, Wissler RW. Stimulation of proliferation in stationary primary cultures of monkey and rabbit aortic smooth muscle cells. I. Effects of lipoprotein fractioning of hyperlipidemic serum and lymph. *Exp Molec Pathol* 1976; **24**:346–59.
67. Carvalho AC, Colman RW, Lees RS. Platelet function in hyperlipoproteinemia. *N Engl J Med* 1974; **290**:434–8.
68. Quinn MT, Parthasarathy S, Fongg LG, Steinberg D. Oxidatively modified low density lipoproteins: A potential role in recruitment and retention of monocyte/macrophages during atherogenesis. *Proc Natl Acad Sci USA* 1987; **84**:2995–8.
69. Quinn MT, Parthasarathy S, Steinberg D. Endothelial cell derived chemotactic activity for macrophages and the effects of modified forms of LDL. *Proc Natl Acad Sci USA* 1985; **82**:5949–53.
70. Benditt EP, Benditt JM. Evidence for a monoclonal origin of human atherosclerotic plaques. *Proc Natl Acad Sci USA* 1973; **70**:1753.
71. Pearson TA, Dillman JM, Heptinstall RH. The clonal characteristics of human aortic intima. Comparison with fatty streaks and normal media. *Am J Pathol* 1983; **113**:33–40.
72. Benditt EP, Barrett T, McDougall JK. Virus in the etiology of atherosclerosis. *Proc Natl Acad Sci USA* 1983; **80**:6386–6389.

73. Majesky MW, Reidy MA, Benditt EP, Juchau MR. Focal smooth muscle proliferation in the aortic intima produced by an initiation-promotion sequence. *Proc Natl Acad Sci USA* 1985; **82**:3450.
74. Fabricant CG. Atherosclerosis: The consequence of infection with a herpes virus. *Adv Vet Sci Comp Med* 1985; **30**:39–66.
75. Penn A, Garte SJ, Warren L, Nesta D, Mindich B. Transforming gene in human atherosclerotic plaque DNA. *Proc Natl Acad Sci USA* 1986; **83**:7951–5.

SUMMARY

Although the precise pathogenesis of atherosclerosis remains to be established, advances in cell and molecular biological techniques and in our understanding of the abnormalities of lipid metabolism have greatly increased our knowledge of the mechanisms involved. Any concepts of atherogenesis must account for the role of the major risk factors (particularly hyperlipidemia, hypertension and smoking); mechanisms of smooth muscle proliferation; the presence of lipid in most lesions; and the focal nature of lesions and their localization to the intima. The concept of atherosclerosis as a response to injury is discussed. Endothelial denudation can lead to smooth muscle proliferation, probably through the release of platelet-derived growth factor from platelets. Even without denuding endothelial injury, endothelial cells may react to stimuli by alterations in function or induction of new properties. For example, adhesion of monocytes, increased permeability of endothelium and disturbances in growth-control properties can occur. Smooth muscle cells produce collagen, elastin and proteoglycans that form part of the atheromatous plaque. The possibility that smooth muscle proliferation may occur without endothelial injury is also considered. Some of the possible mechanisms, including loss of growth control, direct smooth muscle injury and autonomous mutagenic proliferation, are examined. Monocytes and macrophages form an important component of atheromatous plaques, and their role in the initiation and evolution of lesions, as well as the effects of hyperlipidemia on interactions between endothelium, smooth muscle and macrophages are discussed.

RÉSUMÉ

Bien qu'il reste à établir la pathogenèse précise de l'athérosclérose, des progrès dans les techniques biologiques cellulaires et moléculaires et dans notre compréhension des anormalités du métabolisme des lipides ont beaucoup amélioré nos connaissances des mécanismes impliqués. Tout concept d'athérogenèse doit justifier le rôle des facteurs de risques principaux (en particulier l'hyperlipidémie, l'hypertension et le tabac); les mécanismes de prolifération des muscles lisses; la présence de lipides dans la plupart des lésions; et la nature focale des lésions et de leur localisation dans les parois des artères. Le concept de l'athérosclérose à la suite d'une blessure est discuté ici. La dénudation de l'endothélium peut amener à une prolifération de muscles lisses, probablement par l'intermédiaire d'un dégagement de facteurs de développement des plaquettes. Même sans dénuder la blessure endothéliale, les cellules endothéliales peuvent réagir à des excitations par des modifications dans la fonction ou l'induction de nouvelles propriétés. Par exemple une adhésion de monocytes, une perméabilité accrue de l'endothélium et des perturbations dans les propriétés de contrôle du développement peuvent se produire. Les cellules des muscles lisses produisent du collagène, de l'élastine et des protéoglycanes qui forment une partie de la plaque athéromateuse. On examine aussi la possibilité d'une prolifération de muscles lisses sans pour cela qu'il y ait de blessure endothéliale. On étudie quelques-uns des mécanismes possibles, y compris la perte de contrôle du développement, la blessure directe de muscles lisses et la prolifération mutagénique autonome. Les monocytes et les macrophages forment une composante importante des plaques athéromateuses, et leur rôle dans l'initiation et l'évolution des lésions, ainsi que les effets de l'hyperlipidémie sur les interactions entre l'endothélium, les muscles lisses et les macrophages sont aussi discutés.

ZUSAMMENFASSUNG

Obwohl die präzise Pathogenese der Atherosklerose noch ergründet werden muß, haben Fortschritte in zellularen und molekülaren biologischen Verfahren und unser Wissen über die Abnormalitäten des Lipidstoffwechsels unsere Kenntnis der betroffenen Mechanismen sehr bereichert. Jegliche Auffassung der Atherogenese muß die Rolle der Hauptrisikofaktoren (im besonderen Hyperlipämie, Hypertonie und Rauchen), Mechanismen der Glattmuskel-Wucherung, das Vorhandensein von Lipid in den meisten Läsionen, und die fokale Natur der Läsionen und ihrer Lokalisation zu der Intima berücksichtigen. Die Auffassung von Atherosklerose als Reaktion auf Verletzung ist diskutiert. Die Entblößung des Endothels kann zur Wucherung glatter Muskel führen, wahrscheinlich durch die Freigabe des von Plättchen abgeleiteten Wachstumsfaktors der Plättchen. Selbst ohne entblößende Verletzung des Endothels, können Endothelzellen auf Reize durch Funktionsveränderungen oder Induktion von neuen Eigenschaften reagieren. Zum Beispiel, Adhäsion von Monozyten, erhöhte Durchdringbarkeit des Endothels und Störungen der Wachstumskontrolleigenschaften können auftreten. Glattmuskelzellen produzieren Kollagen, Elastin und Proteoglykane, die einen Teil des atheromatösen Belags bilden. Die Möglichkeit, daß die Glattmuskelwucherung auch ohne Verletzung des Endothels auftreten kann, ist auch berücksichtigt. Einige der möglichen Mechanismen, einschließlich Verlust von Wachstumskontrolle, direkter Glattmuskelverletzung und autonomer mutagenischer Wucherung sind untersucht. Monozyten und Makrophagen formen einen wichtigen Teil der atheromatösen Beläge und ihre Rolle in dem Beginn und der Entwicklung von Läsionen, sowohl als auch die Einwirkung von Hyperlipämie auf Wechselwirkungen zwischen Endothel, Glattmuskel und Makrophagen sind diskutiert.

SOMMARIO

Anche se si deve ancora dimostrare la precisa patogenesi dell'aterosclerosi, il progresso nella tecnica della biologia cellulare e moleculare e la nostra comprensione delle anormalità del metabolismo lipido hanno aumentato vastamente la nostra conoscenza dei meccanismi in questione. Per una comprensione completa dell'aterogenesi si deve spiegare il ruolo dei maggiori fattori rischio (particolarmente l'iperlipidemia, l'ipertensione e il fumo); meccanismi della proliferazione del muscolo liscio; la presenza di lipidi nella maggior parte delle lesioni; e la natura focale delle lesioni e la loro localizzazione verso l'intima. È anche discusso il concetto dell'aterosclerosi come una risposta alla ferita. Denudazione endoteliale porta verso la proliferazione del muscolo liscio, probabilmente attraverso il rilascio da piastrine del fattore di crescita derivato di piastrine. Anche senza la denudazione della ferita endoteliale, le cellule endoteliali possono reagire agli stimuli tramite cambiamenti in funzione oppure tramite l'induzione di proprietà nuove. Per esempio, l'adesione di monociti, un aumento della permeabilità dell'endotelio, e disturbi nelle proprietà che controllano la crescita potrebbero occorrere. Cellule di muscolo liscio producono collageno, elastina e proteoglicani che formano parte della placca ateromata. Viene anche considerata la possibilità che la proliferazione del muscolo liscio possa succedere senza ferita endoteliale. Vengono esaminati dei meccanismi possibili, come la perdita del controllo della crescita, la diretta ferita del muscolo liscio e la proliferazione autônoma e mutagênica. I monociti e i macrofagi formano un componente importante di placche ateromate e i loro ruoli nell'iniziativa ed evoluzione di lesioni, vengono discussi; come pure gli effetti dell'iperlipidemia sull'azione reciproca fra l'endotelio, il muscolo liscio e i macrofagi.

SUMÁRIO

Embora a patogénia precisa da aterosclerose ainda não está estabelecida, avanços nas técnicas de biologia celular e molecular e no nosso entendimento das anormalidades do metabolismo de lípidos têm aumentado muito o nosso conhecimento dos mecanismos envolvidos. Quaisquer conceitos sobre aterogênese devem explicar; o papel dos fatores maiores de risco (especialment hiperlipidemia, hipertensão e fumar); os mecanismos da proliferação de músculos lisos; a presença de lípidos na maior parte das lesões; e o caráter focal das lesões e a sua localização na íntima. O conceito de aterosclerose como reação à injúria é examinado. Denudação do endotélio pode resultar em proliferação de músculos lisos, provavelmente através da libertação do fator de crescimento tirado das plaquetas. Mesmo sem uma injúria de denudação do endotélio, células do endotélio podem reagir a estímulos por alterações na função ou na indução de novas qualidades. Por exemplo, adesão de monocitos, permeabilidade aumentada do endotélio e distúrbios nas qualidãdes de contrôle de crescimento podem acontecer. Células de músculos lisos produzem colagênio, elastina e proteoglucanos que formam parte da placa ateromatosa. A possibilidade de que a proliferação de músculos lisos pode acontecer sem injúria do endotélio é também considerada. Alguns dos mecanismos possíveis, incluindo a perda de contrôle de crescimento, injúria direta de músculos lisos, e a proliferação autônoma mutagénica são examinados. Monocitos e macrófagos formam um componente importante de placas ateromatosas e o seu papel na iniciação e na evolução de lesões, como também os efeitos de hiperlipidemia sobre interações entre endotélio, músculo liso e macrófagos são discutidos.

RESUMEN

Aunque la patogénesis precisa de la aterosclerosis todavía no se ha establecido, los avances logrados en las técnicas de biología celular y molecular, y nuestra comprensión de las anormalidades del metabolismo de los lípidos, han incrementado grandemente nuestro conocimiento de los mecanismos involucrados. Todo concepto sobre aterogénesis debe explicar: el papel de los principales factores de riesgo (particularmente hiperlipidemia, hipertensión y tabaquismo); los mecanismos de proliferación del músculo liso; la presencia de lípidos en la mayoría de las lesiones; y la naturaleza focal de las lesiones y su localización en la íntima. Se analiza el concepto de la aterosclerosis como una respuesta a la injulia. La denudación endotelial puede conducir a la proliferación de músculo liso, probablemente a través de la liberación de factor de crecimiento plaquetario. Incluso sin lesiones de denudación endotelial, las células endoteliales podrían reaccionar a los estímulos mediante la alteración de funciones o la inducción de nuevas propiedades. Por ejemplo, adhesión a los monocitos, mayor permeabilidad del endotelio y trastornos en las propiedades de control del crecimiento. Las células del músculo liso producen colágeno, elastina y proteoglicanos que forman parte de la placa ateromatosa. También se considera la posibilidad de que la proliferación del músculo liso ocurra sin lesiones endoteliales. Se examinan algunos de los posibles mecanismos, incluyendo la pérdida de control del crecimiento, lesiones directas en el músculo liso y proliferación mutagénica autónoma. Los monocitos y macrófagos son un componente importante de la placa ateromatosa, y se discute su papel en la iniciación y evolución de las lesiones, así como los efectos de la hiperlipidemia en las interacciones entre el endotelio, músculo liso y macrófagos.

The Role of Cholesterol in Atherosclerosis:
New Therapeutic Opportunities, edited by S. M. Grundy
and A. G. Bearn, Hanley & Belfus, Inc., Philadelphia.

Discussion

LASAGNA: Are there any chemicals which make monocytes less sticky?

COTRAN: Monoclonal antibodies against the leukocyte CDW 18 antigens inhibit leukocyte-dependent adhesion. It is theoretically possible that monoclonal antibodies against the endothelial leukocyte adhesion molecules might be effective.

LEWIS: You asked whether modification of LDL can be shown to occur *in vivo* as well as *in vitro*. My colleague Dr. Shaikh and I may have a partial answer to that. We have done studies in which autologous labeled LDL is injected into patients prior to vascular surgery. If one then extracts LDL-like material from the atherosclerotic plaque, this shows an autoradiographic image in the position of a modified LDL with faster mobility than LDL.

COTRAN: There is also a study by Morton *et al.* (*J Lipid Res* 1986; **27**:1124) from the Cleveland Clinic in which they extracted modified LDL from atheromatous plaques and found that also accumulated in macrophages in culture, very much like some of the other modified LDLs, but not through the acetyl LDL receptor.

DOLLERY: I would like to know where the initiating events lie. Macrophages are such efficient fighting machines that when you have stimulated them they do all sorts of things, and whether you believe the reaction-to-injury hypothesis or put a primary role for the macrophage, one still has to ask what starts it.

COTRAN: Once monocytes adhere and become activated there is no dearth of theoretical mechanisms by which the macrophage alters endothelial function or causes "injury" to start things off. In hypercholesterolemia it might be an effect of the chronic hypercholesterolemic state either on the monocyte or on the endothelium or both. From studies on other systems we know that when monocytes become activated they make more oxygen-free radicals, enzymes and biologically active compounds, and it seems likely that this will cause endothelial injury.

BEARN: Do we know what the proto-oncogenes activate?

COTRAN: Benditt's monoclonal hypothesis postulates that smooth muscle proliferation is primary and all the other effects may be secondary. This autonomous smooth muscle proliferation may possibly be due to putative mutagens which trigger events similar to those of oncogenesis. A recent paper in the Proceedings of the National Academy of Science (*Proc Natl Acad Sci USA* 1986; **83**:7951) identifies the presence of transforming genes in human atheromatous plaques.

ASSCHER: Why should there be *one* initiating factor? We know that irritation can accentuate atheromatous damage, and so can hypertension, presumably by producing endothelial damage. Smoking and the oncogenes might trigger the process in totally different ways.

COTRAN: There is probably not one single answer. The present feeling is that atherogenesis is multifactorial. There is a large number of initiating and overlapping factors such as hyperlipidemia, hypertension, smoking, immune disease, irradiation, environmental toxins, and viruses.

DOLLERY: I accept that macrophages may be an important common pathway, and we have been looking for evidence of macrophage activation in man by measuring urinary thromboxane B2. Platelets produce large amounts of thromboxane but so do macrophages. You can attempt to distinguish the two by giving low-dose aspirin, which will tend to inhibit platelet-derived thromboxane more than that produced by macrophages, because macrophages can resynthesize the cyclo-oxygenase. In acute smoking, and in early studies of chronic smoking, we have been unable to replicate the Nashville findings of increased thromboxane B2 excretion in the urine. Using this rather indirect index of macrophage activation, we have been able to find such evidence in smokers.

COTRAN: We know that macrophages are present in experimental hypercholesterolemia and after other modes of experimental endothelial injury. They are clearly present in human atheromatous lesions. In fatty streaks the preponderant cells are macrophages, and in fibro-fatty plaques they make up to 60% of cells, depending on the location. We know that they have many *potential* effects in atherosclerosis, as I explained, but *in vivo* proof of these effects is more difficult to obtain. It is not possible to keep the monocyte count down for any length of time in experimental animals without complications arising.

MAHLEY: Each model will be different in its cellular response. We need to remember that one of the important initiating factors in many of the models is hyperlipidemia. Within a short time of inducing hypercholesterolemia, monocytes are attracted and attach to the endothelial surface and can enter the subintimal space. The role of oxidized LDL is becoming a stronger possibility as one of the elements of hypercholesterolemia important in atherosclerosis. At recent meetings two different groups (Steinberg and associates of the University of California, San Diego, and Dr. Tora Kita of Japan) have suggested that probucol markedly retards the development of atherosclerosis in the Watanabe heritable hyper-lipidemic rabbit, which has abnormal LDL receptors. These rabbits typically develop very severe atherosclerosis from birth, but when they were treated with probucol the atherosclerosis was virtually eliminated in some cases and markedly decreased in others. One of the effects demonstrated by Steinberg's group was that these LDLs were very resistant to oxidation and difficult to modify. This is the mechanism through which probucol may be having its effect in these rabbits. Modification of LDL could be one of the ways in which low density lipoproteins are atherogenic, but we need to remember that diet-induced changes in lipoproteins, especially chylomicron remnant lipoproteins, can probably cause foam cell formation through the direct uptake by macrophages of these native lipoproteins. The remnant lipoproteins, referred to as beta-VLDL, are naturally occurring lipoproteins that appear to be able to cause foam cell production. Beta-VLDL are induced by diets high in fat and cholesterol.

COTRAN: There was not time to stress the beta-VLDL receptor in my talk, but let me review again the effects of oxidized LDL. Steinberg's group performed many experiments with oxidized LDLs. It seems to play a role in several steps of atherogenesis. Oxidized LDL is chemotactic to monocytes and will recruit them to the intima. LDL can be oxidized more readily in the presence of endothelial cells, smooth muscle cells, and macrophages, and this oxidatively-modified LDL is taken up by macrophages, which become foam cells. Oxidized LDL decreases macrophage mobility thus keeping them from emigrating out of the intima. It is chemo-attractant to circulating monocytes but also decreases the motility of the resident macrophages. Oxidatively-modified LDL also causes endothelial injury and therefore increases endothelial permeability.

The Role of Cholesterol in Atherosclerosis:
New Therapeutic Opportunities, edited by S. M. Grundy
and A. G. Bearn, Hanley & Belfus, Inc., Philadelphia.

Chronology of Cholesterol Biosynthesis

Konrad E. Bloch

Stories often told do not necessarily improve on repetition; yet points of view, emphases and perspectives differ even when the facts are widely accepted and not in dispute. In my brief review of cholesterol biosynthesis I will emphasize the circumstances and accidental findings which led to the elucidation of what is surely one of the most complex biochemical pathways. To have participated in this venture almost from its beginnings and to have seen the story unfold has been an extraordinary experience.

It is fair to say that the history of cholesterol is nearly as long as the history of chemistry and biochemistry; in fact, for nearly 200 years the sterol molecule has held the attention of chemists and life scientists without any signs of that interest abating. The reasons for this continuing attention are many, chiefly the intriguing complexity of cholesterol structure and function and its Janus-faced character that has entered public consciousness increasingly in recent years. Next to DNA it is probably the substance most cited in the media.

Crystallized at the end of the 18th century and available in ample supply, the cholesterol molecule provided the training ground for generations of organic chemists throughout the 19th and early 20th century (Table I). Structural organic chemistry, the design of new reagents and degradative procedures, and especially stereochemical principles such as conformational analysis, all owe much of their success to cholesterol research. This molecule was also the most complex tackled by the early x-ray crystallographers, a challenge they met successfully when the sterol structure was still tentative and under dispute.

It is rare that chemical structure *per se* provides an insight into the biological origin of a molecule produced by nature. It is equally uncommon that the total chemical synthesis of complex natural products as devised by chemists offers any clues to the reactions that a biosynthetic pathway employs. In fact, from a purely chemical perspective the pathways nature chooses are more often crooked than rational. The elucidation of cholesterol biosynthesis is no exception. It has followed an erratic, not a systematic, course.

By the early 1920s, given the fact that cholesterol is found in large amounts both in herbivorous and carnivorous species, it could be inferred that the animal body produces this substance rather than relying on dietary sources. More direct evidence

TABLE I. *Chronology of cholesterol and cholesterol-related chemical research*

1789	Cholesterol crystallized from gallstones
1816	"Unsaponifiable," cholesterine
1888	$C_{27} H_{46} O$
1919	Cholesterol and bile acids share tetracyclic ring system
1928	Tentative Windaus-Wieland structure
1932	Corrected structure
	● Bernal, Rosenheim and King
	● Windaus, Wieland
1929 ⎫	Isolation and structures of steroid hormones:
1940 ⎭	estrone, androsterone, progesterone, cortisone
1947	3-D structure (x-ray diffraction)
1950	Conformational analysis
1952	Structure of lanosterol
1954	Ecdysones (insects)
1966	Ecdysones (plants)
1957	Vitamin D structure
1968	Hormonal forms of vitamin D
1978	Brassinolides, plant growth hormones

for endogenous synthesis came in 1935 when Schoenheimer and Breusch performed careful balance studies comparing intake and output.[1] Yet final proof had to await the advent of isotopic tracers, first the stable isotopes in the 1930s and then radioactive isotopes after World War II. R. Schoenheimer immediately saw the potential of this tool and was the first to apply it to the cholesterol problem. In an early seminal study he and David Rittenberg demonstrated the efficient uptake of deuterium from heavy water in mice,[2] leading to the conclusion that "Formation of cholesterol in the animal body involves the coupling of a large number of small molecules." That this small molecule was acetic acid[3] and acetate is in fact the source of all the carbon and hydrogen atoms of the sterol structure was readily established,[4] which was the essential preliminary for the more demanding task of assigning the origin of each of the 27 carbon atoms of cholesterol to the methyl and carboxyl groups of acetate, respectively.[5–7]

This laborious research covering a period of 15 years was successful in that it provided the first clues for an assembly mechanism of molecules from small to large. In essence the labeling pattern of acetate-derived cholesterol implicated a branched-chain intermediate built from three acetate molecules and perhaps related to the isoprene unit, which according to Ruzicka[8] forms the structural element or monomeric unit of numerous natural products of the terpene family. However, the direct testing of plausible acetate-derived intermediates led nowhere. The identity of branched-chain precursors for the biological isopentenyl unit remained a mystery. Fortunately at that time (1956), the Merck Laboratories, searching for potential new vitamins, identified mevalonic acid (MVA) as an acetate-replacing factor for *Lactobacillus* mutants[9]. Speculating that MVA might arise reductively from acetate by way of β-hydroxy β-methyl glutaric acid, then known to occur in plants, the Merck investigators tested the new growth factor as a sterol precursor. The results were dramatic; conversion to sterol in rat liver was quantitative. It was a classical serendipitous discovery. Logically, lactobacilli were the most improbable source of cholesterol precursors since these organisms do not produce sterols. Later this riddle was solved when bactoprenol, the polyprenol side chains of ubiquinone and isopentenyladenine, were all found to be derived from MVA. It was Merck's continued, active interest in MVA that led in time to effective inhibitors of cholesterol biosynthesis.

Very generously the Merck laboratories shared both information and labeled mevalonic acid with other workers in the field, giving those interested a free hand in pursuing the further steps on the route to cholesterol. There followed, in rapid succession, the discoveries of the three phosphorylating steps that take MVA to isopentenylpyrophosphate, the long-sought biological isoprene unit, and from there to geranylpyrophosphate (C_{10}), farnesylpyrophosphate (C_{15}) and squalene (C_{30}).[7,10] These were exhilarating developments not only because they filled a large gap in the pathway to cholesterol but also because they uncovered novel and unpredicted mechanisms for the formation of carbon-carbon bonds, namely by elimination of pyrophosphate as the driving force.

Once a biosynthetic pathway is established and enters the textbooks, the actual chronology tends to be forgotten. Yet an historical account instructs, if only by underlining the fundamentally different approaches to a problem taken by biological scientists and by the engineer. The engineer follows a blueprint of his design, the biologist takes his cues from unexpected, unintentional observations. Squalene is a case in point. Thirty years before MVA ushered in the new era in cholesterol research, there was some interest in the chemistry of squalene, a hydrocarbon abundant in shark liver. In 1926 the chemist I. Heilbron[11] persuaded H. J. Channon, a nutritionist, to feed squalene to rats. This regimen raised the cholesterol content of the animals' tissues substantially.[12] At the time squalene and cholesterol were known to be large molecule (C_{30} and C_{27}, respectively) containing numerous branched methyl groups, but otherwise their structures were not sufficiently characterized to suggest a precursor-product relationship. Perhaps for this reason Channon's experiments received little attention. However, once solved, the structure of squalene and cholesterol inspired Sir Robert Robinson (1934) to propose a cyclizing mechanism for transforming one into the other.[13] It was a daring proposal not diminished in significance by the later demonstration that squalene cyclization produces lanosterol—not cholesterol.[14] Eventually, in 1952, lanosterol was shown to be a trimethyl derivative of cholesterol,[15] a structure much more attractive as a direct cyclization product of squalene. An alternative to Robinson's scheme was therefore proposed and experimentally documented.[14] By the late 1950s all the gaps in the pathway from acetate to lanosterol had finally been filled and lanosterol shown to be the steroidal precursor of cholesterol in animal tissues.[16] While the major pieces now seemed in place (Table II), one important detail was clearly missing. The clue was that yeast, when grown anaerobically, accumulates squalene instead of converting it into lanosterol or ergosterol. Clearly, oxygen itself, or some equivalent cationic species as Eschenmoser et al.[17] had postulated, seemed to be required for these

TABLE II. *Cholesterol biosynthesis*

1926	Conversion of squalene to cholesterol?
1934	Hypothetical scheme for cyclization of squalene to cholesterol
1935	Net synthesis of cholesterol in animals
1937	Cholesterol synthesized from small molecules arising in intermediary metabolism
1942	Acetate, the carbon source for cholesterol
1953	Acetate-[C_5] → squalene → lanosterol → cholesterol
1956	Discovery of mevalonic acid (MVA)
	MVA → cholesterol
1957	HMG-CoA → mevalonic acid
1958	MVA → isopentenylpyrophosphate (C_5)
	$C_5 → C_{10} → C_{15}$; $2C_{15} →$ squalene
1960	HMG-CoA reductase control site in cholesterol biosynthesis
1977	The LDL pathway, relation to atherosclerosis

transformations. Corey and Russey[18] and van Tamelen *et al.*[19] substantiated this hypothesis by isolating squalene 2,3 epoxide, which now became the immediate substrate for cyclization. Dioxygen also takes part in the final streamlining steps of cholesterol synthesis that involve the oxidative removal of three methyl groups from the tetracyclic nucleus, presumably by way of hydroxymethyl, aldehyde and carboxylate intermediates. The order in which these methyl groups are removed: 14α-methyl, 4β-methyl, 4α-methyl[20] may be viewed as a striking example of the "Wisdom of Nature." As these methyl groups depart, in the order given, the "fitness" of the sterol structure for membrane function improves, reaching perfection with cholesterol itself.[20] In view of the absolute requirement for oxygen in its synthesis, it is reasonable to date cholesterol as a late-comer in evolution, to an era during or after which aerobic cells first appeared.

The central issue in cholesterol research today is perhaps no longer cholesterol synthesis *per se* but the elucidation of the modes of control operating in this molecule's formation and degradation. Whatever the processes, they have to be finely controlled, because the cholesterol molecule and also mevalonic acid serve in numerous essential functions (Table III). Clearly, knowledge of the various biosynthetic steps is a necessary but not a sufficient condition for locating sites and devising means of control.

The literature is replete with nutritional experiments describing the consequences of feeding cholesterol to various animal species. These began in 1913 with the classical studies of Anitschkow[21] showing that dietary cholesterol induces massive fatty deposits in the rabbit aorta.* When cholesterol feeding was combined with the administration of labeled acetate half a century later,[22] the incorporation of isotopes into cholesterol was seen to decrease dramatically. The effect was attributed to end-product or negative feedback control, a phenomenon revealed by earlier research in bacterial physiology. Significantly, since no such inhibition occurred in analogous experiments with labeled mevalonate, the control point could be located at some step between acetate and mevalonate.[23] Thus HMG-CoA reductase emerged

---

*The choice of rabbits was fateful; the pathological response would not have been seen in rats or other rodents. Species differences have remained a vexing problem in atherosclerosis research.

TABLE III. *Biological functions of cholesterol*

1. Physical
   Constituent of eukaryotic plasma membrane
   Stabilizes phospholipid bilayer

2. Precursor of:
   Vertebrate sex hormones and glucocorticoids
   Bile acids
   Vitamin D and oxygenated derivatives, regulators of Ca^{++} metabolism
   Ecdysones, developmental invertebrate hormones
   Ecdysones in plants?
   Brassinolides in plant pollen
   Plant growth hormones

3. Metabolic signalling functions?
   Control of phospholipid biosynthesis
   Protein kinases?

as the probably major regulated enzyme in the cholesterol biosynthetic pathway.[24] The story might end here if one were concerned only with the control of sterol biosynthesis in unicellular organisms. The more primitive forms of life, however, are not endowed with arteries and do not seem to suffer from an excess of cholesterol or whatever sterol they accumulate. Mainstream cholesterol research today, therefore, must deal with the fate of cholesterol during and after absorption, its transport in the circulatory system, and the receptor-mediated transfer of cholesterol-carrying proteins from extra- to intracellular space; in short, the balance between dietary uptake, endogenous synthesis, and removal. These are all subjects in the domain of cell biology and molecular biology[25] as well as biochemistry.

Less in the lime-light, but by no means of secondary importance, are the control processes that channel mevalonic acid into non-steroidal products, the polyprenol side-chains of ubiquinone, into dolichol, a key molecule for glycoprotein synthesis, and into isopentenylated nucleic acid bases.[26] It is interesting to note that evidence is emerging for isopentenylation of protein, post- or co-translationally. Finally, much remains to be learned about the regulation of cholesterol catabolism and anabolism, the conversion to bile acids and to steroid hormones, including those derived from vitamin D, all processes that represent the "good" side of this Janus-faced molecule. Perhaps we can include in this category events controlled by membrane-resident cholesterol *per se*, such as the biosynthesis of membrane-associated processes. For example, a role for sterol in phospholipid biosynthesis is indicated by current investigations in my laboratory.[27]

REFERENCES

1. Schoenheimer R, Breusch F. Synthesis and destruction of cholesterol in the organism. *J Biol Chem* 1933; **103**:439–448.
2. Rittenberg D, Schoenheimer R. Deuterium as an indicator in the study of intermediary metabolism. *J Biol Chem* 1937; **117**:485–490.

3. Bloch K, Rittenberg D. On the utilization of acetic acid for cholesterol formation. *J Biol Chem* 1942; **145**:625–636.
4. Ottke, RC, Tatum EL, Zabin I, Bloch K. Isotopic acetate and isovalerate in the synthesis of ergosterol by neurospora. *J Biol Chem* 1951; **189**:429–433.
5. Cornforth JW, Hunter DG, Popjak G. Studies of cholesterol biosynthesis. 1. A new chemical degradation of cholesterol. *Biochem J* 1953; **54**:590–597.
6. Cornforth JW, Gore IY, Popjak G. Studies on the biosynthesis of cholesterol. 4. Degradation of rings C & D. *Biochem J* 1957; **65**:94–109.
7. Bloch K. Biological synthesis of cholesterol. *Science* 1965; **150**:19–28.
8. Ruzicka L. The isoprene rule and the biogenesis of terpenic compounds. *Experientia* 1953; **9**:357–396.
9. Folkers K. Discovery and elucidation of mevalonic acid. *In:* Wolstenholme GEW and O'Conner M, eds. *CIBA Foundation Symposium on the Biosynthesis of Terpenes and Sterol.* London, Churchill, 1959:4–16.
10. Lynen F, Agranoff BW, Eggerer H, Henning U, Moeslein EM. γ.γ-Dimethyl-allyl-pyrophosphat und Geranyl-pyrophosphat biologische vorstufen des squalens. *Angew Chem* 1959; **71**:657–663.
11. Heilbron IM, Kamm ED, Owens WM. The unsaponifiable matter from the oils of Elasmobranch fish. I. A contribution to the study of the constitution of squalene (Spinacene). *J Chem Soc* 1926; 1630–1644.
12. Channon HJ. Liv. The biological significance of the unsaponifiable matters of oils. 1. Experiments with the unsaturated hydrocarbon, squalene (Spinacene). *Biochem J* 1926; **20**:400–408.
13. Robinson R. Structure of cholesterol. *Chem Ind* 1937; **53**:1062–1063.
14. Woodward RB, Bloch K. The cyclization of squalene in cholesterol synthesis. *J Am Chem Soc* 1953; **75**:2023–2024.
15. Voser W. *et al.* Uber die Konstitution des Lanostadienols (Lanosterins) und seine Zugehorigkeit zu den Steroiden. *Helv Chim Acta* 1952; **35**:2414–2430.
16. Clayton RB, Bloch K. The biological conversion of lanosterol to cholesterol. *J Biol Chem* 1956; **218**:319–32.
17. Eschenmoser A, Ruzicka L, Jeger O, Arigoni D. Eine stereochemische interpretation der biogenetische isoprenregel bei den triterpenen. *Helv Chim Acta* 1955; **38**:1890–1904.
18. Corey EJ, Russey WE. Metabolic fate of 10,11-Dihydrosqualene in sterol-producing rat liver homogenate. *J Am Chem Soc* 1966; **88**:4751–4752.
19. Van Tamelen EE *et al.* Enzymatic conversion of squalene 2,3-oxide to lanosterol and cholesterol. *J Am Chem Soc* 1966; **88**:4752–4754.
20. Bloch K. Sterol structure and membrane function. *Crit Rev Biochem* 1983; **14**:47–92.
21. Anitschkow ND. Veranderungen der Kaninchen-aorta by experimenteller cholesterin steatase. *Beitr Pathol Anat* 1913; **56**:379–404.
22. Taylor CB, Gould RG. The effect of dietary cholesterol on the synthesis of cholesterol in dogs. *Fed Proc* 1950; **9**:179.
23. Bucher NL, Overath P, Lynen F. β-Hydroxy- β-methyl glutanyl-coenzyme A reductase. *Biochim Biophys Acta* 1960; **40**:491–501.
24. Rodwell VW, McNamara DJ, Shapiro DJ. Regulation of β-hydroxy- β-methyl glutanyl-CoA reductase. *Adv Enzymol* 1973; **38**:373–412.
25. Goldstein IL, Brown MS. The low-density lipoprotein pathway and its relation to atherosclerosis. *Ann Rev Biochem* 1977; **46**:897–930.
26. Rudney H, Sexton RC. Regulation of cholesterol biosynthesis. *Ann Rev Nutr* 1986; **6**:245–272.
27. Bloch K. *Lipid Structure and Function in Lipids and Membranes, Past, Present, and Future. In:* Op den Kamp JAF, *et al.*, eds. Amsterdam: Elsevier 1986; 45–59.

SUMMARY

The cholesterol molecule has been studied for over 200 years. Its complexity has continued to intrigue scientists, while more recently it has become the focus of public and media attention. The chemical structure and synthesis of cholesterol have provided few, if any, clues to its origin and biosynthetic pathways. Direct evidence for its endogenous synthesis came in 1935; cholesterol formation was shown to be achieved by the coupling of large numbers of acetate molecules. The task of identifying the origin of each of the 27 carbon atoms took a further 15 years. In 1956, the discovery of an acetate-replacing factor in Lactobacillus mutants led to mevalonic acid (MVA) being identified as a key cholesterol precursor. This chance finding was the start of a new era of cholesterol research. Today, the central issue in cholesterol research is not its synthesis *per se* but the elucidation of the modes of control operating during the molecule's formation and degradation. Much still remains to be learnt about this molecule.

RÉSUMÉ

On étudie la molécule du cholestérol depuis plus de 200 ans. Les chercheurs n'ont jamais cessé d'être intrigués par la complexité de cette molécule, alors que ce n'est que récemment qu'elle a attiré l'attention du public et des média. La structure chimique et la synthèse du cholestérol n'ont fourni que peu d'indications, si on peut dire, sur son origine et ses voies de biosynthèse. C'est en 1935 que l'on a eu des preuves directes de sa synthèse endogène; on a montré que la formation de cholestérol venait de l'accolement en grand nombre de molécules d'acétate. Il a fallu encore 15 ans avant d'arriver à identifier l'origine de chacun de ces 27 atomes de carbone. En 1956 la découverte d'un facteur de remplacement d'acétate dans les mutantes du Lactobacille a amené à identifier l'acide mélavonique comme un précurseur clé du cholestérol. Cette découverte faite au hasard a entamé une nouvelle ère de recherche sur le cholestérol. Aujourd'hui ce n'est pas la synthèse à proprement parler mais plutôt l'élucidation des modes de contrôle qui interviennent lors de la formation et de la dégradation de la molécule qui fait l'objet principal des recherches sur le cholestérol. Il nous reste encore beaucoup à apprendre sur cette molécule.

ZUSAMMENFASSUNG

Das Cholesterinmolekül ist schon seit über 200 Jahren wissenschaftlich untersucht worden. Seine Kompliziertheit hat unaufhörlich Wissenschaftler gefesselt, während es in letzter Zeit zum Mittelpunkt der öffentlichen und Media-Aufmerksamkeit geworden ist. Die chemische Struktur und Synthese von Cholesterin haben wenige, wenn überhaupt einige Anhaltspunkte hinsichtlich seines Ursprungs und seiner biosynthesischen Bahnen geliefert. Direkter Beweis für sein endogene Synthese gelang im Jahre 1935. Die Cholesterinbildung wurde durch die Verbindung von einer grossen Anzahl von Acetat-molekülen nachgewiesen. Die Aufgabe der Identifizierung des Ursprungs von jedem der 27 Kohlenstoffatome bedurfte weiterer 15 Jahre. Im Jahre 1956 führte die Entdeckung eines Acetat-ersetzenden Faktors in Lactobacillus-Mutanten zu Mevalonsäure (MVA), die als Hauptvorläufer des Cholesterins identifiziert wurde. Dieser Zufallsfund war der Beginn einer neuen Epoche der Cholesterinforschung. Heute ist die Hauptaufgabe der Cholesterinforschung nicht sein Synthese *per se*, sondern die Erklärung der Art und Weise der Regulierung, die während der Bildung des Moleküls und dessen Abbau wirksam wird. Über dieses Molekül gibt es noch viel zu lernen.

SOMMARIO

Lo studio sulla molecola del colesterolo è già in progresso da ben piú di 200 anni. La sua complessità ha continuato ad incuriosire gli scienziati, mentre piú recentemente è diventato il focus dell'attenzione pubblica e della stampa. La struttura chimica e la sintesi del colesterolo hanno provvisto pochi, se alcuni, indizi verso la sua origine e la sua traiettoria biosintetica. Evidenza diretta della sua sintesi endogena è arrivata nel 1935; è stato dimostrato che la formazione del colesterolo avviene tramite l'accoppiamento di numerose molecule acetate. Il compito di identificare l'origine di ognuno dei 27 atomi carbonici impiegò altri 15 anni. Nel 1956, la scoperta di un fattore rimpiazzando l'acetate nei mutanti di Lactobacillus portò all'identificazione dell'acido mevalonico come fattore chiave precursore del colesterolo. Questa scoperta, avvenuta quasi per caso, segnò l'inizio di una nuova epoca per la ricerca del colesterolo. Oggi il problema centrale nella ricerca del colesterolo non è la sua sintesi per sé, ma è l'elucidazione dei modi di controllo operanti durante la formazione e degradazione della molecola. C'è ancora molto studio da fare su questa molecola.

SUMÁRIO

A molécula de colesterol tem sido estudada por mais de 200 anos. A sua complexidade tem continuado a intrigar cientistas, enquanto mais recentemente tem vindo a ser o foco de attenção do público e dos méios de comunicação. A estrutura química e a síntese de colesterol têm fornecido poucos indícios, se quaisquer, sobre a sua origem e os seus caminhos biosintéticos. Evidência direta da sua síntese endógena veio em 1935; a formação de colesterol foi mostrada a ser conseguida pela união de grandes números de moléculas de acetato. A tarefa de identificar a origem de cadaum dos 27 átomos de carbônio levou mais 15 anos. Em 1956 o descobrimento dum fator da suplantação de acetato em mutantes do Lactobacillus levou à ácido mevalônico (MVA) ser identificado como um antecessor essencial do colesterol. Este descubrimento por acaso foi o começo duma era nova de pesquisa sobre colesterol. Hoje, o tema central na pesquisa sobre colesterol não é a sua síntese per se mas o esclarecimento dos modos de contrôle funcionando durante a formação e a degradação da molécula. Muito ainda fica para aprender sobre esta molécula.

RESUMEN

La molécula de colesterol se ha estudiado por más de 200 años. Su complejidad ha continuado intrigando a los científicos y recientemente ha sido el foco de atención del público y de los medios de comunicación. La estructura química y la síntesis del colesterol han proporcionado muy pocos indicios con respecto a su origen y a las vías de síntesis orgánica. En 1935 se obtuvo evidencia directa de su síntesis endógena; se demostró que la formación del colesterol se logoraba mediante la unión de un gran número de moléculas de acetato. La labor de identificación del origen de cada uno de los 27 átomos de carbono tomó otros 15 años. En 1956, el descubrimiento de un factor reemplazante del acetato en mutantes de Lactobacillus condujo a la identificatión del ácido mevalónico (MVA) como un precursor clave del colesterol. Este descubrimiento accidental marcó el comienzo de una nueva era en las investigaciones sobre el colesterol. Hoy en día, el foco principal de las investigaciones sobre el colesterol no es su síntesis misma, sino el descubrimiento de los mecanismos de control que operan durante la formación y degradación de la molécula. Todavía tenemos mucho que aprender con respecto a esta molécula.

The Role of Cholesterol in Atherosclerosis:
New Therapeutic Opportunities, edited by S. M. Grundy
and A. G. Bearn, Hanley & Belfus, Inc., Philadelphia.

HMG-CoA Reductase Inhibitors

Eve E. Slater, Alfred W. Alberts and Robert L. Smith

The intense scientific interest surrounding cholesterol derives in large part from the fact that formation of the atheromatous plaque is accompanied by the localized deposition of plasma lipids, primarily cholesterol esters, in the intima of the arterial wall.[1] Growth of the atheroma can lead eventually to obliteration of the coronary arterial lumen and to resultant myocardial infarction. Atherosclerosis is the major pathogenetic determinant of coronary heart disease (CHD), which is the foremost cause of death and disability in Western countries and which accounts for approximately 600,000 deaths annually in the United States alone.

The compelling epidemiological evidence implicating hypercholesterolemia as a primary risk factor for CHD has stimulated research on the development of therapeutic agents for the prevention and treatment of atherosclerosis based on the attenuation of plasma cholesterol levels.[2] The results of the recently completed Lipid Research Clinics Coronary Primary Prevention Trial (LRC-CPPT) provide strong support for the basis of this approach.[3,4] The LRC-CPPT clearly demonstrated that reduction of low density lipoprotein cholesterol (LDL-C) through dietary modification and treatment with the bile acid sequestrant cholestyramine, either alone or in combination, diminished the incidence of CHD morbidity and mortality in hypercholesterolemic men at high risk for CHD. Nevertheless, the reduction of dietary cholesterol and saturated fat intake and the use of bile acid sequestrants often fail to lower elevated plasma LDL-C levels to the desired extent, particularly in patients with familial hypercholesterolemia.

Since approximately two-thirds of total body cholesterol in individuals on a typical Western diet is of endogenous origin, an attractive and potentially more effective way to lower plasma cholesterol levels is to control *de novo* cholesterogenesis by inhibiting an early biosynthetic step. A major rate-limiting step in this pathway is at the level of the microsomal enzyme 3-hydroxy-3-methylglutaryl-coenzyme A reductase [HMG-CoA reductase; mevalonate: $NADP^+$ oxidoreductase (CoA acylating), EC 1.1.1.34], which catalyzes the conversion of HMG-CoA to mevalonic acid and has been considered to be a prime target for pharmacological intervention for several decades[5] (Figure 1).

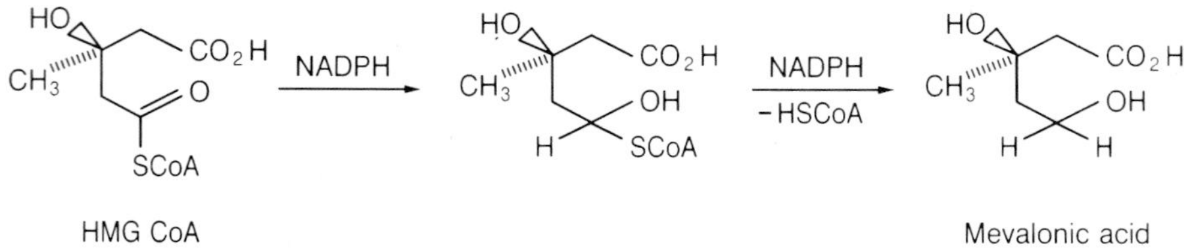

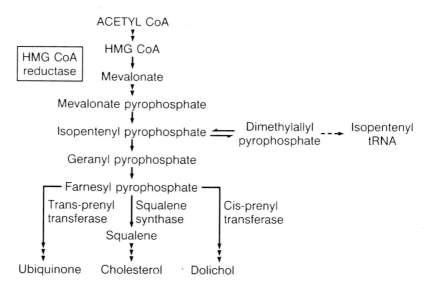

FIG. 1. The reaction catalyzed by the enzyme HMG-CoA reductase: the reduction of HMG-CoA to mevalonic acid.

ROLE OF HMG-CoA REDUCTASE IN CONTROL OF CHOLESTEROL BIOSYNTHESIS

The role of HMG-CoA reductase in control of cholesterol biosynthesis and indeed its selection as a target for pharmacologic intervention derived not only from its location early in the biosynthetic pathway but also from appreciation of the extreme sensitivity of reductase to feedback inhibition by cholesterol and related sterols. HMG-CoA reductase occurs early in the biosynthetic pathway and is among the first committed steps to cholesterol formation (Figure 2). Note that inhibition could lead to accumulation of HMG-CoA, an intermediate which then can be broken down into simpler molecules by a lyase. Thus, inhibition of reductase does not lead to accumulation of intermediates having a formal sterol ring, an effect observed

FIG. 2. A schematic representation of some of the principal steps in cholesterol formation: HMG-CoA reductase is located early in the biosynthetic pathway.

in earlier attempts by others to inhibit cholesterol biosynthesis and presumed responsible for the toxicities observed, for example, with Mer-29 (triparanol). It should also be noted that the *in vivo* consequence of enzyme inhibition for the synthesis of mevalonate and its nonsterol products, the polyisoprenoids, ubiquinones and dolichols, can be quantitated by measurement of mevalonate levels in plasma or urine.

The exquisite sensitivity of HMG-CoA reductase to inhibition by sterols was predicted first in the early 1950s by experiments in which animals fed cholesterol reduced their rate of [^{14}C] acetate incorporation into hepatic cholesterol.[6] Later, this action was linked to a reduction in reductase activity in response to cholesterol, oxygenated sterols (such as 25-hydroxycholesterol), and mevalonate-derived products *in vivo* and in tissue culture systems.[7,8] Not all lipoproteins suppressed reductase activity. Of the two major cholesterol-carrying lipoproteins in human plasma, LDL and HDL, only LDL was effective. This specificity provided Brown and Goldstein with the first clue that a receptor might be involved in pathway-mediated feedback inhibition.[1] This receptor was subsequently identified as the receptor for low density lipoprotein, LDL.

Both the sensitivity of HMG-CoA reductase activity measured in cultured skin fibroblasts to regulation by cholesterol and its resistance to regulation in patients with homozygous familial hypercholesterolemia (FH) are depicted in Figure 3 from the elegant work of Brown and Goldstein. When grown in serum that contained lipoprotein, fibroblast reductase activity from normal patients was reduced, whereas it remained elevated 50- to 100-fold above normal in FH cells. Similarly, this latter activity did not increase significantly when lipoproteins were removed from the serum and there was no suppression when LDL was returned to the medium.[8]

In response to the inhibition of endogenous cholesterol biosynthesis by a reductase inhibitor, however, normal cells, FH cells, or those containing only one copy of the defective LDL receptor gene, as in heterozygous FH, increase HMG-CoA reductase activity in response to enzyme inhibition.[9,10] As will be discussed, both reductase and LDL receptor induction can be demonstrated in response to reductase inhibition *in vivo*.

The HMG-CoA reductase enzyme is a 97 kDa membrane-bound glycoprotein, the only membrane-bound enzyme early in the cholesterol biosynthetic pathway. Its complete nucleotide sequence has been determined from its cDNA clone in hamster and man.[11,12] The amino-terminal hydrophobic domain is conserved between the two species and contains a membrane-spanning region that crosses the endoplasmic reticulum seven times (Figure 4). Interestingly, a configuration containing seven transmembrane segments has been proposed for a number of other membrane-bound molecules, including bovine rhodopsin and the mammalian beta$_2$-adrenergic receptor.[13] The 50–55 kDa carboxyl-terminal active site domain of reductase, which projects into the cytoplasm, is also highly conserved between species.

More recent studies have identified a segment at the 5′ end of the reductase gene that mediates control of transcription by sterols.[14] These experiments involved

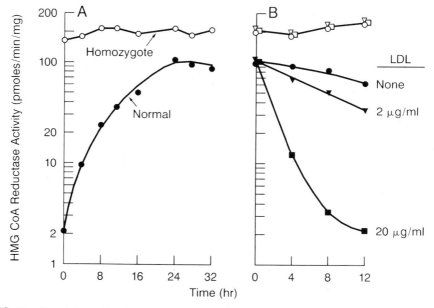

FIG. 3. Regulation of HMG-CoA reductase in fibroblasts from a normal subject (●) and from an FH homozygote (○). *A*, After removal of lipoproteins. Monolayers of cells were grown in dishes containing 10% fetal calf serum. On day 6 of cell growth (zero time), the medium was replaced with fresh medium containing 5% human serum from which the lipoproteins had been removed. At the indicated time, extracts were prepared and HMG-CoA reductase activity was measured. *B*, After addition of LDL. At 24 hours after addition of 5% human lipoprotein-deficient serum, human LDL was added to give the indicated cholesterol concentration. HMG-CoA reductase activity was measured in cell-free extracts at the indicated time. (Reproduced with permission from Goldstein JL, Brown MS. *Proc Natl Acad Sci USA* 1973; **70**:2804–08.)

expression in mouse L-cells of the chimeric gene for reductase joined to the coding region for chloramphenicol acetyltransferase (CAT), and demonstration of its regulation by sterols. Any sizable deletion within a 500 bp region extending 300 bp upstream of the reductase transcription initiation site interfered with sterol effects on CAT expression and reductase mRNA transcription. These studies have enabled the elegant demonstration that one site of control of HMG-CoA reductase occurs at the level of gene transcription.

Utilizing a monoclonal antibody directed against reductase and a cDNA to reductase mRNA, Liscum *et al.* showed that in rats hepatic reductase activity was increased 45-fold when they were fed cholestyramine and lovastatin.[15] Under these conditions, the amount of immunodectable reductase rose by 33-fold and the reductase mRNA became visible by blot hybridization. Cholesterol feeding reversed these changes.

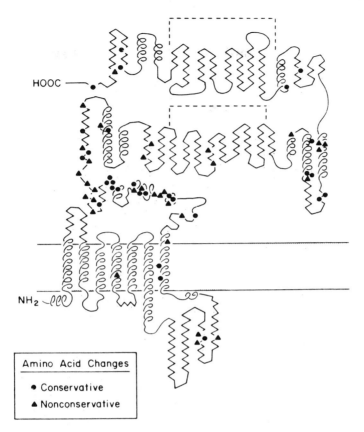

HOOC ———

NH₂

Amino Acid Changes

● Conservative

▲ Nonconservative

FIG. 4. Schematic representation of the secondary structure of HMG-CoA reductase. The proposed structure of hamster reductase is drawn as described by Liscum et al.[34] The membrane of the endoplasmic reticulum is shaded with the seven transmembrane segments of reductase traversing this region. The sites of amino acid substitutions in the human reductase relative to the hamster enzyme are indicated. Each replacement is marked as to whether it is conservative (●) or nonconservative (▲). (Reproduced with permission from Liscum et al. J Biol Chem 1985; **260**: 522–530.)

THE DISCOVERY OF LOVASTATIN*

The first breakthrough in efforts to find a potent, specific, competitive inhibitor of HMG-CoA reductase occurred in 1976 when Endo and coworkers reported the discovery of mevastatin (ML-236B, CS-500, compactin) a highly functionalized fungal metabolite first isolated from cultures of *Penicillium citrinum*[16] (Figure 5).

Subsequent to the first reports describing the structure and biological activity of mevastatin, two lines of investigation were initiated in our laboratories: (1) the rational design and synthesis of structurally novel inhibitors based upon an analysis

---

*Merck & Co., Inc. received U.S. FDA approval for sale of lovastatin on August 31, 1987.

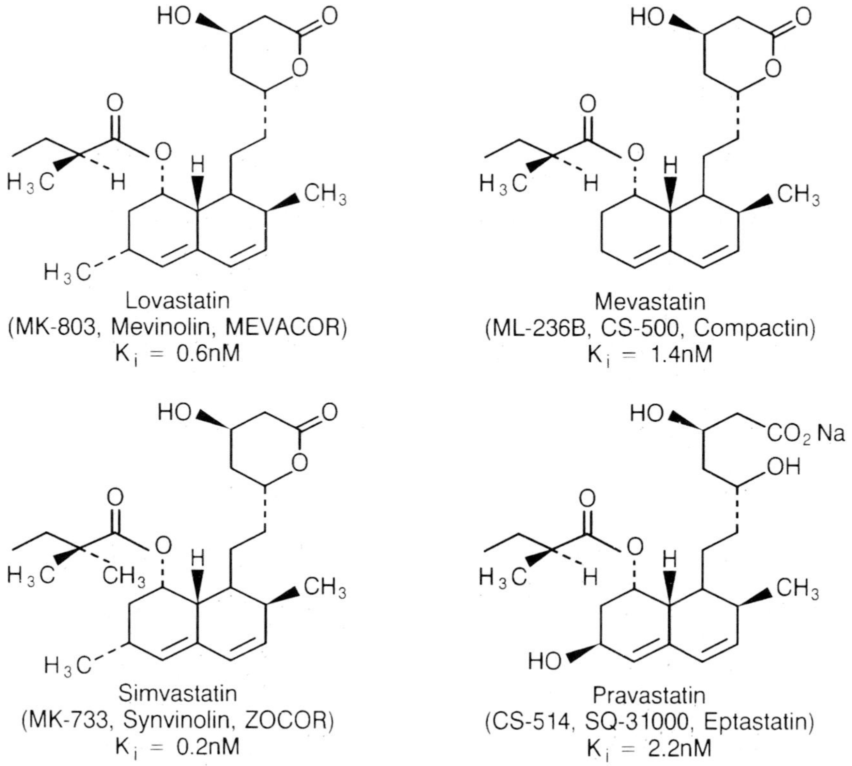

FIG. 5. Structures and inhibitory constants of four HMG-CoA reductase inhibitors: lovastatin, mevastatin, pravastatin, and simvastatin.

of the structural features of mevastatin and the existing information concerning the enzyme-mediated conversion of HMG-CoA to mevalonic acid, and (2) screening fermentation broths against mammalian HMG-CoA reductase. Although both lines of investigation have proved successful, only the latter will be described below.

The screening effort, led by our colleague Art Patchett and one of us (AWA), quickly resulted in the discovery that a strain of *Aspergillus terreus* (ATCC 20542), obtained from a soil isolation program at the Centro de Investigacion Basica (CIBE) Laboratories in Madrid, Spain, produced the novel fungal metabolite lovastatin (MK-803, mevinolin, MEVACOR®).[17] The structure of lovastatin was found to be different from that of mevastatin only by the presence of a 6α-methyl group in the hexahydronaphthalene ring and, based on the physical data reported by Endo, appeared to be identical or very similar to that of monacolin K isolated from *Monascus ruber*[18] (Figure 5). Like mevastatin, the active or ring-opened dihydroxycarboxylate form of lovastatin proved to be a potent, specific, competitive inhibitor of HMG-CoA reductase, and to inhibit cholesterol synthesis in rats and

®Mevacor is a trademark of Merck & Co., Inc., Rahway, N.J., U.S.A.

to lower plasma cholesterol in dogs after oral administration. Interestingly, the intrinsic inhibitory activity of lovastatin (K_i = 0.6 nM) was superior to that of mevastatin (K_i = 1.4 nM), as was its cholesterol inhibitory activity in rats.[17,18]

The availability of lovastatin allowed one of us (RLS) to launch a third line of investigation directed toward two goals: (1) delineation of the structural features of lovastatin responsible for its HMG-CoA reductase inhibitory activity and (2) use of the resulting structure/activity relationships to develop semisynthetic inhibitors with improved biological activity. Achievement of these goals first required the design and development of synthetic strategies for selectively modifying the key structural features of lovastatin.[19,20] Having accomplished this objective, we determined that: (a) saponification of the sidechain ester moiety to afford the corresponding 8α-alcohol was attended by a marked loss in activity as was introduction of an equatorial methyl group into the lactone β-position to afford the mevalonolactone analog, (b) removal of the carbonyl group in the sidechain ester moiety afforded ether analogs with decreased activities, (c) insertion of a methylene unit between the lactone carbinol and carbonyl groups totally ablated activity, (d) reduction of either or both double bond(s) in the hexahydronaphthalene moiety minimally reduced activity (the only exceptions were the markedly less active derivatives bearing a cis-fused A/B ring juncture) and (e) full activity was maintained upon inversion of the asymmetric center in the sidechain ester acyl group. The last observation prompted the preparation of a diverse array of sidechain ester analogs and culminated in the development of simvastatin (MK-733, synvinolin, ZOCOR®), the 2,2-dimethylbutyrate analog of lovastatin.[21] Simvastatin is superior to lovastatin in both intrinsic inhibitory potency (K_i = 0.2 nM) and oral hypocholesterolemic activity (Figure 5).

More recently, pravastatin (CS-514,SQ 31,000, eptastatin), the 6-hydroxy openacid form of compactin, first identified as a urinary metabolite of compactin in dog, was introduced into clinical development.[22] This drug is produced by microbial transformation of compactin using *Nocardia autotrophica* and is a somewhat weaker inhibitor of reductase *in vitro* (K_i = 2.2 nM) and *in vivo*.[23]

Lovastatin and simvastatin, like mevastatin but not pravastatin, are prodrugs that are hydrolyzed *in vivo* to the corresponding ring-opened dihydroxycarboxylates, the principal active metabolites. The hydroxyacid form bears a key structural resemblance to an intermediate in the two-step conversion of the substrate HMG-CoA to the product mevalonate and, thus, these inhibitors may be thought of as transition state inhibitors.

PROPERTIES OF LOVASTATIN

The IC_{50}'s for lovastatin in a variety of cell culture systems are presented in Figure 6.[24] As can be seen, lovastatin is active *in vitro* in the nanomolar range. *In vivo* potency in rat and dog is also presented. In the rat, the orally administered sodium salt of the dihydroxy open-acid form of lovastatin was an active inhibitor of cho-

---

®ZOCOR is a trademark of Merck & Co., Inc., Rahway, N.J., U.S.A.

- Inhibition of sterol synthesis in cultured cells

	IC_{50} (nM)
L-M cells	8.7
Rat hepatoma	3.7
Human hepatoma	37.5

- *In vivo* inhibition of cholesterol synthesis

  Rat: ID_{50} = 46 μg/kg p.o. (open-acid form)

- Plasma cholesterol lowering

Dog:	8 mg/kg/day	29.3 ± 2.5% ↓
Rabbit (WSC Fed):	2 mg/kg/day	37% ↓
	6 mg/kg/day	48% ↓

FIG. 6. Inhibitory effects of lovastatin on sterol synthesis *in vitro* and cholesterol synthesis *in vivo*; effects of lovastatin on plasma cholesterol in dog and rabbits.

lesterol synthesis in an acute assay (50% inhibitory dose = 46 μg/kg). Treatment of dogs for 3 weeks with lovastatin at 8 mg/kg per day resulted in a 29.3 ± 2.5% lowering of plasma cholesterol.[17] Similarly, in the wheat-starch casein-fed rabbit, a model of hypercholesterolemia in this species (average cholesterol concentration of 310 mg/dl over a 66-day period), treatment with lovastatin at a dose of 2 mg/kg per day lowered serum cholesterol levels by an average of 37%, whereas a dose of 6 mg/kg per day resulted in a 48% decrease when compared to control, the observed change being reversed upon discontinuation of drug.[25]

The action of lovastatin is specific for the reductase enzyme. No inhibition of HMG-CoA synthase, HMG-CoA lyase, beta-ketothiolase, or inhibition of the conversion of mevalonate to cholesterol or isoprenoids occurred. In addition, no inhibition of general metabolic pathways, including fatty acid synthesis, protein synthesis, and nucleic acid synthesis, was observed.[24]

As predicted by the work of Anderson *et al.*, the consequence of inhibition of endogenous cholesterol biosynthesis upon the induction of reductase can be appreciated in a study of hepatocyte morphology.[26] Elegant studies by Singer and colleagues have utilized the techniques of immunofluorescence and electron microscopy to study normal and drug-treated rats.[27-29] Rats given 0.075% lovastatin alone in the diet exhibited a striking induction of HMG-CoA reductase localized in periportal hepatocytes. These cells had a homogeneous distribution of reductase staining in their cytoplasm. A combination of exceedingly high doses of lovastatin (0.25%) and cholestyramine (3%) produced a 150-fold increase in enzyme activity and induced prominent juxtanuclear immunofluorescent globules of HMG-CoA reductase in all hepatocytes[27] (Figure 7). Electron microscopy revealed that these

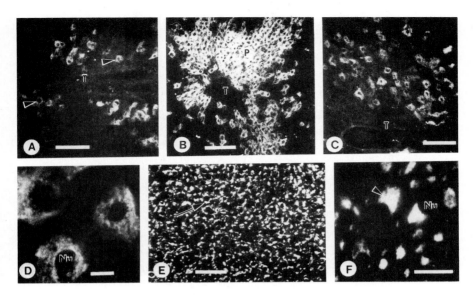

FIG. 7. Immunofluorescent microscopic distribution of HMG-CoA reductase in livers from normal or lovastatin-treated rats. *A,* HMG-CoA reductase-containing hepatocytes (arrowheads) are scattered randomly about the portal triad (T) in untreated rats (Bar = 100 μm). *B,* Lovastatin treatment (0.075%, 20 days) induces an intense staining for reductase in the periportal hepatocytes (P) surrounding the triad (T) (Bar = 100 μm). *C,* A normal pattern of HMG-CoA reductase localization is observed 8 days after cessation of the lovastatin regimen (0.075%, 12 days); T = portal triad (Bar = 100 μm). *D,* A mottled pattern of reductase staining is distributed throughout the cytoplasm of untreated hepatocytes; their nuclei (Nu) are unstained (Bar = 10 μm). *E,* All hepatocytes exhibit granules (arrow) of intense HMG-CoA reductase staining in rats given 3% cholestyramine for 9 days followed by 0.25% lovastatin and 3% cholestyramine for 3 days (Bar = 50 μm). *F,* High magnification of hepatocytes from E. Brilliant globules of reductase (arrowhead) are found in a juxtanuclear location; Nu = nucleus (Bar = 25 μm). (Reproduced with permission from Singer II, *et al. Proc Natl Acad Sci USA* 1984; **81**:5556–60.)

reductase-containing globules appeared to correspond to characteristic whorls of smooth endoplasmic reticulum induced by lovastatin/cholestyramine (Figure 8). These membranes were demonstrated to contain reductase identified by immuno-electronmicroscopy using anti-reductase antibody and anti-IgG colloidal gold conjugate.[28] A similar study has demonstrated that high dose lovastatin (180 mg/kg/day) in rats or dogs resulted in reductase induction in the ileum.[29]

To determine whether reductase inhibition by lovastatin resulted in an increase in the fractional catabolic rate of LDL, Chao *et al.* turned to the wheat-starch casein-fed rabbit model described above, which has been demonstrated to have a slower rate of removal of plasma ^{125}I-labeled LDL.[30] Perfused livers from rabbits treated with lovastatin (20 mg per animal) showed a 3.3-fold increase in the rate of receptor-dependent catabolism of ^{125}I-labeled LDL (4.6%·h^{-1}) when compared with that of livers from non-treated rabbits (1.45%·h^{-1}). Thus, in this model lovastatin treatment appears to have increased the levels of LDL-binding sites and the rate of receptor-dependent catabolism of LDL by the liver (Figure 9).

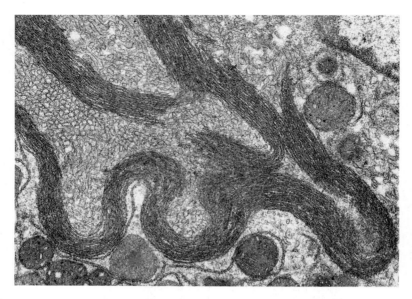

FIG. 8. A juxtanuclear smooth endoplasmic reticulum (SER) aggregate often found in hepatocytes of rats given cholestyramine and lovastatin. Wavy stacks of SER membranes are located peripherally and merge with rough endoplasmic reticulum cisternae, SER vesicles fill the interior, and a paracrystalline SER array is also present (Bar = 50 nm). (Reproduced with permission from Singer II, *et al. Proc Natl Acad Sci USA* 1984; **81**:5556–60.)

Interestingly, in human studies similarly designed to assess LDL-catabolism, Bilheimer *et al.* demonstrated increased fractional catabolic rates in six FH heterozygote patients after treatment with lovastatin.[31] On the other hand, Grundy and Vega were unable to show a statistically significant change in fractional catabolic rate for LDL in 12 patients with moderate hypercholesterolemia but not heterozygous FH, who were treated with low-dose lovastatin (10 mg b.i.d.).[32]

One specific feature of lovastatin is worthy of note. As demonstrated by metabolic studies, lovastatin is targeted to the liver, the organ primarily responsible for regulation of cholesterol biosynthesis. For lovastatin, 70% of the absorbed lactone is sequestered by the liver during its first pass.[24] Only modest levels (approximately 60 ng/ml after a 100 mg p.o. dose) were observed in the systemic circulation.[33] This study by Parker *et al.* went on to demonstrate that lovastatin at a dose of 200 mg (2.5 times the anticipated maximal human dose) did not suppress mevalonate synthesis, as measured by changes in 24-h urinary mevalonate outputs, to levels that would be expected to limit polyisoprenoid biosynthesis.

CONCLUSIONS

The pharmacologic inhibition of endogenous cholesterol biosynthesis can be accomplished effectively by the inhibition of HMG-CoA reductase, a rate-limiting

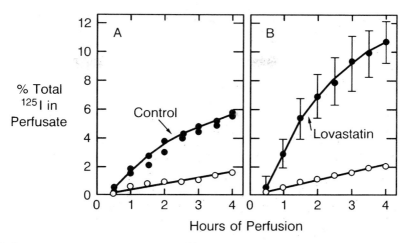

FIG. 9.   Production of nonprotein-bound ¹²⁵I during perfusion of livers from rabbits fed a wheat starch-casein diet (*A*) and from rabbits fed the wheat starch-casein diet and lovastatin (*B*), with rabbit ¹²⁵I-labeled LDL (●) and rabbit ¹²⁵ I-labeled cyclohexanedione-modified LDL (○). Rabbits were fed the diets for 30–40 days. For studies of catabolism of ¹²⁵I-labeled LDL, individual values of perfused livers from two wheat starch-casein-fed rabbits and mean value (± S.D.) of perfused livers from six lovastatin-treated rabbits are shown. For studies of ¹²⁵I-labeled cyclohexanedione-modified LDL, individual data from a paired experiment are shown. Pool size of rabbit LDL or cyclohexanedione-modified LDL apolipoproteins in the perfusate was between 0.2 and 0.3 mg. (Reproduced with permission from Chao YS, *et al. Biochim Biophys Acta* 1983; **754**:134–41.)

step in the cholesterol biosynthetic pathway. This inhibition results in an induction of both reductase activity and LDL receptor number. The increase in LDL receptor number mediates the rate of removal of LDL from the circulation in patients with heterozygous familial hypercholesterolemia. These actions can be demonstrated to normalize cholesterol levels in those individuals in whom defective regulation has resulted in hypercholesterolemia. It should be emphasized that our objective in the use of lovastatin is to normalize elevated plasma cholesterol in man, not to achieve the profound reduction observed, for example, when normocholesterolemic animals such as dogs are treated with the high doses of drug required by systematic toxicological assessment.

REFERENCES

1. Brown MS, Goldstein JL. A receptor-mediated pathway for cholesterol homeostasis. *Science* 1986; **232**:34–47.
2. Prugh JD, Rooney CS, Smith RL. Progress in atherosclerosis therapy: hypolipidemic agents. *Annu Rep Med Chem* 1983; **18**:161–170.
3. The Lipid Research Clinics Coronary Primary Prevention Trial Results. I. Reduction in incidence of coronary heart disease. Lipid Research Clinics Program. Lipid Metabolism-Atherogenesis Branch. National Heart, Lung and Blood Institute. *JAMA* 1984; **251**:351–364.
4. The Lipid Research Clinics Coronary Primary Prevention Trial Results. II. The relationship of reduction in incidence of coronary heart disease to cholesterol lowering. Lipid Research Clinics

Program. Lipid Metabolism-Atherogenesis Branch. National Heart, Lung and Blood Institute. *JAMA* 1984; **251**:365–374.

5. Rodwell VW, Nordstrom JL, Mitschelen JJ. Regulation of HMG-CoA reductase. *Adv Lipid Res* 1976; **14**:1–74.

6. Gould RG. Lipid metabolism and atherosclerosis. *Am J Med* 1951; **11**:209–227.

7. Bucher NLR, Overath P, Lynen F. β-Hydroxy-β-methylglutaryl coenzyme A reductase, cleavage and condensing enzymes in relation to cholesterol formation in rat liver. *Biochim Biophys Acta* 1960; **40**:491–501.

8. Goldstein JL, Brown MS. Familial hypercholesterolemia: identification of a defect in the regulation of 3-hydroxy-3-methyl-glutaryl coenzyme A reductase activity associated with overproduction of cholesterol. *Proc Natl Acad Sci USA* 1973; **70**:2804–2808.

9. Goldstein JL, Helgeson JAS, Brown MS. Inhibition of cholesterol synthesis with compactin renders growth of cultured cells dependent on the low density lipoprotein receptor. *J Biol Chem* 1979; **254**:5403–5409.

10. Cuthbert, JA, East CA, Bilheimer DW, Lipsky PE. Detection of familial hypercholesterolemia by assaying functional low-density lipoprotein receptors on lymphoctyes. *N Eng J Med* 1986; **314**:879–883.

11. Chin DJ, Gil G, Russell DW, *et al*. Nucleotide sequence of HMG CoA reductase, a glycoprotein of the endoplasmic reticulum. *Nature* (London) 1984; **308**:613–617.

12. Luskey KL, Stevens B. Human 3-hydroxy-3-methylglutaryl coenzyme A reductase. *J Biol Chem* 1985; **260**:10271–10277.

13. Dixon RAF, Kobilika BK, Strader DJ, *et al*. Cloning of the gene and cDNA for mammalian β-adrenergic receptor and homology with rhodopsin. *Nature* 1986; **321**:75–79.

14. Osborne TF, Goldstein JL, Brown MS. 5′ End of HMG CoA reductase gene contains sequences responsible for cholesterol-mediated inhibition of transcription. *Cell* 1985; **42**:203–212.

15. Liscum L, Luskey KL, Chin DJ, Ho YK, Goldstein JL, Brown MS. Regulation of 3-Hydroxy-3-methylglutaryl coenzyme A reductase and its mRNA in rat liver as studied with a monoclonal antibody and a cDNA probe. *J Biol Chem* 1983; **258**:8450–8455.

16. Endo A, Kuroda M, Tsujita Y. ML-236A, ML-236B, and ML-236C, new inhibitors of cholesterogenesis produced by *Penicillium citrinum*. *J Antibiot* 1976; **29**:1346–1348.

17. Alberts AW, Chen J, Kuron G, *et al*. Mevinolin: A highly-potent competitive inhibitor of hydroxymethylglutaryl-coenzyme A reductase and a cholesterol-lowering agent. *Proc Natl Acad Sci USA* 1980; **77**:3957–3961.

18. Endo A. Monakolin K—A new hypocholesterolemic agent produced by a *Monascus* species. *J Antibiot* 1979; **32**:852–854.

19. Lee T-J, Holtz WJ, Smith RL. Structural modification of mevinolin. *J Org Chem* 1982; **47**:4750–4757.

20. Kuo CH, Patchett AA, Wendler NL. Reductive transformation and cyclopropanation of mevinolin (6α-Methylcompactin). Generation of chirality in the 1,4-Hydrostannation of a cyclic diene. *J Org Chem* 1983; **48**:1991–1998.

21. Hoffman WF, Alberts AW, Anderson PS, Chen JS, Smith RL, Willard AK. 3-Hydroxy-3-methylglutaryl-coenzyme A reductase inhibitors. 4. Sidechain ester derivatives of mevinolin. *J Med Chem* 1986; **29**:849–852.

22. Haruyama H, Kuwano H, Kinoshita T, Terahara A, Nishigaki T, Tamura C. Structure elucidation of the bioactive metabolites of ML-236B (Mevastatin) isolated from dog urine. *Chem Pharm Bull* 1986; **34**:1459–1467.

23. Nakaya N, Homma Y, Tamachi H, Shigematsu H, Hata Y, Goto Y. The effect of CS-514 on serum lipids and apolipoproteins in hypercholesterolemic subjects. *JAMA* 1987; **257**:3088–3093.

24. Lovastatin, new drug application, 1986.

25. Kroon PA, Hand KM, Huff JW, Alberts AW. The effects of mevinolin on serum cholesterol levels of rabbits with endogenous hypercholesterolemia. *Atherosclerosis* 1982; **44**:41–48.

26. Anderson RGW, Orci L, Brown MS, Garcia-Segura LM, Goldstein JL. Ultrastructural analysis of crystalloid endoplasmic reticulum in UT-1 cells and its disappearance in response to cholesterol. *J Cell Sci* 1983; **63**:1–20.

27. Singer II, Kawka DW, Kazazis DM *et al*. Hydroxymethylglutaryl-coenzyme A reductase-containing hepatocytes are distributed periportally in normal and mevinolin-treated rat livers. *Proc Natl Acad Sci USA* 1984; **81**:5556–5560.

28. Singer II, personal communication.

29. Singer II, Kawka DW, McNally SE, *et al*. Hydroxymethylglutaryl-coenzyme A reductase exhibits graded distribution in normal and mevinolin-treated ileum. *Arteriosclerosis* 1987; **7**:144–151.
30. Chao YS, Kroon PA, Yamin TT, Thompson GM, Alberts AW. Regulation of hepatic receptor-dependent degradation of LDL by mevinolin in rabbits with hypercholesterolemia induced by a wheat starch-casein diet. *Biochim Biophys Acta* 1983; **754**:134–141.
31. Bilheimer DW, Grundy SM, Brown MS, Goldstein JL. Mevinolin and colestipol stimulate receptor-mediated clearance of low density lipoprotein from plasma in familial hypercholesterolemia heterozygotes. *Proc Natl Acad Sci USA* 1983; **80**:4124–4128.
32. Grundy SM, Vega GL. Influence of mevinolin on metabolism of low density lipoproteins in primary moderate hypercholesterolemia. *J Lipid Research* 1985; **26**:1464–1475.
33. Parker TS, McNamara DJ, Brown CD, *et al*. Plasma mevalonate as a measure of cholesterol synthesis in man. *J Clin Invest* 1984; **74**:795–804.
34. Liscum L, Finer-Moore J, Stroud RM, Luskey KL, Brown MS, Goldstein JL. Domain structure of 3-hydroxy-3-methylglutaryl coenzyme A reductase, a glycoprotein of the endoplasmic reticulum. *J Biol Chem* 1985; **260**:522–530.

SUMMARY

Since approximately two-thirds of total body cholesterol in individuals on a typical Western diet is endogenous in origin, a potentially more effective way of lowering plasma cholesterol levels is to control *de novo* cholesterologenesis. The microsomal enzyme 3-hydroxy-3-methylglutaryl-coenzyme A reductase (HMG-CoA reductase) is the major rate-limiting step early in cholesterol biosynthesis and thus suitable for pharmacologic intervention. Inhibition of HMG-CoA reductase results in an induction of both reductase activity and LDL receptor number. Induction of LDL receptor number by an HMG-CoA reductase inhibitor increases the rate of removal of LDL from the circulation in patients with heterozygous familial hypercholesterolemia, and has been shown to result in lower cholesterol levels in these individuals.

The first breakthrough in the search for a specific, competitive inhibitor of HMG-CoA reductase came in 1976 with the discovery of mevastatin. Subsequent screening efforts with fermentation broths against mammalian HMG-CoA reductase resulted in the discovery of a strain of *Aspergillus terreus* which produced the novel metabolite lovastatin. This paper discusses the structure, inhibitory properties, and resulting cholesterol-lowering effects of lovastatin in some detail. It is stressed that the objective in the use of lovastatin is to normalize elevated plasma cholesterol levels in man, and not to achieve the profound reductions in cholesterol observed, for example, when normocholesterolemic animals are treated with high doses of the drug, as required for toxicological assessment.

RÉSUMÉ

Puisqu'environ deux-tiers du cholestérol total du corps chez les êtres humains soumis à un régime alimentaire occidental typique est endogène à l'origine, une façon plus efficace de diminuer les niveaux de cholestérol dans le plasma est de contrôler à nouveau la cholestérologenèse. L'enzyme microsomal réductase 3-hydroxy-3-methylglutaryl-coenzyme A est le principal élément limitateur de taux dans les premières phases de la biosynthèse du cholestérol et de ce fait donc susceptible d'une intervention pharmacologique. L'inhibition de la réductase HMG-CoA a pour résultat une induction à la fois de l'activité de la réductase et du nombre récepteur de lipoprotéines de faible densité. L'induction du nombre récepteur de lipoprotéines de faible densité par un inhibiteur de réductase HMG-CoA augmente le taux de suppression des lipoprotéines de faible densité de la circulation chez les patients atteints d'hypercholestérolémie familiale hétérozygueuse et on a constaté chez ces patients un abaissement des niveaux de cholestérol.

En 1976 la découverte de la mevastatin a constitué un véritable premier pas dans la recherche d'un inhibiteur spécifique, compétitif de la réductase HMG-CoA. Par la suite des examens de bouillons de culture contre la réductase mammifère HMG-CoA ont amené à la découverte d'une souche d'*Aspergillus terreus* qui ont produit le nouveau métabolite lovastatin. On discute ici la structure et les propriétés inhibitoires du lovastatin dans le détail, ainsi que le fait que ce médicament provoque une diminution des taux de cholestérol. On insiste sur le fait que le but du lovastatin c'est de ramener à la normale les taux élevés de cholestérol chez l'homme et non de parvenir aux réductions importantes de cholestérol relevées par exemple, chez des animaux normocholestérolémiques prenant des doses élevées du médicament pour satisfaire aux exigences d'évaluation toxicologique.

ZUSAMMENFASSUNG

Da ungefähr zwei Drittel des gesamten Körpercholesterins von der Herkunft her in Personen, die eine westliche Diät zu sich nehmen, endogen ist, stellt die Kontrolle von *de novo* Cholesteringenese einen potentiell wirksameren Weg zur Erniedrigung der Plasma-Cholesterin-Spiegel dar. Das mikrosomale Enzym 3-Hydroxy-3-Methylglutaryl-Koenzym A Reduktase (HMG-CoA Reduktase) ist der wichtigste Ratebegrenzende Schritt früh in der Cholesterinbiosynthese; es ist daher für den pharmakologischen Eingriff geeignet. Hemmung der HMG-CoA Reduktase resultiert in einer Induktion der Reduktase-Tätigkeit sowie der Zahl der LDL-Rezeptoren. Induktion der LDL-Rezeptoren durch einen HMG-CoA Reduktasehemmer erhöht die LDL-Eliminierungsrate von der Zirkulation bei Patienten mit heterozygöser familiärer Hypercholesterolämie und es hat sich erwiesen, daß diese Induktion niedrigere Cholesterinspiegel in diesen Personen zur Folge hat.

Der erste Erfolg in der Suche nach einem spezifischen, konkurrierenden Hemmer der HMG-CoA Reduktase kam im Jahre 1976 mit der Entdeckung von Mevastatin. Darauffolgende Durchsiebensversuche mit Gärmittelbrühen gegen Säugetier-HMG-CoA Reducktase resultierten in der Entdeckung eines Stamms von *Aspergillus terreus*, der zum dem neuartigem Stoffwechselprodukt Lovastatin führte.

Dieser Vortrag diskutiert ausführlich die Struktur, die hemmenden Eigenschaften und die resultierenden Cholesterin-Erniedrigungswirkungen des Lovastatins. Es wird betont, daß das Ziel beim Gebrauch von Lovastatin die Normalisierung der erhöhten Plasma-Cholesterin-Spiegel im Menschen ist und, daß das Ziel nicht die ausgeprägten Erniedrigungen des Cholesterins ist, wie zum Beispiel bei Versuchen mit Tieren mit normalen Cholesterin-Spiegeln beobachtet, die mit hohen zur toxikologischen Bewertung benötigten Dosen des Medikamentes behandelt werden.

SOMMARIO

Dato che approssimativamente due-terzi del colesterolo totale in individui con una tipica dieta occidentale è endogeno in origine, un metodo potenzialmente piú effettivo di abbassare i livelli del colesterolo nel plasma è quello di controllare, di novo, la colesterologenesi. Le'enzima microsomale 3-idrossi-3 metilglutarile-coenzima A riduttasa (IMC-CoA) è il maggior passo della limitazione di tasso al inizio della biosintesi del colesterolo e quindi adatto a intervenzione farmaceutica. L'inibizione del IMG-CoA riduttasa si risolve in una induzione di entrambe le attività riduttasa e di un numero di ricettori di LBD. L'induzione del numero del ricettore LBD con un inibitore IMG-CoA riduttasa aumenta il tasso dell'eliminazione del LBD dalla circolazione per pazienti con ipercolesterolemia familiare eterozigote ed ha causato l'abbassamento del livello del colesterolo in questi individui. La prima scoperta decisiva nella ricerca per uno specifico e competitivo inibitore del IMG-CoA riduttasa successe nel 1976 con la scoperta del mevastatin. Ulteriore prove, tramite la fermentazione di brodi contro l'IMG-CoA riduttasa mammale, portò alla scoperta di un tipo dell' ''Aspergillus terreus'' che produsse il nuovo metabolito lovastatin. Questo saggio discute nei particolari la struttura, le proprietà inibitrici e gli effetti finali del lovastatin nell'abbassamento del colesterolo. Viene rinforzata l'idea che lovastatin viene usato per normalizzare lo stato elevato del livello del colesterolo nell'uomo e non ad arrivare a riduzioni profonde del colesterolo come, ad esempio, quando animali normocolesterolemici vengono curati con alte dosi della droga, com'è richiesto dall'assessamento tossicologico.

SUMÁRIO

Desde que aproximadamente dois-tercos de todo o colesterol do corpo de pessoas num regime alimentar típico do Ocidente é endógeno na sua origem, uma maneira potenciālmente mais eficaz de baixar os níveis de colesterol no soro é de controlar a formação de colesterol. A enzima microsomal, 3-hidroxi-3-metilglutaril-coenzima-A-reductasa (HMG-CoA-reductasa), é a etapa principal na limitação de taxa cedo na biosíntese de colesterol e assim apropriado para intervenção farmacológica. A inibição de HMG-CoA-reductasa resulta numa indução não só dé atividade da reductasa mas também do númeró de receptores LDL. A indução do número de receptores LDL pelo inibidor HMG-CoA-reductasa aumenta a taxa de afastamento de LDL da circulação em pacientes com hipercolesterolemia familiar heterocigótica e tem sido demonstrada a resultar em níveis de colesterol mais baixos nestas pessoas.

A primeira brecha na pesquisa dum inibidor específico e competidor para HMG-CoA-reductasa veio em 1976 com a descoberta de mevastatina. Os esfôrços subseqüentes com caldos de fermentação contra HMG-CoA-reductasa de mamíferos resultaram na descoberta duma variedade de Aspergillus terreus que produziu o novo metabolito lovastatina. Este documento trata detālhadamente da estrutura, das propriedades inibitórias e dos efeitos resultantes de baixar ó colesterol da lovastatina. E dado ênfase que o objetivo no emprêgo de lovastatina é de normālizar os níveis elevados de colesterol no soro no homen, e não de conseguir as reduções profundas no colesterol observadas, por exemplo, quando os animais normocolesterolémicos são tratados com doses altas do remédio, como é exigido para a avaliação toxicológica.

RESUMEN

Ya que aproximadamente dos tercios del colesterol corporal total en individuos alimentados con una dieta occidental típica es de origen endógeno, una manera potencialmente más eficaz para lograr la disminución de los niveles séricos de colesterol es controlar la formación de colesterol. La enzima microsomal 3-hidroxi-3-metilglutaril-coenzima-A-reductasa (HMG-CoA-reductasa) constituye el principal paso de limitación de la velocidad en las primeras etapas de la biosíntesis del colesterol y es por lo tanto apropiada para la intervención farmacológica. La inhibición de la HMG-CoA-reductasa resulta en una inducción tanto de la actividad de la reductasa como del número de receptores de LDL. La inducción del número de receptores de LDL por medio de un inhibidor de HMG-CoA-reductasa incrementa el índice de extracción de LDL de la circulación de pacientes con hipercolesterolemia familiar heterocigótica, y se ha demostrado que resulta en niveles más bajos de colesterol en estos individuos.

El primer adelanto importante en la búsqueda de un inhibidor específico competitivo de la HMG-CoA-reductasa se logró en 1976 con el descubrimiento de la mevastatina. Esfuerzos posteriores con cultivos de fermentación contra la HMG-CoA-reductasa de mamíferos resultó en el descubrimiento de una cepa de Aspergillus terreus que producía el nuevo metabolito lovastatina. En este estudio se examina con algun detalle la estructura, propiedades inhibitorias y los resultantes efectos de disminución del colesterol producidos por la lovastatina. Se enfatiza el hecho de que el objetivo del empleo de la lovastatina es normalizar los niveles séricos elevados de colesterol en el hombre, y no lograr las profundas reducciones en los niveles de colesterol observadas, por ejemplo, cuando se trata a animales normocolesterolémicos con altas dosis del fármaco, en base a los requisitos de la evaluación toxicológica.

The Role of Cholesterol in Atherosclerosis:
New Therapeutic Opportunities, edited by S. M. Grundy
and A. G. Bearn, Hanley & Belfus, Inc., Philadelphia.

Discussion

LASAGNA: I am concerned about this simplistic statement that a 1% reduction in cholesterol produces a 2% saving in CHD. Does this mean, for example, that by reducing serum cholesterol levels by 50%, all coronary heart disease can be eliminated?

GRUNDY: A 50% reduction probably would greatly reduce CHD as seen in epidemiological studies. Populations with plasma cholesterol levels 50% lower than those in high risk populations have very low rates of CHD.

LASAGNA: That is not the same thing. If a hypertensive person is made normotensive by drug therapy, the life-history of that person does not become the same as that of an untreated normotensive.

GRUNDY: I accept that if you do not lower patients' cholesterol levels until late on, after severe atherosclerosis has already developed, there will not be such a great reduction in CHD.

LANGMAN: We know that serum cholesterol levels vary to an apparently trivial extent according to the ABO blood group, and these changes are associated with differences in the frequency of CHD. How far you can go on depressing serum cholesterol to reduce still further the incidence of CHD is not at all clear.

BLOCH: Are the two effects of lovastatin (the inhibition of HMG-CoA reductase and the increase in LDL catabolism) linked or are they independent?

SLATER: In certain human studies performed by Brown and Goldstein there is a link, and I find their data convincing. They have looked at the fractional catabolic rate for LDL in heterozygous FH patients, and there is a definite increase in that rate induced by reductase inhibition—so there is *de facto* a link. But I don't believe the data are as strong for patients with non-familial hypercholesterolemia (non-FH) and/or for patients with somewhat more modest elevations of cholesterol treated with lower doses of inhibitor.

DOLLERY: It is always helpful when looking at any pharmacological action to try and envisage all the bad things that might happen because some probably will. Suppose you were giving this drug chronically, and you reduced HMG-CoA reductase to a very considerable extent, what happens if you suddenly stop the drug?

SLATER: Induction of the enzyme in man has not been demonstrated to occur. Enzyme induction has been reported in normocholesterolemic rats treated with exceedingly high doses of inhibitor. It is completely reversible on discontinuation of the drug.

DOLLERY: How long does it take the enzyme to down-regulate?

SLATER: It appears to happen within about 24 hours and there are no consequences which can be directly associated with that down-regulation, so far as I am aware.

CORVOL: In hepatoma cells is it possible to measure the level of gene expression of HMG-CoA reductase during its inhibition? Also, what happens to the other enzymes of cholesterol biosynthesis and what happens at the level of gene expression to the LDL receptor under chronic HMG-CoA reductase inhibitor treatment?

SLATER: There is a study by Liscum *et al.* in the Brown and Goldstein laboratory (*J Biol Chem* 1983; **258**:8450–8455) using a monoclonal antibody directed against reductase and a cDNA to reductase mRNA. She measured reductase activity in rat liver and induced it approximately 50-fold when rats were fed a combination of cholestyramine and lovastatin at an exaggeratedly high dose. Under those conditions the amount of immunodetectable reductase increased 33-fold. She stated that reductase mRNA became visible by blot hybridization. I have no information on gene expression for any of the other enzymes in the biosynthetic pathway.

MAHLEY: Brown and Goldstein's laboratory have shown that the LDL receptor number is increased with lovastatin, as is the receptor mRNA in animals.

MEZEY: In view of the importance of the liver in the metabolism of lovastatin, how is its metabolic disposition affected in chronic alcoholics?

SLATER: Alcoholism is a contraindication to the use of lovastatin, as will be discussed later. There is some indication that heavy alcohol users who are prescribed the drug may have a higher incidence of the adverse consequence of asymptomatic transaminase elevation.

GANTEN: Cholesterol is important in many other tissues besides the liver and the arteries. What are your views on the effects of HMG-CoA reductase inhibitors in other tissues, and would you expect any effects there?

SLATER: The aim in the use of these inhibitors is to normalize an abnormal situation, i.e., to lower elevated cholesterol to normocholesterolemic levels. One would assume this normalization to have no effect on steroidogenesis or on incorporation of cholesterol into tissue membranes. In the clinical studies about which Dr. Moncloa will report, we have demonstrated no effect on adrenal steroidogenesis using a therapeutic dose of lovastatin. There have been no toxicological observations using therapeutic dosages of lovastatin directly attributable to the concerns that you are expressing. However, at exceedingly high doses in rats, 800 times the anticipated human dose, teratologic effects have been observed which may well be due to the effect of the drug on cholesterol incorporation in newly-formed membrane.

LANGMAN: There is an epidemiological relationship between fat intake and cancer of the colon. As yet we do not know whether this is a systemic effect or the result of feeding fat to the gastrointestinal bacteria. If you give an experimental animal a carcinogen and fat, you are more likely to produce tumors. Has anyone done any work on carcinogenesis in the presence of lovastatin?

SLATER: Experiments to assess the direct effect of these compounds on genetic material have all proved negative. With regard to bile, human experiments have shown that lovastatin had no apparent effect on bile composition. With respect to certain FH patients, who have now been treated under a compassionate-use protocol for five years, the rate of occurrence of adenomas and carcinomas is not dissimilar to that of untreated patients of comparable sex and age.

LANGMAN: If you gave lovastatin to an animal together with something that caused cancer of the colon you might even get less cancer.

SLATER: There are some intriguing studies by Dr. William Maltese at Columbia University who transplanted neuroblastoma cells into mice and then treated them with lovastatin (Maltese WA, *et al.* *J Clin Invest* 1985; **76**:1748–1754). He found that the tumors shrank dramatically.

LEWIS: Which of the untoward effects that have been observed in animals and human subjects treated with the drug are mode-of-action related?

SLATER: The array of side-effects thus far observed in animals and men treated with lovastatin appear to be mechanism-based, i.e., derived specifically from the inhibition of cholesterol biosynthesis, and this observation would be expected to apply to HMG-CoA reductase inhibitors as a class. We have observed no obvious effects idiosyncratic to lovastatin. If you deliver lovastatin orally in the hydroxyacid form to experimental animals, there is a gastric irritation. This influenced our decision to administer the drug as the lactone.

COTRAN: How much more do you have to give experimental animals to lower normal cholesterol levels?

SLATER: Cholesterol lowering is species-dependent. In a rodent one sees an acute lowering of cholesterol. The consequent induction of enzyme activity prevents one from seeing further cholesterol lowering in rodent species. In dog, by contrast, one sees a logical dose-dependent lowering of cholesterol by the drug. In experiments conducted by our animal safety group, using doses 150 times the predicted human dose, a lowering of LDL cholesterol to virtually zero was seen in certain dogs. This was sustained for periods in excess of one year, and for the most part these animals lived without any obvious consequence. In man, regardless of the starting cholesterol level, there is an approximately 33% reduction in total circulating cholesterol with drug administration.

CORVOL: When you lower LDL cholesterol to almost zero by drug treatment, what happens to steroid hormones produced in the liver?

SLATER: These experiments have not been done.

IMURA: You stressed the importance of increased LDL degradation with lovastatin. What is the effect of this drug on LDL receptors in the homozygous FH patients? We cannot expect the increased degradation of LDL, but it still inhibits HMG-CoA reductase.

SLATER: If one uses the drug in a homozygous FH patient, one can detect some lowering in cholesterol, but these effects are minimal. This presumably implicates the LDL receptor in mediating the plasma cholesterol lowering.

IMURA: Does this suggest that receptor-mediated degradation is very important?

SLATER: Certainly in the FH patients.

The Role of Cholesterol in Atherosclerosis:
New Therapeutic Opportunities, edited by S. M. Grundy
and A. G. Bearn, Hanley & Belfus, Inc., Philadelphia.

Worldwide Clinical Experience with Lovastatin/Simvastatin

Federico Moncloa

A key step in the early biosynthesis of cholesterol is the conversion of hydroxy-methylglutarate (HMG) to mevalonate. HMG-CoA reductase is the enzyme that catalyzes this reaction. Lovastatin and simvastatin are both lactones that, after hydrolysis to their respective open hydroxy acid, become potent and selective competitive inhibitors of HMG-CoA reductase.[1] The inhibition of the enzyme reduces production of cholesterol. In addition, there is probably a secondary increase in the number of LDL receptors, which become the most important factor in decreasing serum cholesterol by removing LDL cholesterol from the circulation.[2]

High levels of serum cholesterol are clearly associated with cardiovascular mortality[3] and relatively modest decreases through diet and resins have resulted in lower mortality and morbidity.[4]

The availability of HMG-CoA reductase inhibitors makes possible therapeutic intervention that will result in important decreases in LDL cholesterol and other positive changes in the lipid profile. This chapter summarizes the published data on efficacy and safety.

EFFICACY OF LOVASTATIN AND SIMVASTATIN

Table I summarizes the efficacy data published on lovastatin and simvastatin. In most studies, the efficacy of these drugs in reducing LDL cholesterol is of the order of 30 to 42%.[5-15] This reduction in LDL cholesterol corresponds to reductions of total cholesterol of about 30%. The effect is obtained rather rapidly and is maintained during long-term treatment.[5,13]

In terms of percent reduction, the response is proportional to the dose in both FH and non-FH hypercholesterolemia.[11,13] The recommended dose range of lovastatin is 20–80 mg daily, taken either once in the evening or in a twice daily regimen. The twice daily regimen results in a somewhat greater response.[16] Table II summarizes the results of the four multicenter studies conducted during the evaluation of lovastatin.

In addition to lowering LDL cholesterol, HMG-CoA reductase inhibitors also increase HDL cholesterol. This increase in HDL cholesterol is of the order of 10%.

TABLE I. *Effect of lovastatin and simvastatin on plasma lipids in patients with familial (heterozygous) and non-familial hypercholesterolemia*

Reference	No. of Patients	Duration of Treatment	Daily Dose (mg)	Percent Changes					
				Total-C	LDL-C	VLDL-C	HDL-C	Apo B	TG
Lovastatin									
Illingworth et al.[5]	11	2–3 yrs.	40–80		–40				
Illingworth et al.[6]	13	4 wks.	10–80	–17 to –33	–20 to –38		+2 to –8		–6 to –34
Illingworth[7]	12	5–9 wks.	80	–33	–38				–25
Vega & Grundy[8]	15	4 wks.	40–80	–26	–34		+16		
Hoeg et al.[9]	24	4 wks.	40	–29	–34	–41	+6	–33	–35
Hoeg et al.[10]	31	4 wks.	40	–24	–31	–31	+16		–17
Hunninghake et al.[11]	101	6 wks.	10–80	–21 to –32	–25 to –39	–2 to –31	+4 to +13	–12 to –32	–21 to –27
DuJovne et al.[12]	170	12 wks.	40–80	–27 to –34	–32 to –42	–31 to –34			
Havel et al.[13]	101	6 wks.	10–80	–14 to –34	–17 to –39		+1 to +18	+1 to –23	+6 to –16
Simvastatin									
Moll et al.[14]	11	4 wks.	40–80	–32 to –36	–37 to –42		+21 to +9		–34 to –11
Olsson et al.[15]	20	4 wks.	2.5–80	–23	–28		+8	–24	–26

TABLE II. *Results of multicenter studies in relation to dose and dosage schedule*

Daily Dosage	Schedule	Total-C	LDL-C	HDL-C
20 mg	Once-a-day*	−17%	−21%	+11%
40 mg	Once-a-day	−24%	−28%	+8%
	Twice-a- day	−27%	−32%	+10%
80 mg	Once-a-day	−30%	−37%	+11%
	Twice-a-day	−33%	−41%	+9%

* Once-a-day doses were given in the evening.

Epidemiological data have indicated that HDL cholesterol is a protective factor against coronary heart disease,[17] possibly facilitating the removal of cholesterol from peripheral tissues.

Additionally, there is a decrease in apoliprotein B ranging from 24% to 33%, which indicates that the reduction in LDL cholesterol is the result of an actual decrease in the lipoproteins.

Both lovastatin and simvastatin have been shown to produce decreases in very low density lipoproteins (VLDL) and triglycerides, which are positive results for the prevention of coronary heart disease.

Concomitant Use with Other Lipid-lowering Agents

Table III summarizes the results obtained when lovastatin was concomitantly administered with other lipid-lowering agents. The use of lovastatin and resins[7,8] resulted in an additive effect on the reduction of LDL cholesterol and total cholesterol.

The addition of neomycin to lovastatin resulted in only slightly greater decreases in LDL and total cholesterol, but the effect on VLDL was attenuated and the positive effect of lovastatin on HDL cholesterol was reversed, since neomycin decreases HDL cholesterol.[10]

It has been reported that lovastatin used concomitantly with colestipol plus niacin produces an impressive mean reduction of LDL cholesterol of 67%.[18]

EVALUATION OF SAFETY

Lovastatin has been tested in about 900 patients in clinical trials sponsored by Merck. This number includes more than 100 patients with two or more years of treatment. Overall the incidence of side effects is low, with a discontinuation rate of about 2%. Special emphasis has been given to certain areas, which will be discussed in some detail. The long-term experience with simvastatin is still too limited to evaluate safety.

TABLE III. *Percent changes in lipids in patients treated with lovastatin alone or with lovastatin plus colestipol or neomycin, or with lovastatin, colestipol and niacin*

	Total-C	LDL-C	VLDL-C	HLD-C	TG
Lovastatin 20 mg b.i.d. 7 patients	−26	−34		+16	0
Lovastatin 20 mg b.i.d. + colestipol 10 gr b.i.d. 7 patients	−36	−53		+37	−8
Lovastatin 40 mg b.i.d. 10 patients	−33	−38		0	−25
Lovastatin 40 mg b.i.d. + colestipol 20 gr/ day 10 patients	−45	−54		−2	+7
Lovastatin 20 mg b.i.d. 31 patients	−24	−31	−25	+16	−17
Lovastatin 20 mg b.i.d. + neomycin 1 g b.i.d. 31 patients	−28	−34	−14	−7	−10
Colestipol + niacin	−31	−37	−21	+28	
Lovastatin 40–60 mg/day + colestipol + niacin 22 patients	−55	−67	−68	+36	

Liver Enzyme Elevations

From a clinical perspective, lovastatin is associated with two types of elevation of liver enzymes. The first type is trivial elevations, which are less than three times the upper limit of normal; may occur at any time during treatment; are present at any given point in about 5% of the patients; are transient and do not require discontinuation of drug therapy. The second type of transaminase elevation, more than three times the upper limit of normal, occurs in about 2% of the patients; usually occurs between 3–12 months of treatment; tends to be persistent; is asymptomatic and is not associated with increases in alkaline phosphatase or in bilirubin.

In two-thirds of patients who were rechallenged, elevation of transaminases occurred after a lag period of 1–8 months.

Lenses

MER-29 gave a bad reputation to cholesterol-lowering agents in relation to lens opacities. This, together with the toxicologic findings that doses about 50 times higher than those used in humans produced cataracts in dogs, prompted an extensive evaluation of the data regarding lens opacities in clinical trials of lovastatin. Quantification of lens opacities in clinical trials has several methodologic problems, most notably that the results of the lens examinations are not reproducible. Some opacities noted at baseline "disappear" in subsequent examinations whereas others not seen at baseline appear in subsequent examinations. This "noise" in the examination of the lens precludes a valid determination of incidence; thus it is more appropriate to present the data in terms of prevalence on the reasonable assumption that the noise in the lens examinations remains the same before and after treatment.

The distribution of opacities according to their localization was similar among the "new," the "lost," and the baseline opacities (Fig. 1). It is unlikely, therefore, that a drug effect on the lenses will result in a distribution of opacities similar not only to baseline but also to the distribution of "lost" opacities. Furthermore, there was no increase in the proportion of patients with subcapsular opacities; this is a relevant negative finding since the opacities reported in dogs at high toxic doses were subcapsular.

During the Phase II development program, the participating investigators were informed about toxicologic findings that lovastatin causes lens opacities in dogs. This introduced a bias that resulted in an apparent increase in prevalence. During Phase III, all observations took place after the toxicologic report. The data of Phase III are presented in Table IV. It can be seen that there were no important changes

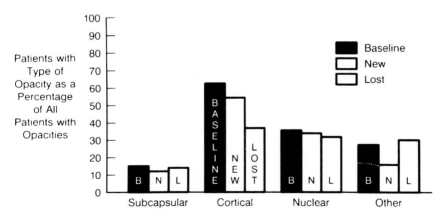

FIG. 1. Lens opacities in phase IIB and phase III studies (total patients = 477).

TABLE IV. *Prevalence of lens opacities in 431 patients treated with lovastatin*

	Baseline	Last Available Examinations
As per Dr. Chylack's classification*	23.4%	23.4%
As per Dr. Fraunfelder's classification	34.1%	31.5%

* The ophthalmologic reports included several terms to refer to lens abnormalities. Drs. Chylack and Fraunfelder were asked independently to indicate which of those terms should be classified as lens opacities.

in prevalence of lens opacities before and after treatment. Furthermore, there was no clinically significant change in visual acuity in the patients who had new opacities reported, and no patient has been withdrawn from therapy because of a lens opacity. Only three patients have had cataract surgery; all were in their sixties and had lens opacities at baseline.

Increases in Creatine Phosphokinase

During clinical trials of lovastatin, there were elevations of creatine phosphokinase in about 9% of the patients. A significantly lower incidence was observed in the control group treated with cholestyramine. Most of these elevations are transient and asymptomatic. However, myositis requiring discontinuation of therapy occurred in 0.5% of patients. In about half of these cases, the patients were also receiving gemfibrozil.

CONCLUSIONS

There are some adverse effects of lovastatin on liver enzymes that require periodical monitoring. Furthermore, full ophthalmologic examinations are recommended periodically. On the other hand, lovastatin and simvastatin have an efficacy profile that combines a large effect in decreasing the plasma concentration of LDL cholesterol with a decrease in apolipoprotein B, triglycerides and VLDL cholesterol, plus an increase in HDL cholesterol. All these changes are positive. Therefore, when the role of hypercholesterolemia is considered in the pathogenesis of atherosclerosis in general, and of coronary atheroma in particular, the benefit/risk evaluation is positive.

REFERENCES

1. Alberts AW, Chen J, Kuron G. Mevinolin: A highly potent competitive inhibitor of 3-hydroxy-3-methylglutaryl coenzyme A reductase, and a cholesterol-lowering agent. *Proc Natl Acad Sci USA* 1980; **77**:3957.
2. Kovanen PT, Bilheimer DW, Goldstein JL. Regulatory role for hepatic low density lipoprotein receptors in vivo in the dog. *Proc Natl Acad Sci USA* 1981; **78**:1194–1198.

3. Anderson KM, Castelli WP, Levy D. Cholesterol and mortality. 30 years of follow-up from the Framingham Study. *JAMA* 1987; **257**:2176–2180.
4. Lipids Research Clinics Program. The Lipid Research Clinics Coronary Primary Prevention Trial Results. I. Reduction in incidence of coronary heart disease II. The relationship of reduction in incidence of coronary heart disease to cholesterol lowering. *JAMA* 1984; **251**:351–374.
5. Illingworth DR, Pappu AS, Bacon SP. Metabolic and clinical effects of mevinolin in familial hypercholesterolemia. *In*: Fidge NH, Nestel PJ, eds. *Atherosclerosis VII*. Amsterdam: Elsevier (Biomedical Division), 1986, 611.
6. Illingworth DR, Sexton GJ. Hypocholesterolemic effects of mevinolin in patients with heterozygous familial hypercholesterolemia. *J Clin Invest* 1984; **74**:1972–1978.
7. Illingworth DR. Mevinolin plus colestipol in therapy for severe heterozygous familial hypercholesterolemia. *Ann Intern Med* 1984; **101**:598–604.
8. Vega GL, Grundy SM. Treatment of primary moderate hypercholesterolemia with lovastatin (mevinolin) and colestipol. *JAMA* 1987; **257**:33–38.
9. Hoeg JM, Maher MB, Zech LA *et al*. Effectiveness of mevinolin on plasma lipoprotein concentrations in type II hyperlipoproteinemia. *Am J Cardiol* 1986; **57**:933–939.
10. Hoeg JM, Maher MB, Bailey KR, Brewer Jr HB. The effects of mevinolin and neomycin alone and in combination on plasma lipid and lipoprotein concentrations in type II hyperlipoproteinemia. *Atherosclerosis* 1986; **60**:209–214.
11. Hunninghake DB, Miller VT, Palmer RH *et al*. (The Lovastatin Study Group II). Therapeutic response to lovastatin (mevinolin) in nonfamilial hypercholesterolemia. *JAMA* 1986; **256**:2829–2834.
12. DuJovne CA, Feldman EB, Frost PH, *et al*. A comparison of lovastatin and cholestyramine for the treatment of primary hypercholesterolemia. Sixtieth Scientific Session of the American Heart Association, 1987.
13. Havel RJ, Hunninghake DB, Illingworth DR, *et al*. A multicenter study of lovastatin (mevinolin) in the treatment of heterozygous familial hypercholesterolemia. *Ann Intern Med* 1987; **107**:609–615.
14. Mol MJTM, Erkelens DW, Gevers Leuven JA, Schouten JA, Stalenhoef AFH. Effects of synvinolin (MK-733) on plasma lipids in familial hypercholesterolemia. *Lancet* 1986; **2**:936–939.
15. Olsson AG, Molgaard J, von Schenk H. Synvinolin in hypercholesterolemia. *Lancet* 1986; **2**:390–391.
16. Illingworth DR. Comparative efficacy of once versus twice daily mevinolin in the therapy of familial hypercholesterolemia. *Clin Pharmacol Ther* 1986; **40**:338–343.
17. Gordon T, Castelli WP, Hjortland MC, Kannel WB, Dawber TR. High density lipoprotein as a protective factor against coronary heart disease. *Am J Med* 1979; **62**:707–714.
18. Malloy MG, Kane JP, Kunitake ST, Tun P. Complementarity of colestipol, niacin, and lovastatin in treatment of severe familial hypercholesterolemia. *Ann Intern Med* 1987; **107**:616–623.

SUMMARY

The efficacy and safety data of the HMG-CoA reducatase inhibitors lovastatin and simvastatin are reviewed. Studies have shown that both drugs have a marked (decreasing) effect on the plasma concentrations of LDL cholesterol, of the order of 30–42%, while also producing a decrease in apolipoprotein B, triglycerides and very low density lipoprotein (VLDL) cholesterol and an increase in HDL cholesterol. These are all positive results for the prevention of coronary heart disease. The safety of lovastatin has been evaluated in clinical trials of about 900 patients, including over 100 patients in whom the drug has been used for two or more years. Overall, the incidence of side-effects is low, with a discontinuation rate of about 2%. Both trivial and more marked elevations in liver enzymes have been reported in patients treated with lovastatin. Such changes appear to be asymptomatic, but it is recommended that liver enzymes are monitored regularly and treatment discontinued if the elevations are persistent and above three times the upper limit of normal. Lens opacities have been reported in dogs treated with toxicologic doses of lovastatin, but the data from Phase III trials give no indication of important changes in the prevalence of lens opacities before and after treatment. Nevertheless, periodic, full ophthalmologic examinations are recommended. It is concluded that, in view of the association between hypercholesterolemia and CHD and the efficacy profile of lovastatin and simvastatin in treating hypercholesterolemia, the benefit/risk evaluation for these drugs is positive.

RÉSUMÉ

Les données concernant la sécurité d'utilisation et l'efficacité des inhibiteurs de réductase HMG-CoA, lovastatin et simvastatin, sont examinés ici. Des études ont prouvé que ces deux médicaments réduisent d'une façon marquée les concentrations plasmatiques de cholestérol des lipoprotéines de faible densité, de l'ordre de 30 à 42%, tout en produisant aussi une diminution de l'apolipoprotéine B, des triglycérides et du cholestérol des lipoprotéines de très faible densité et une augmentation du cholestérol des lipoprotéines de forte densité. Tous ces résultats sont positifs pour la prévention des maladies coronariennes. Des essais cliniques ont été menés pour évaluer la sécurité d'utilisation du lovastatin: 900 patients ont été traités avec ce médicament, dont plus de 100 sur une période de 2 ans ou plus. Dans l'ensemble, on a noté peu d'effets secondaires, qui d'ailleurs disparaissent à un taux de 2%. On a signalé chez les patients qui prenaient du lovastatin des augmentations plus ou moins marquées des enzymes du foie. Ces changements sont asymptomatiques, toutefois il est recommandé de contrôler régulièrement les enzymes du foie et d'interrompre le traitement si les élévations persistent et atteignent trois fois la limite d'une normale élevée. On a constaté chez les chiens traités avec des doses toxicologiques de lovastatin des opacités de la lentille oculaire, mais les données de la Phase III des essais cliniques n'indiquent aucun changement important dans la prédominance des opacités oculaires avant et après le traitement. Néanmoins, il est recommandé de subir périodiquement des examens ophtalmologiques complets. En conclusion, il apparait que, vu les rapports qui existent entre l'hypercholesterolémie et les maladies coronariennes, le lovastatin et le simvastatin s'avèrent très efficaces pour le traitement de l'hypercholestérolémie. Les avantages de ces médicaments en surpassent les risques.

ZUSAMMENFASSUNG

Die Wirksamkeits- und Gefahrlosigkeitsdaten der HMG-CoA Reduktase Hemmstoffe Lovastatin und Simvastatin sind überprüft. Studien haben gezeigt, daß beide Medikamente einen merklichen (reduzierenden) Einfluß auf die Plasmakonzentrationen des LDL-Cholesterins von etwa 30–42% haben, obwohl sie ebenfalls eine Reduktion des Apolipoproteins B, Triglyzeride und des sehr niedrigdichten Lipoprotein-(VLDL)-Cholesterins und eine Erhöhung des HDL-Cholesterins produzieren. Dies sind alle positive Resultate für die Verhütung von koronarer Herzkrankheit. Die Gefahrlosigkeit von Lovastatin ist in klinischen

Versuchen an ungefähr 900 Patienten überprüft worden, einschließlich über 100 Patienten an denen das Medikament über den Zeitraum von 2 oder mehr Jahren angewandt wurde. Insgesamt gesehen ist das Auftreten Nebenwirkungen niedrig, mit einer Einstellungsrate von ungefähr 2%. Sowohl geringfügige als auch auffälligere Erhöhungen der Leberenzyme sind bei Patienten berichtet worden, die mit Lovastatin behandelt wurden. Solche Veränderungen scheinen asymptomatisch, aber es ist empfohlen, daß die Leberenzyme regelmäßig überwacht werden und, daß die Behandlung eingestellt wird, falls die Erhöhungen hartnäckig bestehen und über der dreifachen Höhe der oberen Grenze des normalen Spiegels sind. Linsenundurchsichtigkeiten in mit toxikologischen Dosen von Lovastatin behandelten Hunden sind berichtet worden, aber die Daten der Phase III-Versuche ergaben keinen Hinweis auf wichtige Änderungen im Vorherrschen der Linsenundurchsichtigkeiten vor oder nach der Behandlung. Trotzdem sind periodische ophthalmologische Gesamtuntersuchungen empfohlen. Man geht dabei davon aus, daß hinsichtlich der Verbindung zwischen Hypercholesterinämie und CHD und des Wirksamkeitsprofils von Lovastatin und Simvastatin bei der Behandlung von Hypercholesterinämie, die Nutzen/Risiko Auswertung dieser Medikamente positiv erscheint.

SOMMARIO

I dati di sicurezza e di efficacia degli inibitori del IMG-CoA riduttasa, Lovastatin e Simvastatin, vengono riesaminati. Gli studi dimostrano che entrambe droghe hanno uno specifico (diminuente) effetto sul concentramento nel plasma del colesterolo LBD, piú o meno fra il 30–42%, anche producendo un ribasso nell'apolipoproteina B, nella trigliceride e nel colesterolo con lipoproteina con densità molto bassa (LDMB) e un aumento nel colesterolo LAD. Questi sono tutti dei risultati positivi per la prevenzione della malattia coronaria del cuore. La sicurezza del lovastatin è stata evaluata in prove cliniche di circa 900 pazienti, 100 dei quali l'hanno usato per due o piú anni. Complessivamente, l'occorrenza di effetti collaterali è minima, con una percentuale di discontinuità del 2%. Sia minime che maggiori elevazioni negli enzima del fegato sono state riportate da pazienti curati con lovastatin. Tali cambiamenti non sembrano recare alcuni sintomi, ma si raccomanda di controllare regolarmente gli enzima del fegato e di non continuare l'uso se le elevazioni sono continue e tre volte superiori al limite normale. Sono state riportate opacità di lenti in cani curati con dosi tossicanti di lovastatin, ma il rapporto dalle ricerche della Fase III, non indica cambiamenti importanti nell'opacità di lenti prima o dopo la cura. In ogni caso, periodiche e complete esaminazioni oftalmologiche sono raccomandate. Vien concluso che, per quanto riguarda l'associazione fra l'ipercolesterolemia e MCC e l'efficacia del lovastatin e il simvastatin come cure per l'ipercolesteremia, l'evalutazione del beneficio/rischio di queste droghe sembra di essere positiva.

SUMÁRIO

Os dados sobre a eficácia e a segurança dos inibidores de HMG-CoA-reductasa, a lovastatina e a simvastatina, são examinados. Os estudos têm mostrado que ambos os remédios têm um efeito marcado (diminuindo) nas concentrações no plasma do colesterol-LDL, da ordem de 30–42%, enquanto também produzem uma redução em apolipoproteína B, triglicéridos e colesterol de lipoproteína de densidade muito baixa (VLDL), e um aumento em colesterol-HDL. Estes são todos resultados positivos para evitar a cardiopátia coronária. A segurança da lovastatina tem sido avaliada em testes clínicos com à volta de 900 pacientes, incluindo mais de 100 pacientes nos quais o remédio foi usado por dois ou mais anos. Em tôda parte, a incidência de efeitos secundários é baixa, com uma taxa de descontinuação em volta de 2%. Tanto subidas sem importância como outras mais marcadas nas enzimas do fígado têm sido noticiadas nos pacientes tratados com lovastatina. Tais mudanças aparecem ser asintomáticas, mas é recomendado que as enzimas do fígado sejam examinadas regularmente e que o tratamento seja terminado se as subidas são persistentes e mais que três vezes o limite superior do normal. Opacidades de cristalino têm sido noticiadas em câes tratados com doses toxicológicas de lovastatina, mas os dados das experiências da Fase III dâo nenhuma indicação de mudanças importantes na prevalência de opacidades do cristalino antes e depois do tratamento. Todavia, as examinações periódicas e completas são recomendādas. A conclusão é que, em vista da associação entre hipercolesterolemia e CHD e o perfil de eficácia de lovastatina e simvastatina no tratamento de hipercolesterolemia, a avaliação de benefício/risco de êstes remédios parece ser positiva.

RESUMEN

Se discuten los datos con respecto a la eficacia y seguridad de los inhibidores de HMG-CoA-reductasa, la lovastatina y la simvastatina. Varios estudios han mostrado que ambos fármacos tienen un marcado efecto (depresor) en las concentraciones plasmáticas de colesterol-LDL de aproximadamente 30 a 42%, al mismo tiempo que producen una disminución en la apolipoproteína B, los triglicéridos y el colesterol de lipoproteínas de muy baja densidad (VLDL) y un incremento en el colesterol HDL. Todos estos resultados son muy positivos para la prevención de cardiopatía coronaria. La seguridad de la lovastatina se ha evaluado en ensayos clínicos con participación de aproximadamente 900 pacientes, incluyendo más de 100 pacientes en los que el fármaco se ha empleado durante dos años o más. Globalmente la incidencia de efectos secundarios es baja, con un índice de abandonos de aproximadamente 2%. Se ha informado de incrementos triviales y marcados en ciertas enzimas hepáticas en pacientes tratados con la lovastatina. Tales cambios parecen ser asintomáticos, pero se recomienda que las enzimas hepáticas se vigilen regularmente y se discontinúe el tratamiento si las elevaciones son persistentes y aproximadamente tres veces mayores que el límite superior normal. Se ha informado de opacidades del cristalino en perros tratados con dosis tóxicas de la lovastatina, pero los datos obtenidos en los ensayos de Fase III no dan indicación de cambios importantes en la prevalencia de opacidades del cristalino antes y después del tratamiento. De todas maneras, se recomienda efectuar exámenes oftalmológicos completos periódicamente. Se concluye que, en vista de la asociación entre la hipercolesterolemia y la CHD y el perfil de eficacia de la lovastatina y la simvastatina en el tratamiento de la hipercolesterolemia, la relación riesgo:beneficio para estos fármacos parece ser positiva.

The Role of Cholesterol in Atherosclerosis:
New Therapeutic Opportunities, edited by S. M. Grundy
and A. G. Bearn, Hanley & Belfus, Inc., Philadelphia.

Discussion

LEWIS: Do you have any indication from the smaller number of studies on simvastatin that the side-effect pattern is different quantitatively or qualitatively?

MONCLOA: No. We think it is quite similar.

LEDINGHAM: You mentioned liver enzymes and transaminases and you have a 0.5% incidence of myositis. Are you quite sure that it is liver and not muscle that those enzymes are reflecting?

MONCLOA: Yes; both transaminases are elevated.

LEDINGHAM: Couldn't they come from muscles as well?

MONCLOA: We don't think so.

LEDINGHAM: Do they go up together or separately?

MONCLOA: Separately; there is no association between the elevations of CPK and the elevations of transaminases.

ASSCHER: In view of this rise in transaminase of liver origin, is there any suggestion of enzyme induction and interaction with oral contraceptives?

MONCLOA: No. In humans there is no evidence of enzyme induction.

LASAGNA: How many of the animals have developed cataracts?

SLATER: With lovastatin, 10% of dogs at 60 mg/kg/day (roughly 60 times the anticipated human dose), and none at any lower dosages, have developed them. With simvastatin, a similar number of dogs have developed cataracts, again with a wide margin between toxic and therapeutic dosage.

POOLE-WILSON: After chronic treatment could you say how quickly the plasma cholesterol returns to normal?

MONCLOA: If we define chronic treatment as two months or so, a four-week washout period is plenty of time for it to return to previous values.

MEZEY: What about the therapeutic benefits after the withdrawal of lovastatin? Is there a smooth carry-over effect or a rebound phenomenon?

MONCLOA: We do not have daily measurements but within two weeks plasma cholesterol levels are almost back to the previous value. There is no obvious rebound effect.

LEDINGHAM: There must be great difficulty in selecting an optimal dosage. It seems surprising, if the mechanism relates to LDL receptor numbers, that you need to give the drug twice a day. Wouldn't less frequent dosage be effective?

65

MONCLOA: We don't want to give lovastatin twice a day but earlier studies performed on normal volunteers showed that twice a day was clearly superior to once a day. In those studies it was given once daily in the morning. In later studies lovastatin was given in the evening because some reports suggested that cholesterol biosynthesis occurred mainly at night. With the nightly dose the difference between once a day and twice a day became less marked.

BAYLISS: I understand you started by modifying the diet. Was this a standard modification for all patients treated, was it continued throughout the whole trial, and how do we know that patients kept to their diets?

MONCLOA: All patients were advised to follow the American Heart Association type I diet and they had diet counseling throughout the study. We saw no evidence of escape in terms of cholesterol lowering. We interpret that as adequate compliance with the diet.

NORTH: You would not observe noncompliance, as the dietary effect on serum cholesterol is likely to be about 4%. If some people altered their diets at different stages in the trial, you would not be able to detect this change.

BEARN: It is probably also true that the response to diet is very variable. In some patients a response of considerably more than 4% can be achieved, whereas others seem to be extraordinarily resistant, again showing the heterogeneity of the population to whom we are introducing the drug. Despite the heterogeneity of the population, however, the response to lovastatin is unambiguous.

The Role of Cholesterol in Atherosclerosis:
New Therapeutic Opportunities, edited by S. M. Grundy
and A. G. Bearn, Hanley & Belfus, Inc., Philadelphia.

Experience with Lovastatin: Studies on Mechanisms of Action

Scott M. Grundy

Lovastatin is a specific inhibitor of 3-hydroxy-3-methylglutaryl-coenzyme A (HMG-CoA) reductase. This enzyme catalyzes the rate-limiting step in the synthesis of cholesterol, namely, the conversion of HMG-CoA into mevalonic acid. Mevalonic acid is converted mainly to cholesterol, although it also is the precursor for ubiquinone, dolichol, and isopentenyl transfer RNA. The major action of lovastatin appears to be in the liver, although it may have some activity in the intestine and other extrahepatic tissues. The liver seemingly extracts lovastatin rapidly from the circulation, and thus the amounts of the drug available for action in extrahepatic tissues may be relatively small. The duration of action of lovastatin in its inhibition of HMG-CoA reductase has not been determined with certainty, but it may be relatively short because of rapid catabolism of the drug within the liver cell. While it is certain that lovastatin is a competitive inhibitor of HMG-CoA reductase, details of its own metabolism remain to be worked out or published in detail.

EFFECTS OF LOVASTATIN ON CHOLESTEROL SYNTHESIS IN HUMANS

Since lovastatin inhibits the conversion of HMG-CoA reductase to mevalonic acid, it should reduce the synthesis of cholesterol in humans. To test its effect in humans, we carried out cholesterol-balance studies in five patients treated with lovastatin[1] (Fig. 1). In three of the patients (MB, JP and CC), lovastatin (mevinolin) produced a distinct reduction in the output of fecal steroids (neutral steroids and/or bile acids). This change strongly suggests that the lovastatin produces a mild-to-moderate inhibition of whole-body cholesterol synthesis. In another patient (JC), lovastatin reduced steroid output near the end of the period, but in yet another (MBa), there was no change in total steroid excretion. Nevertheless, taken as a whole, this study indicates that lovastatin usually causes some reduction in cholesterol synthesis. On the other hand, the drug did not cause a marked decrease in synthesis of cholesterol that might result in a severe depletion of whole-body cholesterol. Thus, the reduction in cholesterol synthesis associated with lovastatin therapy does not appear sufficient to pose a threat to overall health.

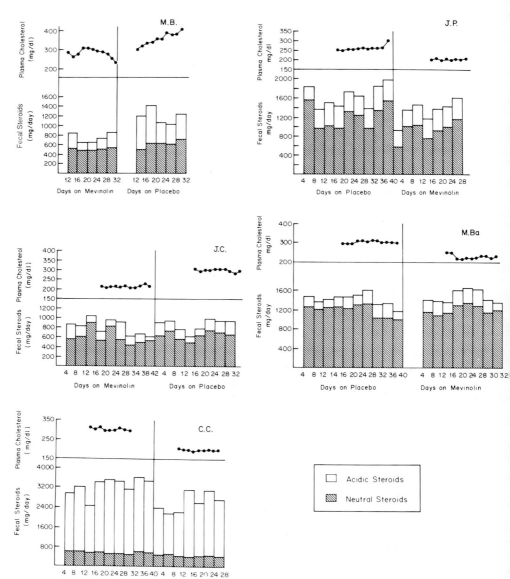

FIG. 1.   Cholesterol-balance studies in five patients treated with lovastatin. Three patients (JP, MBa and CC) received placebo first, and the other two (MB and JC) received lovastatin first. Levels of plasma cholesterol are shown for the period in which LDL turnover was carried out. In this study, acidic steroids are equivalent to bile acids, and neutral steroids represent cholesterol and its bacterial conversion products—coprostanol and coprostanone. (Reproduced with permission from Grundy SM, Bilheimer DW. Inhibition of 3-hydroxy-3-methylglutaryl CoA reductase by mevinolin in familial hypercholesterolemia heterozygotes: Effects on cholesterol balance. *Proc Natl Acad Sci USA* 1984; **81**:2538–2542.)

SECONDARY ACTIONS OF LOVASTATIN

The metabolic consequences of a partial inhibition of cholesterol synthesis are not fully understood. The major effect, however, appears to be the stimulation of synthesis of low density lipoprotein (LDL) receptors. It is known that the production of LDL receptors is metabolically regulated.[2] When the concentration of cholesterol in the liver cell is reduced, the synthesis of receptors is increased. Seemingly, cholesterol (or one of its products) directly suppresses the activity of the gene for LDL receptors, and by inhibiting the synthesis of cholesterol, this leads to an enhanced formation of LDL receptors. For example, lovastatin has been shown to increase the messenger RNA for LDL receptors in laboratory animals.[3]

Another possible action of lovastatin is to inhibit the synthesis of lipoproteins within the liver. If the drug retards the formation of cholesterol, an important component of lipoproteins, then it too might interfere with the hepatic synthesis of lipoproteins containing apolipoprotein B-100 (apo B). To date, however, there are no reports on effects of lovastatin on the synthesis of apo B in hepatocytes.

MECHANISM FOR LDL LOWERING

The effects of lovastatin on concentrations of LDL cholesterol can best be considered by a review of the metabolism of lipoproteins containing apo B. The current concepts of this system are outlined in Figure 2. The liver synthesizes and secretes triglyceride-rich lipoproteins—the very low density lipoproteins (VLDL). The triglycer-

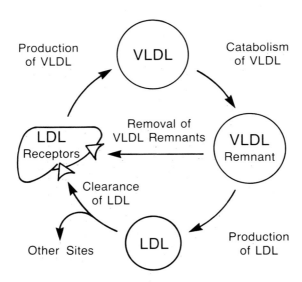

FIG. 2.   Pathways in metabolism of lipoproteins containing apolipoprotein B-100.

ides of VLDL are hydrolyzed by lipoprotein lipase into smaller lipoproteins, named VLDL remnants. These remnants can have two fates: they can either be removed by the liver or be converted to LDL. The LDL are the major cholesterol-carrying lipoproteins of plasma. The LDL are cleared from the circulation mainly by specific LDL receptors, but small quantities of LDL can be removed by nonreceptor mechanisms. Although many tissues of the body contain LDL receptors, most LDL appears to be cleared via the liver.[4] VLDL remnants apparently are removed in large part by LDL receptors as well.[5]

The mechanisms for lowering LDL levels in patients with heterozygous familial hypercholesterolemia (FH) were studied by Bilheimer, Grundy, Brown, and Goldstein.[6] Investigations were carried out in six patients with this disorder. To distinguish between receptor-dependent and receptor-independent pathways of LDL catabolism, the simultaneous clearance rates of native LDL and LDL that had been modified by *in vitro* glycosylation were compared. Previous work[7] had demonstrated that glycosylated LDL does not bind to LDL receptors *in vivo* or *in vitro*, and for this reason, the catabolism of glycosylated LDL can be used to estimate the fractional catabolic rate (FCR) for receptor-independent clearance of LDL. In our study, all six patients with heterozygous FH had markedly elevated concentrations of LDL cholesterol in the control period. After treatment of these patients with lovastatin (20 mg twice daily) for three to six weeks, the mean concentration of LDL cholesterol fell by 27% (Fig. 3). In these patients, the FCRs for native LDL rose by 37%. These results are consistent with an increased activity of LDL receptors during lovastatin therapy.

The data for simultaneous studies of catabolism of ^{131}I-native LDL and ^{125}I-glycosylated LDL in one patient with heterozygous FH during control and lovastatin-treatment periods are presented in Figure 4. Before drug treatment, the FCR for native LDL was 0.29 pools/day, whereas the FCR for glycosylated LDL was 0.16 pools/day. The difference of 0.13 pools/day presumably represented the FCR for the receptor-mediated component. When lovastatin was administered, the FCR for native LDL rose to 0.48 pools/day, while the FCR for glycosylated LDL (i.e., 0.18 pools/day) was basically unaltered. In this patient, it appeared that the FCR for the receptor-mediated pathway increased from 0.13 to 0.30 pools/day on lovastatin, which can be taken to mean that lovastatin stimulated the receptor-mediated clearance of LDL but did not change the nonreceptor-mediated pathway. Thus, one action of lovastatin appears to be to increase the synthesis of LDL receptors.

What are the effects of lovastatin on the production of LDL? In the six patients with heterozygous FH, the drug did not significantly reduce the transport rate (production rate) of LDL. However, a different result was obtained by Grundy and Vega[8] in patients with primary moderate hypercholesterolemia. In this investigation, kinetic parameters of LDL metabolism were determined in 12 patients with plasma total cholesterol levels in the range of 240 to 300 mg/dl (6.2–7.8 mmol/L); in these patients, LDL cholesterol concentrations generally were between 160 and 200 mg/dl (4.1 and 5.2 mmol/L), or in a few patients, somewhat higher. When these patients were treated with lovastatin, a surprising finding was that the drug did not

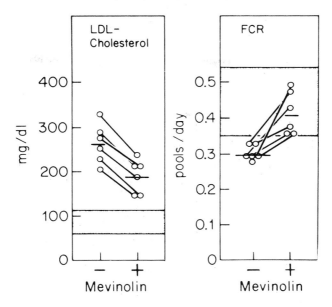

FIG. 3. LDL cholesterol concentrations (left panel) and fractional catabolic rates (FCRs) for plasma LDL-apo B (right panel) in six patients with heterozygous familial hypercholesterolemia before ($-$) and during ($+$) treatment with mevinolin (lovastatin). The mean values for each parameter are indicated by the horizontal bars, and the shaded areas denote the range for normal subjects. (Reproduced with permission from Bilheimer DW, Grundy SM, Brown MS, Goldstein JL. Mevinolin and colestipol stimulate receptor-mediated clearance of low density lipoprotein from plasma in familial hypercholesterolemia heterozygotes. *Proc Natl Acad Sci USA* 1983; **80**:4124–4128.)

significantly increase FCRs for LDL; instead, the major effect of lovastatin was a decrease in production rates for LDL. This finding is contrary to what might have been expected if the primary action of lovastatin is to increase the number of LDL receptors. In these patients, if the number of LDL receptors was not increased by lovastatin, the decrease in LDL levels on drug therapy would have to be explained by a decrease in the production of VLDL, the precursor of LDL. An alternative explanation, however, is that lovastatin enhanced the clearance of VLDL remnants and thereby reduced the number of remnant particles available for conversion to LDL.

To date, it has not been possible to distinguish between these two mechanisms with certainty. It seems likely, however, that at least part of the decrease in production rates of LDL can be explained by an enhanced clearance of VLDL remnants. This conclusion seems almost inescapable, since abundant evidence indicates that the drug increases the activity of LDL receptors.[3] Further data to support this contention are that lovastatin has little effect on LDL concentrations in patients with homozygous FH who are devoid of LDL receptors. A preliminary study from our laboratory[9] was carried out in three such patients. Relatively large doses of lovastatin

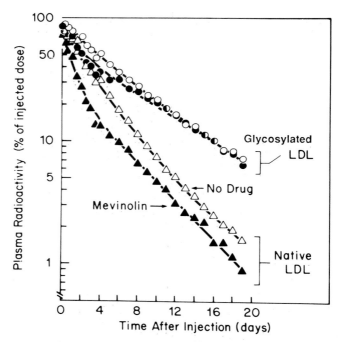

FIG. 4. Plasma decay curves after intravenous injection of radioiodinated native LDL and glycosylated LDL in a patient with heterozygous familial hypercholesterolemia before and during treatment with mevinolin (lovastatin) therapy. The turnover of glycosylated LDL was essentially unchanged by drug therapy, whereas turnover of native LDL was increased on lovastatin. (Reproduced with permission from Bilheimer DW, Grundy SM, Brown MS, Goldstein JL. Mevinolin and colestipol stimulate receptor-mediated clearance of low density lipoprotein from plasma in familial hypercholesterolemia heterozygotes. *Proc Natl Acad Sci USA* 1983; **80**:4124–4128.)

were given to all the patients, and in none did the drug cause a significant reduction in LDL concentrations. This finding is consistent with the concept that lovastatin acts mainly to lower LDL concentrations by promoting the synthesis of LDL receptors. Nevertheless, we have not ruled out the possibility that the drug has an additional action of inhibiting the formation of apo B-containing lipoproteins by the liver.

METABOLISM OF VERY LOW DENSITY LIPOPROTEINS

If the major action of lovastatin is to enhance the activity of LDL receptors, then it might be expected that the drug would have few effects on the metabolism of VLDL. There is, nevertheless, evidence that lovastatin does affect VLDL metabolism. The observation that lovastatin reduces the influx of LDL in patients with hypercholesterolemia implies that it alters the metabolism of VLDL, the precursor of LDL. As indicated above, this effect could be due either to an inhibition of synthesis of VLDL or to increased clearance of VLDL remnants.

To date, there are no extensive studies on the kinetics of VLDL in patients treated with lovastatin. Several studies, however, have suggested that VLDL metabolism is affected significantly by lovastatin. First, the drug often causes a lowering of plasma triglycerides; and second, in patients with familial dysbetalipoproteinemia, who have an increase in beta-VLDL (a form of VLDL remnants), lovastatin causes a significant reduction in concentrations of VLDL-cholesterol.[10] The latter finding in particular suggests that the clearance of VLDL remnants is enhanced by lovastatin therapy. And third, as mentioned above, lovastatin reduces production rates for LDL in many patients, which is consistent with the concept that the drug has a significant effect on VLDL metabolism. All of these lines of evidence are indirect, and more studies will be required to determine the full extent of lovastatin and other reductase inhibitors on the metabolism of triglyceride-rich lipoproteins.

METABOLISM OF HIGH DENSITY LIPOPROTEINS (HDL)

In our investigation of patients with primary moderate hypercholesterolemia,[8] we obtained the first evidence that lovastatin can raise plasma levels of HDL-cholesterol. In 11 patients with this condition, we observed that lovastatin (20 mg twice daily) caused a rise in HDL cholesterol levels of 23%, from 40 ± 4 (SEM) mg/dl to 48 ± 3 mg/dl (1.0 to 1.2 mmol/L). When 10 patients with primary moderate hypercholesterolemia were given the combination of lovastatin and colestipol, a rise in HDL-cholesterol from 39 ± 4 to 52 ± 5 mg/dl (1.0–1.3 mmol/L) likewise was observed. Further, in eight patients with heterozygous FH who were treated with the combination of lovastatin and colestipol, the HDL cholesterol concentration rose from 27 ± 3 to 35 ± 5 mg/dl (0.7 to 0.9 mmol/L). The HDL-raising action of lovastatin has subsequently been confirmed in other studies,[11] although it is not a consistent response for all patients.

The mechanisms by which lovastatin often raises HDL cholesterol levels have not been determined. This response may be related to the effects of the drug on VLDL metabolism. An inverse relationship between concentrations of VLDL and intermediate density lipoproteins (IDL) is well recognized, and when lovastatin reduces plasma concentrations of VLDL and IDL, it may simultaneously raise the HDL level. The reasons for an inverse correlation between VLDL/IDL and HDL are not fully understood, but the reduction in concentrations of VLDL and IDL during lovastatin therapy is a reasonable explanation for the rise in HDL levels. However, other factors yet to be determined also may play a role.

CONCLUSIONS

Lovastatin is a promising drug for lowering plasma cholesterol levels in patients with hypercholesterolemia. Our experience with this drug has provided new insights into its actions. The drug seemingly affects the concentrations of all the lipoproteins. Certainly, a major action of lovastatin is the stimulation of the synthesis of LDL receptors. Although we have not ruled out the possibility that lovastatin has other effects, such as inhibition of VLDL synthesis, the argument can be made that all of the observed changes can be explained by a stimulation of LDL receptor synthesis. To confirm or disprove this argument, it will be necessary to carry out more direct studies of the actions of the drug at the cellular and subcellular level. These studies may best be carried out in experimental animals, but investigations on human tissues, such as human liver, are not entirely out of the question.

REFERENCES

1. Grundy SM, Bilheimer DW. Influence of inhibition of 3-hydroxy-3-methylglutaryl CoA reductase by mevinolin in familial hypercholesterolemia heterozygotes: Effects of cholesterol balance. *Proc Natl Acad Sci USA* 1984; **81**:2538–2542.
2. Goldstein JL, Brown MS. The low density lipoprotein pathway and its relation to atherosclerosis. *Ann Rev Biochem* 1977; **46**:897–930.
3. Ma PTS, Gil G, Sudhof TC, Bilheimer DW, Goldstein JL, Brown MS. Mevinolin, an inhibitor of cholesterol synthesis, induces mRNA for low density lipoprotein receptor in livers of hamsters and rabbits. *Proc Natl Acad Sci USA* 1986; **83**:8370–8374.
4. Bilheimer DW, Goldstein JL, Grundy SM, Starzl TE, Brown MS. Liver transplantation to provide low-density-lipoprotein receptors and lower plasma cholesterol in a child with homozygous familial hypercholesterolemia. *N Engl J Med* 1984; **311**:1658–1664.
5. Brown MS, Goldstein JL. Lipoprotein receptors in the liver: Control signals for plasma cholesterol traffic. *J Clin Invest* 1983; **72**:743–747.
6. Bilheimer DW, Grundy SM, Brown MD, Goldstein JL. Mevinolin and colestipol stimulate receptor-mediated clearance of low density lipoprotein from plasma in familial hypercholesterolemia heterozygotes. *Proc Natl Acad Sci USA* 1983; **80**:4124–4128.
7. Kesaniemi YA, Witztum JL, Steinbrecher UP. Receptor-mediated catabolism of low density lipoprotein in man: Quantitation using glycosylated low density lipoproteins. *J Clin Invest* 1983; **71**:950–959.
8. Grundy SM, Vega GL. Influence of mevinolin on metabolism of low density lipoproteins in primary moderate hypercholesterolemia. *J Lipid Res* 1985; **26**: 1464–1475.
9. Uauy R, Vega GL, Bilheimer DW, Grundy SM. Effect of lovastatin on lipoproteins and LDL kinetics in homozygous familial hypercholesterolemia. *Pediatr Res* 1987; **21(II)**:349A.
10. East CA, Grundy SM, Bilheimer DW. Preliminary Report: Treatment of Type III hyperlipoproteinemia with mevinolin. *Metabolism* 1986; **35**:97–98.
11. The Lovastatin Study Group II. Therapeutic response to lovastatin (mevinolin) in nonfamilial hypercholesterolemia: A multicenter study. *JAMA* 1986; **256**:2829–2834.

SUMMARY

Lovastatin is a specific inhibitor of 3-hydroxy-3-methylglutaryl coenzyme A (HMG-CoA) reductase, the enzyme that catalyzes the rate-limiting step in the synthesis of cholesterol. Its major site of action appears to be the liver. Cholesterol-balance studies in humans have shown that lovastatin usually causes some reduction in cholesterol synthesis but not sufficient to lead to severe depletion of whole-body cholesterol. The major effect of this partial inhibition of cholesterol synthesis appears to be the stimulation of synthesis of low density lipoprotein (LDL) receptors. It is also possible that lovastatin inhibits the synthesis of lipoproteins within the liver. The mechanism by which lovastatin lowers LDL cholesterol is outlined: the triglycerides of the very low density lipoproteins (VLDL) are hydrolyzed to smaller lipoproteins—the VLDL remnants, which can either be removed by the liver or converted into LDL. The LDL (the major cholesterol-carrying lipoproteins) are cleared from the circulation mainly by specific LDL receptors. Investigations into the mechanisms for lowering LDL levels in patients with heterozygous familial hypercholesterolemia (FH) and patients with primary moderate hypercholesterolemia are described. In the latter group it appears that lovastatin reduces LDL cholesterol not by increasing the clearance of LDL itself but by enhancing the clearance of VLDL remnants. The investigations described also provide some evidence that lovastatin can cause a rise in plasma levels of HDL cholesterol. Further studies on the direct action of the drug need to be carried out to confirm or disprove these preliminary findings.

RÉSUMÉ

Le lovastatin est un inhibiteur spécifique de la réductase du Coenzyme A 3-hydroxy-3-methylglutaryl (HMG-Co A), enzyme qui catalyse la phase de taux limite dans la synthèse du cholestérol. Son principal site d'action semble être le foie. Des études visant à l'équilibre du cholestérol chez les humains ont montré que le lovastatin provoque généralement une réduction dans la synthèse du cholestérol, insuffisante cependant pour provoquer une grave déplétion du cholestérol du corps entier. L'effet principal de cette inhibition partielle semble être la stimulation d'une synthèse de récepteurs de lipoprotéines de faible densité. Peut-être aussi que le lovastatin inhibite la synthèse de lipoprotéines dans le foie. On décrit le mécanisme par lequel le lovastatin réduit le cholestérol des lipoprotéines de faible densité: les triglycérides des lipoprotéines de très faible densité sont hydrolysées en plus petites lipoprotéines qui peuvent être soit éliminées par le foie soit transformées en lipoprotéines de faible densité. Les lipoprotéines de faible densité (principales lipoprotéines porteuses de cholestérol) sont libérées de la circulation principalement par les récepteurs spécifiques de lipoprotéines de faible densité. On décrit les travaux de recherche pour découvrir les mécanismes qui réduisent les niveaux de lipoprotéines de basse densité chez les malades atteints d'hypercholestérolémie familiale hétérozygueuse et chez les malades atteints d'hypercholestérolémie modérée primaire. Dans ce dernier groupe on a noté que le lovastatin réduit le cholestérol des lipoprotéines de faible densité non pas en augmentant la libération des lipoprotéines de faible densité mais plutôt en facilitant la libération des restes de lipoprotéines de très faible densité. Les travaux de recherche décrits montrent aussie que le lovastatin peut provoquer une élévation dans les niveaux de plasma du cholestérol des lipoprotéines à forte densité. D'autres études sur l'action directe du médicament doivent être menées pour confirmer ou réfuter ces premières constatations.

ZUSAMMENFASSUNG

Lovastatin ist ein spezifischer Hemmstoff der 3-Hydroxy-3-Methylglutaryl-Koenzym A (HGM-CoA)-Reduktase, das Enzym, das den Geschwindigkeit-begrenzenden Schritt der Cholesterinsynthese katalysiert. Der Hauptwirkungsort scheint die Leber zu sein. Cholesteringleichgewichtsstudien an Menschen haben gezeigt, daß Lovastatin im allgemeinen einige Reduktion der Cholesterinsynthese verursacht, aber nicht ausreichend, um zu ernster Entleerung des Cholesterins des ganzen Körpers zu führen. Die Hauptfolge dieser teilweisen Hemmung der Cholesterinsynthese scheint die Anreizung der Synthese der Rezeptoren des niedrigdichten Lipoproteins (LDL) zu sein. Es ist ebenfalls möglich, daß Lovastatin die Synthese der Lipoproteine innerhalb der Leber hemmt. Der Mechanismus, durch den Lovastatin das LDL-Cholesterin erniedrigt, ist umrissen—die Triglyzeride der sehr niedrigdichten Lipoproteine (VLDL) werden in kleinere Lipoproteine (die VLDL-Reste) hydrolysiert, die entweder durch die Leber entfernt oder in LDL umgesetzt werden können. Die LDL (die Hauptträger für Cholesterin) werden hauptsächlich durch spezifische LDL-Rezeptoren von der Zirkulation entfernt. Untersuchungen der Mechanismen zur Erniedrigung der LDL-Spiegel bei Patienten mit heterozygöser familiärer Hypercholesterinämie (FH) und Patienten mit primärer mäßiger Hypercholesterinämie sind beschrieben. Es scheint als ob in der letzten Gruppe Lovastatin LDL-Cholesterin reduziert, jedoch nicht durch erhöhte Eliminierung des LDL an sich, sondern durch gesteigerte Eliminierung des VLDL-Restes. Die beschriebenen Untersuchungen erstellen ebenfalls einiges Beweismaterial, daß Lovastatin erhöhte HDL-Cholesterinspiegel im Plasma verursachen kann. Weitere Forschungen bezüglich der direkten Wirkung des Medikamentes müssen angestellt werden, um diese vorläufigen Befunde zu bestätigen oder zu widerlegen.

SOMMARIO

Lovastatin è uno specifico inibitore del IMG-CoA riduttasa, l'enzima che catalizza il passo della limitazione di tasso nella sintesi del colesterolo. Il piú frequente luogo d'azione sembra essere il fegato. Studi sull'equilibrio del colesterolo dimostrano che, nella razza umana, lovastatin di solito causa qualche abbassamento nella sintesi del colesterolo ma non è sufficiente a ridurre considerevolmente il colesterolo dal corpo intero. L'effetto maggiore di quest'inibizione parziale della sintesi del colesterolo sembra essere la stimolazione della sintesi dei ricettori di lipoproteina con bassa densità (LBD). È inoltre possibile che il lovastatin inibisce la sintesi delle lipoproteine dentro il fegato. Viene tracciato il meccanismo in cui lovastatin abbassa il colesterolo del LBD: le trigliceridi delle lipoproteine con densità molto bassa (LDMB) sono idrolizzate in minori lipoproteine—le LDMB rimanenti—che possono ugualmente essere eliminate dal fegato o convertite in LBD. Le LBD (le lipoproteine maggiore, trasportatrici di colesterolo) sono eliminate, per la maggior parte, dalla circolazione da specifici ricettori LBD. Vengono descritte le investigazioni nei meccanismi per l'abbassamento dei livelli LBD nei pazienti con ipercolesterolemia familiare (IF) eterozigote e pazienti con ipercolesterolemia primaria e moderata. Nell'ultimo gruppo sembra che Lovastatin riduce il colesterolo del LBD senza aumentare la schiaritura del LBD in se stesso, ma con l'intensificazione della schiaritura dei rimanenti del LBD. L'investigazione descritta fornisce anche evidenza che Lovastatin puo' causare un aumento nei livelli plasma del colesterolo del LAD. Ulteriori studi sull'azione diretta di questa droga sono necessari in modo da poter confermare o disapprovare queste scoperte preliminare.

SUMÁRIO

A lovastatina é um inibidor específico da 3-hidroxi-3-metilglutaril-coenzima-A-reductasa (HMG-CoA-reductasa), a enzima que catalisa a etapa que limita a velocidade na síntese de colesterol. O seu lugar principal de ação aparece ser o fígado. Estudos do equilibro do colesterol feitos com pessoas têm mostrado que a lovastatina geralmente causa alguma redução na síntese de colesterol, mas não suficiente para levar ao deploção severa do colesterol do corpo inteiro. O efeito principal da síntese de colesterol aparece ser a estimulação da síntese de receptores de lipoproteínas de baixa densidade (LDL). É também possível que a lovastatina inibe a síntese de lipoproteínas dentro do fígado. O mecanismo através do qual a lovastatina baixa o colesterol-LDL é delineado: os triglicéridos das lipoproteínas de densidade muito baixa são hidrolisados a lipoproteínas mais pequenas—os resíduos VLDL, que podem ou ser afastados pelo fígado ou convertidos em LDL. Os LDL (as lipoproteínas principais que levam o colesterol) são jogados fora da circulação principalmente por receptores de LDL específicos. As investigações sobre os mecanismos para reduzir os níveis de LDL em pacientes com hipercolesterolemia familiar heterocigótica (FH) e pacientes com hipercolesterolemia primária moderada são expostas. Neste último grupo, aparece que a lovastatina reduz colesterol-LDL não por aumentar a eliminação de LDL em si, mas por aumentar a eliminação dos resíduos de VLDL. As investigações traçadas também fornecem alguma evidência de que a lovastatina pode causar um aumento em níveis no soro de colesterol-HDL. Mais estudos sobre a ação direta do remédio precisam de ser feitos para confirmar ou descreditar estes descobrimentos preliminares.

RESUMEN

La lovastatina es un inhibidor específico de la 3-hidroxi-3-metilglutaril-coenzima-A-reductasa (HMG-CoA-reductasa), la enzima catalizadora del paso de limitación de la velocidad de la síntesis del colesterol. Su principal sitio de acción aparentemente es el hígado. Estudios de equilibrio del colesterol realizados en seres humanos han demostrado que la lovastatina usualmente causa cierta reducción en la síntesis del colesterol, pero no la suficiente como para llevar a un agotamiento severo del colesterol total del cuerpo. El efecto principal de esta inhibición parcial de la síntesis del colesterol parece ser la estimulación de la síntesis de los receptores de lipoproteínas de baja densidad (LDL). También es posible que la lovastatina inhiba la síntesis de lipoproteínas dentro del hígado. Se bosqueja el mecanismo por el que la lovastatina disminuy el nivel de colesterol LDL: los triglicéridos de las lipoproteínas de muy baja densidad (VLDL) son convertidos en lipoproteínas más pequeñas por hidrolización—los remanentes de VLDL, que pueden ser extraídos por el hígado o convertidos en LDL. Las lipoproteínas de baja densidad (las lipoproteínas portadoras de colesterol más importantes) son extraídas de la circulación principalmente por receptores específicos de LDL. Se describen las investigaciones con respecto a los mecanismos de disminución de los niveles de LDL en pacientes con hipercolesterolemia familiar heterocigótica (FH) y pacientes con hipercolesterolemia primaria moderada. Parece que en este último grupo la lovastatina reduce el nivel de colesterol LDL, no mediante el incremento en la eliminación de LDL sino mejorando la eliminación de los remanentes de VLDL. Las investigaciones descriptas también proporcionan cierta evidencia de que la lovastatina puede causar una elevación en los niveles séricos de colesterol HDL. Será necesario estudiar más a fondo la acción directa del fármaco para confirmar o desmentir estos hallazgos preliminares.

The Role of Cholesterol in Atherosclerosis:
New Therapeutic Opportunities, edited by S. M. Grundy
and A. G. Bearn, Hanley & Belfus, Inc., Philadelphia.

Discussion

CORVOL: Is there a known genetic predisposition to drug metabolism?

SLATER: We have no indication that there is a wide variation, but metabolism studies have been hampered by the exceedingly low plasma levels of the drug.

CORVOL: Is it possible to assess the degree of HMG-CoA reductase inhibition in a given patient?

GRUNDY: It is difficult to estimate the HMG-CoA reductase activity in humans, but it is possible to measure the metabolism of mevalonic acid in the blood and urine. Lovastatin acutely decreases the formation of mevalonic acid, so formation of mevalonic acid can be monitored throughout the day to see how quickly the drug works. Alternatively, cholesterol balance studies can be used to show the overall effects on cholesterol metabolism over a long period. This is an indirect way to monitor HMG-CoA reductase activity in patients.

BLOCH: About six months ago there was a warning statement in *JAMA* saying that the methodology of cholesterol analysis is not very reliable and that different methods are used in different laboratories. It called for standardization of methods. Were the methods uniform?

GRUNDY: Cholesterol can be measured very accurately, and methods have been standardized.

MONCLOA: For the clinical studies we used a central laboratory.

BLOCH: Does one have to be careful in interpreting reports in the literature?

GRUNDY: Most major laboratories doing research do have accurate methods. It is of concern when private physicians are using hospital-based laboratories where the methodology is not so rigorously standardized.

LEWIS: Not only is there some degree of laboratory inaccuracy and imprecision worldwide, but the technique of blood sampling is a further source of error. Venous stasis and posture, in particular, add to the laboratory variation.

I would like to comment on your mode of action studies and to mention some studies into the kinetics of VLDL and LDL metabolism in rabbits, both normal rabbits and rabbits with a genetic disorder in which there is over-production of VDL and LDL. Like you, we find the fall in LDL concentration is associated with decreased production of LDL as well as some increase in fractional catabolism; in addition there is marked reduction in VLDL production with no change in fractional catabolism. I do not know if this has been directly studied in man, but it should be.

GRUNDY: You are implying that there is a decrease in the production of VLDL, but many of the lipoproteins that come into the circulation are cleared very rapidly. If a drug increases the receptor activity, this will lead to an even more rapid clearance of precursor lipoproteins. It is very difficult by kinetic means to differentiate between changes in production and clearance. To get at what lovastatin does to the synthesis of lipoproteins, we will have to look into the liver itself.

LEWIS: If the concentration of VLDL falls and the fractional catabolic rate is seemingly unchanged, input into the circulation must be the mechanism.

GRUNDY: When input into the system is decreased by enhanced clearance of precursor lipoproteins, the turnover of the particles remaining in the circulation is decreased. A reduced form of lipoproteins as determined by kinetic methods therefore does not necessarily mean the liver is secreting less lipoproteins, because you may have a fraction that you cannot measure because turnover is so fast. This latter fraction may be cleared even more rapidly.

LANGMAN: If fecal sterols go down, which is particularly likely in combination with bile acid resins, it is essential that someone examine biliary secretion in man. You will then be able to predict whether you will get gallstones.

Secondly, there is a close correlation between coronary heart disease mortality and carcinoma of the colon mortality, and a suggestion that the latter is related to fecal sterol output.

GRUNDY: It is commonly believed that drugs that lower cholesterol will increase the risk of gallstones and that is true with fibric acids. It is not true of other drugs like nicotinic acid or bile acid binding resins. Lovastatin did not change the bile saturation in one study specifically designed to examine this question.

LASAGNA: Is there any evidence that age or gender affect the cholesterol response to these drugs?

MONCLOA: No.

ASSCHER: In your cases of familial hypercholesterolemia, does the drug get rid of xanthomata?

MONCLOA: There is a group looking at that and their results after two years of observation should be available soon.

LEDINGHAM: Returning to production versus catabolic rate, I wondered about secondary causes of hyperlipidemia, particularly those that cannot be corrected, such as the nephrotic syndrome. I understood that nephrotic hyperlipidemia was an overproduction problem. Does the drug reduce VLDL production by the liver?

GRUNDY: In the nephrotic syndrome, lovastatin lowers the cholesterol level dramatically. Overproduction of lipoproteins is the underlying cause of hypercholesterolemia, but we also found that the increased triglycerides in nephrotic patients were due to some catabolic defect. Lovastatin increased the catabolism of the VLDL, probably by increasing LDL receptors.

GANTEN: Dr. Moncloa, one of your slides showed that a single dose of lovastatin produced rapid changes in blood biochemistry. On the other hand, maximal action after chronic treatment was achieved after 14 days and took 4 weeks to return to pretreatment levels when the patients were taken off the drugs. The question then is, should you reduce the dose since you have such a prolonged duration of action? You really don't need the maximal effects very rapidly. As with the converting enzyme inhibitors, might high doses produce more rapid onset of action, whereas maximal action with lower doses might be produced more slowly but with fewer side effects?

MONCLOA: The dose studies were of a parallel design not titration studies. Therefore the different effects of different doses was not an effect of time.

IMURA: In our experience probucol lowers LDL cholesterol and HDL cholesterol, whereas lovastatin increases HDL cholesterol. That is a great benefit, but is there any difference in HDL cholesterol response in FH and non-FH patients?

Secondly how does lovastatin increase HDL cholesterol?

MONCLOA: Our FH patients are heterozygous, and there were no differences between them and the non-FH patients in the increased HDL cholesterol.

GRUNDY: There is an inverse relationship between VLDL and IDL, and HDL, and if you reduce the VLDL and IDL levels then the HDL levels usually go up. That may account for the rise.

DOLLERY: In trying to link the cataract findings and the kinetics of the drug, when comparing man and dog, comparative plasma concentrations would be interesting. Secondly, is it worth thinking about local effects? Within a general reduction in cholesterol you might get intense local effects due to local accumulation. Do you have any data on what is happening in the lens of the dog or whether you have been able to put a patient who is to have a cataract extraction on the drug to see what happens in the lens in man?

SLATER: Bear in mind that these are cataracts in animals. The lens opacities Dr. Moncloa referred to in humans are not cataractous and have not compromised vision in any patient so far. In dogs with dose levels at least 60 times the anticipated human dose, we have seen typical cataracts, with an incidence of 10%. We haven't seen cataracts in rodents. Other, synthetic, HMG-CoA reductase inhibitors, which achieve higher plasma inhibitory levels, show a higher incidence of cataracts in dogs.

DOLLERY: Is the incidence of cataracts in controls very low?

SLATER: Yes. For lovastatin specifically, the 10% of dogs who developed the cataracts had exceptionally high plasma levels, much higher than the levels in dogs who did not develop cataracts in orders of magnitude higher than plasma levels at use levels in man. We are analyzing several dog lenses with cataracts. No gross difference in cholesterol or lipid content has yet emerged.

The Role of Cholesterol in Atherosclerosis:
New Therapeutic Opportunities, edited by S. M. Grundy
and A. G. Bearn, Hanley & Belfus, Inc., Philadelphia.

Use of Hypolipidemic Strategies to Halt Atherosclerosis: Evidence for Alteration in Clinical Course

Peter H. Stone, Frank M. Sacks, and Thomas W. Smith

Coronary atherosclerosis is a slowly progressive process that begins in early adulthood and usually culminates in clinical manifestations in the fifth and later decades of life. Myocardial ischemia generally does not result, however, even under conditions of stress and increased myocardial oxygen demands, until the luminal diameter of the coronary artery is obstructed by at least 50%, corresponding to a reduction in luminal cross-sectional area of at least 75%.[1-6] The relationship between diameter obstruction and reduction in coronary flow is exponential, such that once a vessel diameter is obstructed by 70% (90% reduction in area), small additional increments in diameter obstruction ($\leq$5%) are associated with dramatic 3–4 fold reductions in coronary flow.[5] Morbidity and mortality in an individual with coronary disease may therefore result from even a small increase in luminal obstruction; conversely, stability or resolution of manifestations may result from even small decrements or at least halting of progression of the atherosclerotic process.

Although there is no relationship between the clinical status and degree of coronary luminal obstruction observed on a single coronary arteriogram,[7,8] there is nevertheless evidence that progression of clinical symptoms is associated with progression of anatomic obstructions. Of 313 consecutive medically treated patients who underwent coronary angiography twice, a mean of 39 months apart, 139 patients (44%) demonstrated progression of stenoses, which was associated with a significantly higher incidence of angina at rest, worsening stable angina, interim myocardial infarction, and unstable angina compared with the 174 patients (56%) who did not exhibit progression.[9]

RELATIONSHIP BETWEEN LIPID PROFILE AND ATHEROGENESIS

Epidemiologic studies have clearly established that the incidence of atherosclerosis and the manifestations of coronary artery disease are related to plasma cholesterol levels. The risk is primarily associated positively with total cholesterol and the low-density lipoprotein (LDL) fraction and associated inversely with the high-density lipoprotein (HDL) fraction. Observations from the Framingham Study suggest that the ratio of plasma total cholesterol to HDL cholesterol is the most powerful predictor of the development of coronary artery disease.[10] Cross-cultural studies of industrial nations confirm the significant impact of the total cholesterol level, HDL cholesterol level, and the ratio of total to HDL cholesterol on coronary artery disease mortality, especially among men (Figs. 1 and 2).[11]

The severity of atherosclerotic obstructions in individual patients has similarly been related to cholesterol fractions. In a recent study comparing levels of several components of plasma lipoproteins and the angiographic severity of coronary artery disease in 65 men and 42 women, Reardon and colleagues found that in men the severity of atherosclerosis was strongly related to total cholesterol, LDL cholesterol, and apolipoprotein B concentrations, whereas in women it was related to triglyceride concentrations in intermediate-density lipoproteins (IDL) and LDL and to the cholesterol and apolipoprotein B concentrations in IDL.[12] No statistically significant relationships were found between the severity of atherosclerotic lesions and HDL or apolipoprotein A–I concentrations in either group.

Serial coronary angiographic studies have confirmed the importance of plasma lipids in the progression of existing atherosclerotic obstructions and in the development of new lesions. Campeau *et al.* examined serial angiograms performed 10 years apart in 82 patients who underwent coronary bypass surgery at the beginning of the study[13] and evaluated the obstructions both in the grafts and the native vessels. They observed that progression of obstructions (in the grafts, native vessels, or both) occurred in 67 (82%) patients, whereas there were no new lesions in 15 (18%) patients. Although there was no significant difference between the two groups in the incidence of hypertension, diabetes, or cigarette smoking, there were highly significant differences in the plasma lipid profile. Using univariate analysis, patients with progression of coronary disease exhibited a significantly higher total cholesterol, triglycerides, LDL, and LDL apoprotein B, and a significantly lower HDL. Multivariate analysis demonstrated that LDL apoprotein B and HDL were the principal factors associated with the presence or absence of atherosclerosis.

An association between coronary artery disease and a plasma lipoprotein now known as Lp(a) was first noted in the early 1970s. Dahlen and associates[14] have recently reported an association between Lp(a) levels and coronary artery disease among 307 patients who underwent coronary angiography. Levels of Lp(a), which resembles LDL in several respects but can be distinguished and quantified by electroimmunoassay, were associated significantly, and by multivariate analysis independently, with the presence of coronary artery disease ($p < 0.02$) and tended to correlate with the severity of coronary stenosis ($p = 0.06$). The authors concluded that plasma Lp(a), at least in white patients, is a coronary risk factor with an importance approaching that of LDL or HDL cholesterol levels.

REVERSAL OF ATHEROSCLEROSIS BY LOWERING PLASMA CHOLESTEROL LEVELS

The positive association between plasma lipids and atherosclerosis has led to an extensive body of work using a variety of interventions to lower cholesterol with

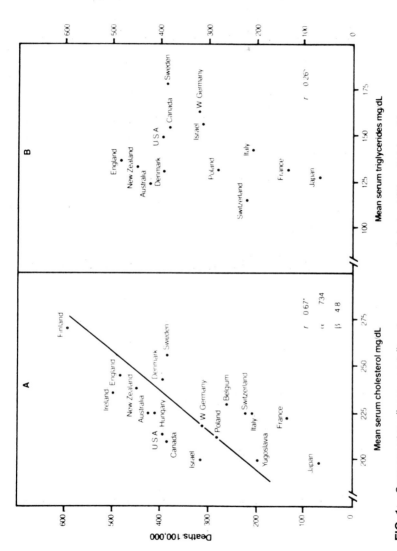

FIG. 1. Coronary artery disease mortality rate versus serum cholesterol (A) and triglyceride concentrations (B) in men. NS = not significant; alpha = intercept; beta = slope. (Reproduced with permission from Simons LA. Interrelations of lipids and lipoproteins with coronary artery disease mortality in 19 countries. *Am J Cardiol* 1986; **57**:5G–10G.)

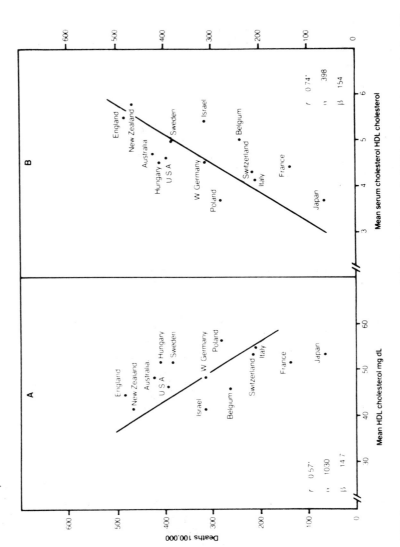

FIG. 2. Coronary artery disease mortality rate versus high density lipoprotein (HDL) cholesterol concentration (A) and serum cholesterol/HDL cholesterol (B) in men. (Reproduced with permission from Simons LA. Interrelations of lipids and lipoproteins with coronary artery disease mortality in 19 countries. *Am J Cardiol* 1986; **57**:5G–10G.)

the hopes of effecting a regression of atherosclerotic obstructions or at least of halting or slowing its progression.

Dietary Interventions

Nonhuman primates have served as an important model for the study of human atherogenesis. Monkeys rarely acquire atherosclerosis when fed low-fat chow in the laboratory. Widespread atherosclerosis that is morphologically similar to human disease occurs when these monkeys are fed diets high in saturated fat or cholesterol for 1–2 years.[15] Regression of coronary and peripheral atherosclerosis by returning the animals to a standard laboratory chow diet was demonstrated by the experiments of several groups of researchers.[16–20] Nearly complete removal of atheroma cholesterol occurred over the ensuing 6 months, and elastin and calcium decreased during the next 12 months. Mean coronary stenosis decreased from 60% to 20%.[18] Since monkeys have a greater sensitivity of plasma LDL to diet and under these experimental conditions a much more rapid induction of atherosclerosis than humans, it cannot be assumed that human plaque will respond similarly to dietary changes. However, these studies are useful in demonstrating that fibrous, mineral, and lipid elements of complex plaque can be removed by a hypolipidemic diet and in defining (at least for this experimental model) the time course of mobilization of plaque elements.

Very few studies in man have investigated the effects of a lipid-lowering diet on coronary obstructions using serial angiography, and the majority of these studies have included only patients with hyperlipoproteinemia. The extrapolation of the results to the general population with "normal" serum cholesterol, therefore, remains conjectural.

The Leiden Intervention Trial[21] was a prospective study of 39 patients with stable angina pectoris (mean serum cholesterol at baseline 267 mg/dl) in whom coronary angiography demonstrated at least one vessel with 50% obstruction before intervention. The intervention consisted of a two-year vegetarian diet containing less than 100 mg of cholesterol per day and in which the ratio of polyunsaturated to saturated fatty acids was at least 2. Repeat angiography after 2 years demonstrated a lack of lesion growth in 18 patients (46%); the progression of disease was correlated with the ratio of total/HDL cholesterol but not with blood pressure, smoking status, alcohol intake, weight, or drug treatment. Disease progression occurred only in patients whose ratio of total/HDL cholesterol was 6.9 throughout the study period; there was no progression in patients with a ratio <6.9 throughout the trial or in those who initially had a ratio >6.9 and who reduced it below that level by dietary intervention.

Pharmacologic Interventions

Early studies evaluating the concept of regression of atherosclerosis in man utilized serial femoral angiograms analyzed by digital imaging processing to yield a computer estimate of atherosclerosis.[22] Twenty-five patients with Type II or Type IV hyperlipoproteinemia were treated with a variety of hypolipidemic agents such as clofibrate, neomycin sulfate, and tibric acid, and were evaluated angiographically an average of 13 months later. Nine patients showed a regression of atherosclerosis area, three showed no change, and thirteen showed progression. Although there was no difference in coronary risk factors before the first angiogram, at the end of the study the only significant difference between those who had regression compared to those who had progression was a lower cholesterol in the former group. These non-controlled observations were followed by a randomized controlled trial in hyperlipidemic patients which similarly demonstrated that an effective lipid-lowering regimen (cholestyramine, nicotinic acid, or clofibrate) for a mean of 19 months reduced total cholesterol, LDL, and triglycerides compared with control hyperlipidemic patients and halted progression of existing obstructions in the femoral artery and promoted regression of luminal irregularities.[23]

More recent studies have investigated the reversibility of coronary atherosclerosis but have been somewhat limited by inadequacies of study design and by reliance on visual, and therefore crude, assessments of coronary luminal diameter (Table I). Using a non-randomized study design, Nash and coworkers found that of 36 patients with a cholesterol $\geq$250 mg/dl (6.5 mmol/L) who responded to colestipol (mean change in serum cholesterol 21.4%, in triglycerides -7.5%), 30 patients (83%) had stable lesions by angiography after a 23-month follow-up, while only 6 patients (17%) exhibited progression.[24] In contrast, of 21 similar patients who did not respond to colestipol and who were then put on placebo, mean cholesterol was reduced by only -2.5%, triglycerides increased by $+13.8\%$, and progression of coronary lesions occurred in 10 patients (48%, $p < 0.02$ for comparison of progression in responders vs non-responders to colestipol).

Nikkila and colleagues compared serial coronary angiograms in 28 patients with serum cholesterol >278 mg/dl (7.2 mmol/L) treated with diet and drugs (clofibrate or nicotinic acid or both) with 20 similar patients who received no treatment to reduce lipid concentrations and served as non-randomized controls (Table I).[25] The initial levels of coronary risk factors and the angiographic appearance of obstructions were comparable in the two groups. In the patients receiving active treatment, total cholesterol, total triglyceride, and LDL concentrations were reduced by an average of 18%, 38%, and 19% respectively, and HDL was increased an average by 10%. By all visual criteria coronary lesions progressed significantly less in the patients receiving active therapy than in the controls: the angiographic state remained completely unchanged in nine patients (32%) compared with only one (8%) of the surviving controls; of the arterial segments at risk, 46 (16.5%) progressed in the patients compared with 50 (38.2%) in the controls ($p < 0.001$), and the coronary obstruction increased less in patients than in controls (74.3% vs 141.1%, $p < 0.05$). Within the group receiving active treatment there was also a positive correlation between the elevation of total cholesterol and LDL/HDL ratio and the degree of progression of coronary obstructions, and an inverse correlation with the elevation of HDL.

TABLE I. The effect of lipid-lowering drugs on progression of coronary atherosclerosis (all patients with hyperlipidemia and coronary disease)

Study (year)	No. of patients	Drug	Duration of Follow-up	Reduction in serum lipids				Arteriographic status: Percentage of Patients with Progression	Comments
				Chol	LDL	HDL	TG		
Nash (1984)[24]	36 active drug	colestipol	23 months	−21%***	—	—	−8%	17% of colestipol patients vs 48% of "controls"**	Not blinded, randomized, or controlled. "Controls" were those who did not respond to colestipol.
	21 "controls"			−3%	—	—	* +14%		
Nikkila (1984)[25]	28 active drug 20 controls	clofibrate, nicotinic acid, or both	7 years	−18%	−19%	+10%	−38%	16.5% of patients on active therapy vs 38.2% of controls**	Controls not randomly assigned.
NHLBI Type II Trial (1984)[26]	59 active drug	cholestyramine	5 years	−17%**	−26%**	+8%	+28%	32% of cholestyramine patients vs 49% of controls*	Randomized, placebo-controlled, double-blind
	57 placebo			1%	−5%	+2%	+26%		
CLAS (1987)[27]	80 active drug	colestipol and niacin	2 years	−26%**	−43%**	+37%	−22%	38.8% of patients on active therapy vs 61.0% of controls* Regression occurred in 16.2% of patients on active therapy vs 2.4% of controls*	Randomized, placebo-controlled. Included patients with "normal" cholesterol.
	82 placebo			−4%	−5%	** +2%	** −5%		

* p < 0.05
** p < 0.001
*** p < 0.0001

The National Heart, Lung and Blood Institute of the U.S. National Institutes of Health (NHLBI) Type II Coronary Intervention Study has been the most ambitious and best-designed trial to investigate the effect of lipid lowering on progression of coronary angiographic obstructions in hyperlipidemic patients (Table I).[26] One hundred and sixteen patients with Type II hyperlipoproteinemia and coronary disease were placed on a low-fat, low-cholesterol diet and were then randomly allocated to receive either cholestyramine or placebo. Coronary angiography was performed at the beginning of the study and repeated after 5 years of blinded therapy. Total cholesterol was reduced by 17% in the cholestyramine group (n = 59) and by only 1% in the placebo group (n = 57) (p < 0.001), and LDL reduced by 26% in the treatment group compared with only 5% in the placebo group (p < 0.001). There was no significant treatment effect on HDL and triglyceride concentrations. Visual assessment of the serial coronary angiograms (blinded top treatment assignment) demonstrated that coronary obstructions progressed in 49% of the placebo-treated patients compared with 32% of the cholestyramine-treated patients (p < 0.05). Of lesions causing 50% or greater stenosis at baseline, 33% of placebo-treated patients exhibited lesion progression compared with only 12% of cholestyramine-treated patients (p < 0.05). Similar analyses with other endpoints (percent of baseline lesions that progressed, lesions that progressed to occlusion, lesions that regressed, size of lesion change, and all cardiovascular endpoints) all tended to favor the cholestyramine-treated group but were not statistically significant.

Recent results from the Cholesterol-Lowering Atherosclerosis Study (CLAS) have extended the concept that a reduction in lipids favorably influences atherosclerosis for the first time to include individuals with an ostensibly "normal" cholesterol level (mean cholesterol 246 mg/dl (6.4 mmol/L) on entry).[27] Using a randomized, placebo-controlled trial design, an aggressive regimen of lipid-lowering diet and combined colestipol and niacin therapy was compared to a regimen of diet alone in 162 non-smoking men aged 40–59 years with previous coronary bypass surgery (Table I). Individuals underwent coronary angiography at study entry and again after two years of therapy; cineangiograms were analyzed visually by a panel of expert angiographers who assigned each film pair a score representing degrees of progression or regression of luminal obstructions. During two years of treatment there was a 26% reduction in total plasma cholesterol, a 43% reduction in LDL cholesterol, plus a simultaneous 37% elevation of HDL cholesterol. This resulted in a significant reduction in the average number of lesions per subjects that progressed (p < .03) and the percentage of subjects with new atheroma formation (p < .03) in native coronary arteries. Also, the percentage of subjects with new lesions (p < .04) or any adverse change in bypass grafts (p < .03) was significantly reduced. Deterioration in overall coronary status was significantly less in drug-treated subjects than placebo-treated subjects (p < .001). Atherosclerosis regression, as indicated by perceptible improvement in overall coronary status, occurred in 16.2% of colestipol-niacin treated vs 2.4% in the placebo-treated (p = .002). The beneficial effects on atherosclerosis were evident in 78 patients with a "low" cholesterol at study entry (185-240 mg/dl, mean 216 mg/dl; 4.8–6.2 mmol/L, mean

5.6 mmol/L) as well as in the 84 patients with a "high" cholesterol (241–350 mg/dl, mean 270 mg/dl; 6.2–9.0 mmol/L, mean 7.0 mmol/L.) The particularly striking benefit observed in CLAS may have been due to the implementation of a consistent and aggressive lipid-lowering regimen for the entire study duration that led to more dramatic reductions in plasma cholesterol than had been achieved in previous studies, and also to the screening process that excluded patients who did not tolerate or respond to the study medications.

EFFECT OF HYPOLIPIDEMIC REGIMENS ON MANIFESTATIONS OF CORONARY DISEASE

Dietary Interventions (Table II)

A number of large scale trials have investigated the ability of a cholesterol-lowering diet, often in the setting of other risk factor modifications, to reduce cardiovascular morbidity and mortality. The Oslo Diet-Heart Study[28] randomized 412 men, aged 30–64 years, an average of 20 months after a first myocardial infarction, to either an experimental diet or a control group. The experimental diet consisted of a diet low in saturated fats and cholesterol, and high in polyunsaturated fats. The mean serum cholesterol was reduced by 17.6% in the diet group and by 3.7% in the control group. After 5 years there was a 26% reduction in coronary "relapses," including fatal and nonfatal myocardial infarction (MI) in the diet group compared with the control group. (p = 0.05). After 11 years there was a significant reduction in the incidence of fatal infarction among the diet group compared with the control group (32% vs 57%, p = 0.004) and a trend toward reduced total coronary mortality (fatal MI and sudden death, 38% vs 46%, p = 0.097).

Bierenbaum and colleagues compared the 10-year mortality of 100 men with coronary disease and a previous MI who were treated with a diet containing less than 9% of calories as saturated fat and less than 400 mg exogenous cholesterol daily with 100 "matched" controls not under dietary management.[29] After 10 years the diet-managed group had a mortality of 16% compared with 28% in the control group (p < 0.05), although data on the serum lipids during the follow-up period were not noted.

A number of more recent large-scale studies have addressed the role of a cholesterol-lowering diet in the primary prevention of coronary heart disease. Turpeinen and colleagues performed a classic controlled intervention trial in two mental hospitals near Helsinki in 1959–1971.[30] The subjects were 619 hospitalized middle-aged men. For the first six years, one of the hospitals changed its diet so that the dairy fats originally present in the normal diet were almost totally replaced by vegetable oils, mainly soybean oil. The other hospital, serving as the control, was continued on the normal diet. For the second six years the role of the hospitals in the experimental design was reversed by returning the first hospital to the normal diet and by placing the other hospital on the vegetable oil diet. The diet led to a

TABLE II. *Effect of lipid-lowering diet on manifestations of coronary disease (randomized, controlled clinical trials)*

Study (year)	No. of patients	Duration of Follow-up	Diet	Reduction in serum cholesterol	Coronary Events	Comments
Secondary Prevention						
Oslo Diet-Heart Study (1970)[28]	412 men after first MI	5 years	Low in saturated fats and cholesterol, high in polyunsaturated fats	17.6% reduction in diet group vs 3.7% reduction in controls	26% reduction in fatal and non-fatal MI in diet group ($p = 0.05$)	
Bierenbaum (1973)[29]	200 men with previous MI	10 years	<9% of calories as saturated fats, <400 mg cholesterol	not available	mortality 16% in diet group vs 28% in control group ($p < 0.05$)	"matched" controls not randomly allocated
Primary Prevention						
Turpeinen (1978)[30]	619 men	6 years	replaced dairy fats with vegetable oil	17% reduction in diet group	4.2 coronary events/ 1,000 man years in diet group vs 12.7 in controls ($p < 0.001$)	coronary events = coronary death or evidence of coronary disease
Oslo Study Group (1981)[31]	1,232 men with hypercholesterolemia	5 years	cholesterol-lowering diet	13% reduction in diet group vs controls	47% reduction in incidence of fatal and non-fatal MI and sudden death in intervention group ($p = 0.028$)	multiple interventions (cessation of smoking and BP reduction)
MRFIT (1982)[32]	12,866 men at high risk	7 years	<10% of calories as saturated fats, <300 mg cholesterol	2% reduction in intervention group	7.1% reduction in coronary mortality in intervention group (p NS)	multiple interventions (BP reduction, cessation of smoking)
Belgian Heart Disease Prevention Project (1985)[33]	19,409 men at high risk	5 years	cholesterol-lowering diet	15.8% reduction in "coronary risk profile" in intervention group	24.5% reduction in coronary mortality and non-fatal MI in intervention group ($p = 0.038$)	multiple interventions (BP reduction, cessation of smoking)

MI = myocardial infarction; BP = blood pressure.

decrease in serum cholesterol of approximately 17% (p < 0.001) in each hospital. In both hospitals during the experimental diet periods, the incidence of coronary heart disease, as measured by the occurrence of coronary deaths and the appearance of certain ECG patterns, was less than half that during the normal diet periods (4.2 vs 12.7 events/1,000 man years, p < 0.001).

Three other large-scale national studies investigated the role of a cholesterol-lowering diet as part of a multifactorial approach to reducing coronary risk factors. The effect of reduction in serum lipids alone was not addressed in these studies. The Oslo Study Group[31] identified 1232 healthy, normotensive men at high risk for coronary heart disease on the basis of hypercholesterolemia (290–380 mg/dl; 7.5–9.8 mmol/L), coronary risk scores (based on cholesterol levels, smoking habits, and blood pressure) in the upper quartile of the distribution, and systolic blood pressure below 150 mm Hg. The individuals were randomized either to an intervention group, consisting of recommendations to lower their blood lipids by change of diet and to stop smoking, or to a control group, and followed for 5 years. Mean serum cholesterol concentrations were approximately 13% lower in the intervention group than in the control group during the trial, and tobacco consumption fell about 45% more in the intervention group than in the controls. These improvements in risk factors were associated with a 47% improvement in the incidence of myocardial infarction (fatal and non-fatal) and sudden death in the intervention group compared with the controls (p = 0.028). Further analysis of the results suggested that the dietary changes produced two-thirds of the improved incidence of coronary disease and the remaining one-third was due to a reduction in tobacco use.

The Multiple Risk Factor Intervention Trial (MRFIT) was designed to test the hypothesis that special interventions to reduce the risk factors of hypercholesterolemia, hypertension, and cigarette smoking among high-risk men would result in a significant reduction in mortality from coronary disease as compared with usual intervention by practicing physicians.[32] The study included 12,866 men aged 35 to 57 years and free of clinical manifestations of, but at high risk for, coronary artery disease who were randomly assigned to receive either special intervention or usual care. The intervention program included counseling on dietary modification, restricting both saturated fats and caloric intake, treating arterial hypertension, and counseling on cessation of cigarette smoking. At the end of the trial (average follow-up 7 years), patients in both the special intervention and usual care groups experienced reductions in blood cholesterol level, blood pressure level, and cigarette smoking, although reductions were slightly better in the special intervention group. The patients in the special intervention group experienced only a non-significant 7.1% reduction in coronary heart disease mortality; in fact total mortality was 2.1% higher in the special intervention group than in the usual care group. Although the explanation for the lack of benefit in the special intervention group is unknown, the fact that the "usual care" group did much better than expected, due to nationwide dietary changes and more aggressive medical treatment, may have made an incremental benefit from the special interventions more difficult than expected to prove.

The Belgian Heart Disease Prevention Project utilized a similar multifactorial approach to the primary prevention of coronary disease.[33] The study included 19,409 men aged 40–59 years at high risk for coronary disease who were randomly assigned to an intervention or a control group and followed for 5–6 years. The intervention group received health education promoting a cholesterol-lowering diet, smoking cessation, weight control, physical activity, and treatment of arterial hypertension. Using a coronary risk "profile," patients in the intervention group experienced a 21% reduction in the multiple risk factors during the first 4 years ($p < 0.05$), although by the end of the study the average reduction was only 15.8% (p NS). Nevertheless, total mortality showed a gradual divergence in favor of the intervention group, reaching a cumulative difference of 17.5% ($p = 0.038$). The cumulative coronary mortality was reduced by 20.8% at the end of the study, but this difference did not achieve statistical significance. The "coronary incidence" (sum of coronary mortality and non-fatal myocardial infarction) was significantly different after the third year of the study, culminating in a 24.5% reduction in the intervention group ($p = 0.08$).

Pharmacologic Interventions (Table III)

A number of pharmacologic regimens have been investigated to lower cholesterol and thereby improve coronary disease manifestations; although certainly not uniform, the results have generally further strengthened the concept that reductions in blood cholesterol levels are associated with reductions in the incidence of coronary heart disease and mortality.[34]

The Coronary Drug Project[35] was an ambitious study that randomly divided 8,341 patients with a previous myocardial infarction into six different groups: two received conjugated estrogen regimens, one received clofibrate, one dextrothyroxine, one niacin, and one placebo. The niacin group experienced a 9.9% decrease in cholesterol and a 26.1% decrease in triglycerides compared with the placebo group, and the clofibrate group experienced a 6.5% and 22.3% reduction in cholesterol and triglycerides, respectively. The findings at the end of the trial were essentially negative, except for significantly lower incidence of non-fatal myocardial infarction in the niacin group. A recent update almost ten years after termination of the trial indicated that the niacin group experienced a 11% reduction in mortality compared with the placebo group ($p < 0.01$).[36]

The Newcastle-upon-Tyne Study also studied the effects of clofibrate on coronary disease manifestations and found somewhat different results.[37] Four hundred ninety-seven patients with ischemic heart disease were randomly assigned to receive clofibrate or placebo and were then followed for 5 years. Clofibrate caused a modest fall in the mean cholesterol level in men (28 mg/dl; 0.7 mmol/L) and in women (41 mg/dl; 1.1 mmol/L) throughout the course of the study. This was associated with a reduction in total mortality in the active treatment group compared to placebo (3.07 vs 5.34 deaths per 1,200 patient months, $p = 0.02$). Fewer non-fatal infarcts

TABLE III. Effect of lipid-lowering drugs on manifestations of coronary disease (randomized, placebo-controlled, clinical trials)

Study (year)	No. of patients	Duration of Follow-up	Therapy	Reduction in lipids Chol	LDL	TG	Coronary Events	Comments
Coronary Drug Project (1975)[35]	2,840 men with previous MI	5 years	clofibrate niacin	−6.5% −9.9%		−22.3% −26.1%	No significant difference in total mortality or cause-specific mortality. Niacin group had lower incidence of non-fatal MI than control group (8.9% vs 12.2%, $p < 0.005$)	9-year follow-up niacin group showed 11% reduction in mortality compared with placebo group ($p < 0.01$)
Newcastle-upon-Tyne Study (1971)[37]	497 men with coronary disease	5 years	clofibrate	−28 mg/dl in men −41 mg/dl in women			3.07 deaths/1,200 pt months in clofibrate group vs 5.37 in placebo ($p = 0.02$)	no apparent relationship between reduction in lipids and outcome
Lipid Research Clinic Primary Prevention Trial (1984)[38]	3,806 men with hyper-cholesterolemia	7 years	cholestyramine	−13.4%	−20.3%		19% reduction of risk of coronary death or non-fatal MI ($p < 0.05$)	reduction in events appeared proportionate to reduction in cholesterol

also occurred in the clofibrate gorup, although the difference did not reach the accepted statistical significance (3.68 vs 5.76 non-fatal infarcts per 1,200 patient months, p = 0.055). There was no apparent relationship between the reduction in blood lipids and outcome in either group.

The Lipid Research Clinics Coronary Primary Prevention Trial has rekindled a great deal of support in the United States for efforts to reduce hypercholesterolemia. Cholestyramine or placebo was administered to 3,806 asymptomatic middle-aged men with primary hypercholesterolemia for an average of 7.4 years.[38] Both groups followed a moderate cholesterol-lowering diet. The cholestyramine group experienced average reductions of total and LDL cholesterol of 13.4% and 20.3%, respectively, which were 8.5% and 12.6% greater reductions than those obtained in the placebo group. The reductions in cholesterol were associated with a 19% reduction of risk of definite coronary death or non-fatal myocardial infarct in the cholestyramine group compared with the placebo group (p < 0.05). When the cholestyramine group was analyzed separately, a 19% reduction in coronary risk was associated with each decrement of 8% in total cholesterol or 11% in LDL (p < 0.001). Furthermore, the incidence of coronary events in men achieving a 25% reduction in total cholesterol or 35% reduction in LDL (typical responses to the prescribed dosage of cholestyramine, 24 g/day) was half that of men who remained at pre-treatment levels. Thus, the reduction in the incidence of coronary heart disease in the cholestyramine group seemed to have been mediated chiefly by reduction in the total LDL cholesterol levels.

CONCLUSIONS

It must be emphasized that although this chapter has focused primarily on the role of strategies devoted to reducing cholesterol levels, a comprehensive intervention program to reduce the manifestations of coronary disease must also include strategies directed toward blood pressure reduction, cessation of cigarette smoking, and possibly recommendations for physical exercise as well. The positive correlation between levels of serum cholesterol and the incidence of coronary disease in epidemiologic studies is clear, as is the relationship between levels of serum cholesterol and the severity of coronary artery obstructions in individual patients. There are now encouraging data suggesting that interventions that reduce serum cholesterol can halt progression of atherosclerosis as assessed from coronary angiography. Evidence for actual regression of atherosclerotic obstructions is less clear, although the recent findings of Blankenhorn et al.[27] are encouraging. Most of the available regression studies have only included hypercholesterolemic men; additional studies are necessary to confirm whether reductions in serum cholesterol in individuals with ostensibly "normal" cholesterol levels (i.e. <90th percentile) can also lead to improvement in atherosclerotic obstructions in coronary or other vascular beds.

Large-scale clinical trials involving tens of thousands of individuals in industrialized nations have indicated that reductions in cholesterol levels by either diet or pharmacologic means are generally associated with significant reductions in the morbidity and mortality from coronary disease. The design of many of the trials also incorporated concomitant reduction in other coronary risk factors, however, such as smoking and hypertension, so that assessment of the independent contribution of cholesterol reduction in the beneficial outcome in the "intervention" group may be obscured. Many of the trials also included only men at high risk for coronary disease; it therefore remains to be proven that the beneficial outcome observed in these trials can be extrapolated to women and to individuals with "normal" risk factors and a "normal" cholesterol level. The growing body of evidence linking a reduction in blood cholesterol to a reduction in coronary heart disease manifestations has become sufficiently convincing, however, that a recent National Heart, Lung, and Blood Institute Consensus Development Conference recommended that national efforts be expanded to identify cholesterol levels in all individuals and to reduce elevated levels by dietary means if possible, and by pharmacologic means if necessary.[39]

It should also be emphasized that the observed reduction in blood cholesterol from either diet or drugs in many of the trials has been quite modest. Recent calculations using a model based on data from the Framingham Study, for example, indicate that a lifelong program of dietary cholesterol reduction that lowered serum cholesterol by 6.7% (the level achieved by the dietary intervention in MRFIT) would prolong life by only 3 days to 3 months in low-risk individuals and by only 18 days to 12 months in high-risk individuals.[40] Results from the CLAS study indicate, however, that an aggressive lipid-lowering regimen of diet and drugs can achieve much more striking improvements in serum lipids: a 26% reduction in total cholesterol and a 46% decrease in the ratio of total/HDL cholesterol.[27] The improvement in coronary luminal obstructions resulting from such improvements in serum lipids has been demonstrated; the clinical benefit now remains to be determined.

We believe that a careful assessment of the available evidence suggests that "negative" clinical trials that have failed to show benefit of cholesterol-lowering regimens on clinical outcome (particularly survival) have been those in which the cholesterol-lowering effect of the dietary and/or drug intervention has been small in magnitude and the numbers of subjects followed too small to give a substantial probability of showing a modest effect on clinical outcome. Although data from studies in which major effects on serum cholesterol levels were achieved are limited, they support the conclusion of the LRC trial[38] that a predictable quantitative relationship exists such that greater sustained reductions in serum cholesterol levels are associated with greater improvements in clinical outcome statistics. While we regard these matters more as hypotheses in need of testing than as demonstrated facts, advances in dietary and pharmacologic means to effect substantial reductions in serum cholesterol levels now provide enhanced opportunities to design and carry out clinical trials that will provide much-needed data upon which sound recommendations can be based. The potential importance of such recommendations to the public health of industrialized nations can scarcely be overemphasized.

REFERENCES

1. Mates RE, Gupta RL, Bell AC, Klocke FJ. Hemodynamics of coronary artery stenosis. *Circ Res* 1978; **42**:152–62.
2. Gould KL. Pressure-flow characteristics of coronary stenosis in unsedated dogs at rest and during coronary vasodilation. *Circ Res* 1978; **43**:242–53.
3. Selzer A, Pasternak RC. Role of coronary arteriography in the evaluation of patients with coronary artery disease. *Am J Med* 1981: **70**:747–51.
4. Bateman TM, Gray RJ, Raymond MJ, *et al.* Coronary artery stenosis. Relationship between angiographic severity and impact on mean diastolic pressure gradient. *J Thorac Cardiovasc Surg* 1983; **85**:499–507.
5. Klocke FJ. Measurements of coronary blood flow and degree of stenosis: current clinical implications and continuing uncertainties. *J Am Coll Cardiol* 1983; **1**:31–41.
6. Klocke FJ. Clinical and experimental evaluation of the functional severity of coronary stenoses. Newsletter of the Councils on Clinical Cardiology of the American Heart Association 1982; **71**–9.
7. Principal Investigators of CASS and their Associates. The National Heart, Lung, and Blood Institute Coronary Artery Surgery Study (CASS). *Circulation* 1981; (Suppl I): I-1–81.
8. Roberts WC, Jones AA. Quantification of coronary arterial narrowing at necropsy in acute transmural myocardial infarction. Analysis and comparison of findings in 24 patients and 22 controls. *Circulation* 1980; **61**:786–90.
9. Moise A, Theroux P, Taeyamaus Y, *et al.* Clinical and angiographic factors associated with progression of coronary artery disease. *J Am Coll Cardiol* 1984; **3**:659–67.
10. Castelli WP. Epidemiology of coronary heart disease: The Framingham Study. *Am J Med* 1984; **76**(Suppl 2A):4–12.
11. Simons LA. Interrelations of lipids and lipoproteins with coronary artery disease mortality in 19 countries. *Am J. Cardiol* 1986; **57**:5G–10G.
12. Reardon MF, Nestel PJ, Craig IH, Harper RW. Lipoprotein predictors of the severity of coronary artery disease in men and woman. *Circulation* 1985; **71**:881–8.
13. Campeau L, Enjalbert M, Lesperance J, *et al.* The relation of risk factors to the development of atherosclerosis in saphenous-vein bypass grafts and the progression of disease in the native circulation. A study 10 years after aortocoronary bypass surgery. *N Engl J Med* 1984; **311**:1329–32.
14. Dahlen GH, Guyton JR, Attar M, Farmer JA, Kantz JA, Gotto AM Jr. Association of levels of lipoprotein Lp(a), plasma lipids, and other lipoproteins with coronary artery disease documented by angiography. *Circulation* 1986; **74**:758–65.
15. Wagner WD, Clarkson TB. Comparative primate atherosclerosis. II. A biochemical study of lipids, calcium, and collagen in atherosclerotic arteries. *Exp Molec Pathol* 1975; **23**:96–121.
16. Vesselinovitch D, Wissler RW, Hughes R, Borensztajn J. Reversal of advanced atherosclerosis in rhesus monkeys. Part a. Light microscopic studies. *Atherosclerosis* 1976; **23**:155–76.
17. Wagner WD, St Clair RW, Clarkson TB, Conner JR. A study of atherosclerosis regression in Macaca mulatta. III. Chemical changes in arteries from animals with atherosclerosis induced for 19 months and regressed for 48 months at plasma cholesterol concentrations of 300 or 200 mg/dl. *Am J Pathol* 1980; **100**:633–50.
18. Armstrong ML, Warner ED, Conner WE. Regression of coronary atheromatosis in rhesus monkeys. *Circ Res* 1970; **27**:59–67.
19. Armstrong ML, Megan MB. Lipid depletion in atheromatous coronary arteries in rhesus monkeys after regression diets. *Circ Res* 1972; **30**:675–80.
20. Armstrong ML, Megan MB. Arterial fibrous proteins in cynomolgus monkeys after atherogenic and regression diets. *Circ Res* 1975; **36**:256–61.
21. Arntzenius AC, Kromhout D, Barth JD, *et al.* Diet, lipoproteins, and the progression of coronary atherosclerosis. The Leiden Intervention Trial. *N Engl J Med* 1985; **312**:805–11.
22. Blankenhorn DH, Brooks SH, Selzer RH, Barndt R. The rate of atherosclerosis change during treatment of hyperlipoproteinemia. *Circulation* 1978; **57**:355–61.
23. Duffield RGM, Miller NE, Brunt JNH, *et al.* Treatment of hyperlipidaemia retards progression of symptomatic femoral atherosclerosis. *Lancet* 1983; **2**:639–41.
24. Nash DT, Gensini G, Esente P. The progression of coronary atherosclerosis. *J Cardiac Rehab* 1984; **4**:21–26.

25. Nikkila EA, Viikinkoski P, Valle M, Frick MH. Prevention of progression of coronary athero-sclerosis by treatment of hyperlipidemia: a seven year prospective angiographic study. *Br Med J* 1984; **289**:220–3.
26. Brensike JF, Levy RI, Kelsey SF, *et al*. Effects of therapy with cholestryramine on progression of coronary arteriosclerosis: results of the NHLBI Type II Coronary Intervention Study. *Circulation* 1984; **69**:313–24.
27. Blankenhorn DH, Nessim SA, Johnson RL, Sanmarco ME, Azen SP, Cashin-Hemphill L. Beneficial effects of combined colestipol-niacin therapy on coronary atherosclerosis and coronary venous bypass grafts. *JAMA* 1987; **257**:3233–40.
28. Leren P. The Oslo Diet-Heart Study. Eleven-year report. *Circulation* 1970; **42**:935–42.
29. Bierenbaum ML, Raichelson RI, Fleischman AI, Hayton T, Watson PB. Ten-year experience of modified-fat diets on younger men with coronary heart disease. *Lancet* 1973; **1**:1404–7.
30. Turpeinen O, Karvonen MJ, Pekkarinen M, Miiettinen M, Elosuo R, Paavilainen E. Dietary prevention of coronary heart disease: the Finnish Mental Hospital Study. *Int J Epidemiol* 1979; **8**:99–1118.
31. Hjermann I, Velve Byre K, Holme I, Leren P. Effect of diet and smoking intervention on the incidence of coronary heart disease. *Lancet* 1981; **2**:1303–10.
32. Multiple Risk Factor Intervention Trial Research Group. Multiple risk factor intervention trial. Risk factor changes and mortality results. *JAMA* 1982; **248**:1465–77.
33. Kornitzer M, Dramaix M, Thilly C, *et al*. Belgian Heart Disease Prevention Project: incidence and mortality results. *Lancet* 1983; **1**:1066–70.
34. Borhani NO. Prevention of coronary heart disease in practice. Implications of the results of recent clinical trials. *JAMA* 1985; **254**:257–62.
35. Coronary Drug Project Research Group. Clofibrate and niacin in coronary heart disease. *JAMA* 1975; **231**:360–81.
36. Canner PL. Mortality in coronary drug project patients during a nine year post-treatment period (abstract). *J Am Coll Cardiol* 1985; **5**:442.
37. Trial of clofibrate in the treatment of ischemic heart disease. Five year study by a group of physicians of the Newcastle upon Tyne Region. *Br Med J* 1971; **4**:767–75.
38. Lipid Research Clinics Program. The Lipid Research Clinics Coronary Primary Prevention Trial results. *JAMA* 1984; **251**:351–74.
39. The NIH Consensus Development Conference to Lower Blood Cholesterol for Prevention of Heart Disease. *JAMA* 1985; **253**:2080–6.
40. Taylor WE, Pass TM, Shepard DS, Komaroff AL. Cholesterol reduction and life expectancy. A model incorporating multiple risk factors. *Ann Intern Med* 1987; **106**:605–14.

SUMMARY

Epidemiologic studies have clearly established that the incidence of atherosclerosis is related to plasma cholesterol levels, and serial angiographic studies support the importance of plasma lipids in the progression of existing atherosclerotic obstructions and the development of new lesions. This association has led to clinical studies using a variety of cholesterol-lowering interventions in the hope of reversing or at least slowing down the disease process. This review outlines the major dietary and pharmacologic cholesterol-reducing programs that have been reported. The effect of such hypolipidemic regimens on other manifestations of coronary disease, such as myocardial infarction, are also examined. The available data suggest that interventions that reduce serum cholesterol can delay or halt the progression of athero-sclerosis, as assessed from coronary angiography. Evidence for regression of atherosclerotic coronary obstructions is less abundant, but initial findings are encouraging. Large-scale clinical trials have also indicated that reductions in cholesterol, either by dietary or pharmacologic means, are generally associated with significant reductions in morbidity and mortality from coronary disease. The mean reductions in serum cholesterol in most studies have been quite small; recent data suggest that a more aggresive lipid-lowering regimen of diet and drugs should result in greater sustained reduction in serum cholesterol levels and greater improvement in clinical outcome statistics. Strategies directed toward blood pressure control and the cessation of smoking should form an integral part of any coronary prevention program.

RÉSUMÉ

Des études épidémiologiques ont clairement mis en évidence que les incidences d'athérosclérose sont directement liées aux niveaux de cholestérol dans le plasma et des études angiographiques renforcent l'importance des lipides plasmatiques dans la progression des obstructions athérosclérotiques déjà existantes et dans le développement de nouvelles lésions. Cette association a conduit à de nouvelles études cliniques visant á faire baisser le taux de cholestérol dans l'espoir d'inverser ou tout au moins de ralentir le développement de la maladie. On examine ici les principaux programmes institués en vue de faire baisser les taux de cholestérol: programme de régulation alimentaire, programmes pharmacologiques. On examine aussi les résultats de ces régimes hypolipidémiques sur d'autres manifestations des maladies coronariennes, tels les infarctus du myocarde. Les données disponibles suggèrent que les interventions qui réduisent le cholestérol peuvent retarder ou même arrêter la progression de l'athérosclérose, comme l'indique l'évaluation angiographique. On a moins de preuves concernant la régression des obstructions coronaires athérosclérotiques, cependant les premiers résultats sont encourageants. Des essais cliniques à grande échelle ont également permis de constater que des réductions de cholestérol, soit grâce à un régime alimentaire soit grâce à des médicaments, correspondent à d'importantes réductions de morbidité et de mortalité à la suite de maladies coronariennes. Les moyennes de réduction de cholestérol ont été minimes dans la plupart des études; les données récentes suggèrent que des régimes plus agressifs pour faire baisser le cholestérol (nutrition et thérapie) auraient pour résultat un abaissement plus important et plus soutenu des niveaux de cholestérol et de meilleurs résultats statistiques. Des stratégies visant à contrôler l'hypertension et à éliminer l'usage du tabac devraient faire partie intégrante de toute campagne de prévention contre les maladies coronariennes.

ZUSAMMENFASSUNG

Epidemiologische Studien haben deutlich nachgewiesen, daß das Auftreten von Atherosklerose im Zusammenhang mit den Plasma-Cholesterin Spiegeln steht, und reinhenmäßige angiographische Studien bestätigen die Wichtigkeit der Plasma-Lipide im Fortschreiten der existierenden atherosklerotischen Versperrungen und in der Entwicklung von neuen Läsionen. Dieser Zusammenhang hat zu klinischen Studien geführt, die eine Reihe von Eingriffen zur Erniedrigung des Cholesterins benutzen, in der Hoffnung den Krankheitsverlauf aufzuheben oder wenigstens zu verlangsamen. Dieser Überblick umreisst die wichtigsten diätetischen und pharmakiologischen Cholesterinherabsetzungsprogramme, die gemeldet wurden. Der Einfluß solcher hypolipidämischen Behandlungsvorschriften auf andere Symptome der koronaren Krankheit, wie z. B. Myokardinfarkt, wird auch überprüft. Die vorhandenen Daten weisen darauf hin, daß Eingriffe, die Serum Cholesterin erniedrigen, das Fortschreiten von Atherosklerose hinauschieben oder ihm Halt gebieten können, wie durch koronare Angiographie beurteilt. Beweise für die Regression der atherosklerotischen koronaren Versperrungen sind weniger reichlich vorhanden, aber die anfänglichen Befunde sind ermutigend. Großangelegte klinische Versuche haben ebenfalls angedeutet, daß Reduzierungen des Cholesterins entweder durch diätetische oder durch pharmakologische Mittel im allgemeinen mit erheblichen Reduzierungen der Morbidität und der Sterblichkeitsrate durch koronare Krankheit verbunden sind. Die mittleren Reduzierungen des Serum-Cholesterins waren in den meisten Studien ziemlich klein; Daten neueren Datums gehen davon aus, daß eine aggressivere Lipid-erniedrigende Behandlungsvorschrift betreffend Diät und Medikamenten eine anhaltend größere Erniedrigung der Serum-Cholesterin-Spiegel und größere Besserung der klinischen Resultatstatistiken zur Folge haben sollte. Strategien, die auf Blutdruckkontrolle gerichtet sind, und das Einstellen des Rauchens sollten einen wesentlichen Bestandteil jegliches Programmes für die Verhütung der koronaren Herzkrankheit bilden.

Sommario

Studi epidemiologici hanno definitivamente stabilito che l'occorrenza dell'aterosclerosi è connessa ai livelli del colesterolo nel plasma, e studi angiografici in serie appoggiano l'importanza dei lipidi nel plasma nella progressione delle esistenti ostruzioni aterosclerotiche e lo sviluppo di nuove lesioni. Quest'associazione ci ha guidati verso alcuni studi clinici usando una varietà di interventi d'abbassamento del colesterolo con la speranza di invertire o almeno di ritardare l'avanzamento della malattia. Questo sommario tratteggia i maggiori programmi dietari e farmaceutici per la riduzione del colesterolo. Gli effetti di tali regimi ipolipidemici su altre manifestazioni della malattia coronaria, come ad esempio l'infarto miocardiaco, vengono anche esaminati. I dati disponibili suggeriscono che le interventi che riducono il colesterolo nel siero possono ritardare o fermare la progressione dell'aterosclerosi, com'è evidenziato dall'angiografia coronaria. Evidenza per la rigressione di ostruzioni coronarie aterosclerotiche è meno abbondante, ma i risultati iniziali sono incoraggianti. Prove cliniche a grandi proporzioni hanno anche indicato che le riduzioni del colesterolo, sia per mezzi di dieta sia con droghe, sono di solito associate con riduzione significativa di morbosità e di mortalità per causa di malattia coronaria. Le ricerche indicano che, in media, le riduzioni del colesterolo nel siero sono state poche. Dati piú recenti suggeriscono che un regime di dieta e di droga piú aggressivo verso la riduzione-deilipidi dovrebbe risultare in una maggiore riduzione prolungata del livello del colesterolo nel siero e in un miglioramento di statistiche. Strategie dirette verso il controllo della pressione del sangue e la cessazione del fumo, dovrebbero far parte di qualsiasi programma preventivo sulle malattie coronarie.

Sumário

Estudos epidemiológicos têm estabelecido claramente que a incidência de aterosclerose é ligada a niveis de colesterol no soro, e os estudos angiográficos em série suportam a importância de lípidos plasmáticos na progressão de obstruções ateroscleróticas existentes e o desenvolvimento de lesões novas. Esta associação tem levado a estudos clínicos usando uma variedade de intervenções baixandoo colesterol na esperança de invertor ou pelō menos de retardar a marcha da doença. Esta revista esboça os programas principais para um regime alimentar e para a redução farmacológica de colesterol que têm sido noticiados. Os efeitos de tais regimes hiperlipidémicos sobre outras manifestações de doença coronária, tal como o infarto miocárdico, são também examinados. Os dados disponíveis lembram que as intervenções que reduzem o colesterol no soro podem atrasar ou parar a progressão de aterosclerose, como está avaliado de angiográficas coronárias. A evidência de regressão de obstruções ateroscleróticas coronárias é menos abundante, mas as primeiras descobertas são animadoras.

As experiências clínicas em grande escala têm tambêm indicado que as reduções em colesterol, por meio dum regime alimentar ou por meios farmacológicos, são geralmente associadas com reduções significativas em morbidez e mortalidade de doença coronária. As reduções médias em colesterol no soro na maior parte dos estudos têm sido muito pequenas; os dados recentes indiciam que um regime alimentar e de remédios mais agressivo para baixar os lípidos devia resultar numa redução mais prolongada nos níveis de colesterol no soro e um melhoramente maior nos dados estatísticos dos resultados clínicos. Estratégias dirigidas ao contrôle da pressão arterial e à cessação do fumar deviam formar uma parte integral de qualquer programa de prevenção coronária.

RESUMEN

Varios estudios epidemiológicos han establecido claramente que la incidencia de ateroscle-rosis se halla relacionada con los niveles séricos de colesterol, y estudios angiográficos soriados dan apoyo a la importancia de los lípidos plasmáticos en la progresión de obstruc-ciones ateroscleróticas existentes y el desarrollo de nuevas lesiones. Esta relación ha llevado a varios estudios clínicos que emplean una variedad de intervenciones con el propósito de disminuir los niveles de colesterol, con la esperanza de revertir o al menos lograr un enlon-terimiento en el progreso de la enfermedad. Se presenta un bosquejo de los principales programas dietéticos y farmacológicos encaminados a reducir el colesterol de que se ha informado. También se examinan los efectos de tales regímenes hipolipidémicos en otras manifestaciones de cardiopatía coronaria, tal como el infarto miocárdico. Los datos de que se dispone sugieren que la intervención médica para reducir los niveles séricos de colesterol puede retardar o detener el progreso de la aterosclerosis, en base a la evaluación de angio-grafías coronarias. Las evidencias de regresión de las obstrucciones ateroscleróticas coron-arias son menos abundantes, pero los resultados iniciales son alentadores. Varios ensayos clínicos en gran escala también indican que las reducciones en los niveles de colesterol, sea por medios dietéticos o farmacológicos, generalmente se hallan asociadas con reducciones significativas en la morbilidad y mortalidad causadas por la coronariopatía. La reducción promodio en los niveles séricos de colesterol en la mayoría de los estudios ha sido bastante pequeña; datos más recientes sugieren que un régimen más vigoroso encaminado a reducir los niveles de lípidos mediante la dieta y los fármacos disponibles debe resultar en una mayor reducción sostenida de los niveles séricos de colesterol y una mayor mejoría en las estadísticas de los resultados clínicos. Las estrategias dirigidas hacia el control de la presión arterial y la terminación del hábito de fumar deben ser una parte integral de todo programa de prevención de la coronariopatía.

The Role of Cholesterol in Atherosclerosis:
New Therapeutic Opportunities, edited by S. M. Grundy
and A. G. Bearn, Hanley & Belfus, Inc., Philadelphia.

Overview of Quantitative Coronary Angiographic Techniques; Morphology, Densitometry and Standardization of Acquisition

Johan H. C. Reiber

The limitations in the visual interpretation of the morphology of coronary obstructions have been well documented in the literature. These are the large intra- and interobserver variabilities,[1-9] the fact that visually only relative percent diameter and/or area stenosis can be estimated, and thirdly that the physiologic significance is very difficult, if not impossible, to assess. Moreover, the ever increasing application of recanalization techniques in the catheterization laboratory (such as PTCA,[10-12] the use of thrombolytic agents,[12-14] the introduction of the stent,[15] and possibly in the near future laser[16] and/or spark erosion[17] techniques), the need to study the effects of vasoactive drugs,[18,19] and the interest in finding ways to achieve regression or no-growth of coronary artherosclerosis[20] have stimulated research and development toward computer-based techniques for the objective and reproducible quantitative analysis of the coronary morphology. Such techniques should provide, among other information, absolute measurements on the minimal diameter; extent and asymmetry of the obstructions; relative percent diameter and area stenosis; the roughness of the coronary arterial segment; as well as data on the mean diameters of nonobstructed coronary segments, assessed from multiple projections. By combining all stenosis measurements, the functional pressure-flow effects of the stenosis and the coronary flow reserve can be assessed.[21] In situations where the obstructions are very asymmetric, such as post-PTCA where dissections frequently occur, the computation of relative and absolute cross-sectional narrowing by densitometry seems the ultimate goal to achieve.

The majority of the applications of quantitative coronary cineangiography require the comparison of the arterial dimensions either in a control group versus those in a treated group, or pre- versus post-intervention, possibly with the data from some later control-angiogram. The sample size of the number of patients that need to be investigated to demonstrate a certain effect is proportional to the variability of the measurement technique divided by the number of years between the angiograms squared.[22] From the point of view of the population size, duration and cost-effectiveness of a study, it is therefore of great importance to minimize the variability of the angiographic data acquisition and computer analysis procedures.

In general, the quantitative analysis of coronary obstructions is performed from 35 mm cinefilm. However, recent developments in digital cardiac imaging systems have been directed towards obtaining such measurements on-line during the catheterization procedure from video digitized images. With the present limitations in spatial resolution of these on-line digitized images, this approach is particularly of interest as a tool for diagnostic and/or therapeutic decision-making during the catheterization procedure. However, with the use of modern small field-of-view (FOV) image intensifiers (4″ and 5″ FOV) and the increase in data transfer rates such that 1024^2 images at 30 frames/sec will become feasible, it may be possible in the near future to assess the effects of interventions on-line using the diameter and densitometric cross-sectional area measures mentioned above.

At the present time there are about a dozen groups worldwide actively involved in the development of techniques for the objective and reproducible quantitative morphologic and densitometric computer-aided analysis of the coronary obstructions.[23,24] In this chapter an overview will be given of these different techniques. The majority of the approaches has been developed for cinefilm analysis; these are, however, in the same or slightly modified format also applicable to the on-line digitally acquired data.

IMAGE DIGITIZATION

Because of its inherently high resolution, 35 mm cinefilm has continued to be the medium of choice for the registration of interventional coronary angiograms. For the digitization of selected cineframes, basically two approaches have been taken: (1) optical magnification of a region of interest in a cineframe by means of a cine-video projector with different lens systems and a video camera;[24–26] and (2) electronic magnification by means of a cinedigitizer with a high resolution linear array CCD-camera.[24,27]

Following the first approach, a second generation video-based cine-digitizing system has recently been completed in our laboratory. In this unit the cinefilm is mounted on a plateau with a film guiding system that can be moved under computer control left/right and upwards/downwards; the selected portion of the image is then projected onto a high resolution 1″ Pasecon video camera. The camera and the projection lens can be moved independently from each other under computer control, allowing the selection of the appropriate optical magnification (ranging from 0.7 to 4 in steps of $\sqrt{2}$). The light source consists of three light emitting diodes (LEDs) with a narrow light spectrum; the emitted amount of light can be linearly adjusted. A user-controlled, motor-driven diaphragm and automated light control system further provide for optimal image quality in the selected region of interest. The resulting video signal is then digitized with a standard 15 MHz video A/D converter and the image data stored in an image processor. With a 2.0 × optical magnification, the pixel size in the digitized image, referred to the original cineframe (18 × 24 mm), is 17.6 μm. At the usual x-ray system settings of x-ray source and image intensifier (focus-isocenter = 70 cm, isocenter-image intensifier = 20 cm), a 7″ image intensifier, and subtotal overframing of the cinefilm, the true object size of the original pixel at the isocenter is 84 μm at this magnification. For a 5″ image intensifier the true pixel size would be 60 μm.

The GE CAP35 projector modified by the addition of a 1000-line video camera has also been used for cinefilm digitization; this projector uses a halogen light source for the illumination of the selected cineframe.[28]

By the second approach, the CCD-camera based cinefilm digitizer is a standard cineprojector (Tagarno 35CX) with a field-installable modification package for high resolution digitization of a selected cineframe (Fig. 1). This modification package consists of a film-guiding system, a specially developed optical chain, and a linear array (1728 elements) CCD-camera; the array can be moved mechanically over a total of 2846 positions. The monochromatic light source consists of an array of LEDs optimally suitable for densitometric analysis of the cinefilm with the present optical chain. Any area of 6.9 × 6.9 mm in a selected cineframe (size 18 × 24 mm) can be digitized by the CCD-camera with a resolution of 512 × 512 pixels with 8 bits of grey levels. Effectively, this means that the entire cineframe of size

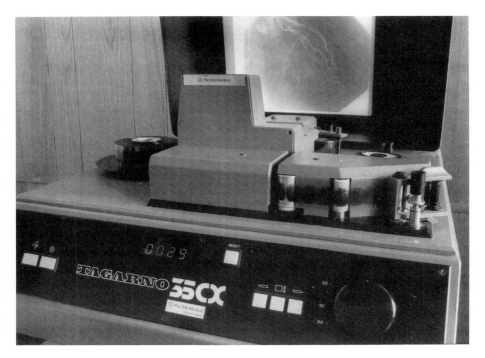

FIG. 1. Photograph of Tagarno 35CX with modification package for high-resolution digitization of a selected cineframe by means of a linear array CCD-camera.

18 × 24 mm can be digitized at a resolution of 1329 × 1772 pixels. A homogeneity in the brightness distribution over the entire digitized image of better than 5% has been achieved.[29]

The currently commercially available digital cardiac imaging systems allow 512 × 512 matrix acquisitions at 30 frames/sec and 1024 × 1024 matrix acquisitions at max. 7 frames/sec, although systems with 30 frames/sec 1024^2 acquisitions have been announced already by a number of manufacturers. In general, plumbicon video tubes with a gamma = 1, with either interlaced or noninterlaced scanning systems, have been used. For high-resolution digitization, noninterlaced (progressive) scanning should be used with preferably 10 bits of density resolution.

To compare the order of magnitude of the pixel size that can be achieved with a digital system with that from cinefilm digitization (71 μm at the isocenter with a 7″ image intensifier), we can make the following calculation. Assume again that a 7″ FOV image intensifier is used and that the 512^2 matrix precisely fits within the 7″ circle. With the heart positioned at the isocenter, and a distance from focus to isocenter of 70 cm and from isocenter to image intensifier of 20 cm, a pixel size of 188 μm is found at the isocenter. For a 5″ FOV image intensifier the true pixel size would be 134 μm. Of course, these pixel sizes should not be confused with the final resolution that one can obtain from these images; however, this simple calculation shows that the sampling density from cinefilm is a factor of 2.6 higher than from direct digital acquisition.

CALIBRATION

To compute absolute sizes of the arterial segment analyzed, a calibration factor needs to be determined. Three different approaches have been used for the coronary arteries: (1) analytically from geometric x-ray system parameters; (2) on the basis of the known diameter of the contrast catheter; and (3) biplane assessment of the distance of cardiomarker rings on the contrast catheter.

Following the first approach, the size of an object in the plane through the center of rotation of the x-ray system (isocenter) and parallel to the image intensifier input screen can be determined based on simple geometric principles from the height levels of x-ray tube and image intensifier. However, for objects above or below the center of rotation, a slightly more complicated analysis must be carried out, requiring a second, preferably orthogonal, view of the object. Wollschlaeger *et al.* have developed a method to calculate the exact radiological magnification factors for each point in the fields of view of biplane multidirectional isocentric x-ray equipment.[30] By this approach they avoid two error sources: (1) contour detection of the catheter segment, and (2) the differential magnification of the scaling device and the arterial segment.

If the catheter is used as the scaling device (second approach), the contours of a short segment of the tip or shaft may either be manually defined with a writing tablet,[31] or contour detection techniques similar to those used for the coronary segments may be applied. In our routine practice, the catheter is magnified optically or electronically with a factor of $2\sqrt{2}:1$ or 2:1, respectively, and *a priori* information is included in the iterative edge detection procedure, based on the fact that the selected part of the catheter is the projection of a cylindrical structure (Fig. 2). It should be realized that the size of the catheter as given by the manufacturer, in general, will deviate from its true size, especially for disposable catheters. For intervention studies, therefore, it may be advisable to measure the size of the catheter following the catheterization procedure with a micrometer.[32,33] Recently, new catheters have been developed with flat metallic markers of precisely known size positioned near the tip of the catheter. Advantages of this approach are (1) good image contrast of the markers, resulting in precise edge definition; and (2) since the size of the marker is well-known, remeasurement with a micrometer following the catheterization procedure is not necessary.

If the known size of the catheter in a single angiographic view is used for calibration purposes, the computed calibration factor is only applicable to objects in the plane of the catheter parallel to the image intensifier input screen. The change in magnification for two objects located at different points along the x-ray beam axis is about 1.5% for each centimeter that separates the objects axially (based on the commonly used focus-image intensifier distances). For coronary segments lying in other planes, corrections to the calibration factor can be assessed from other views.

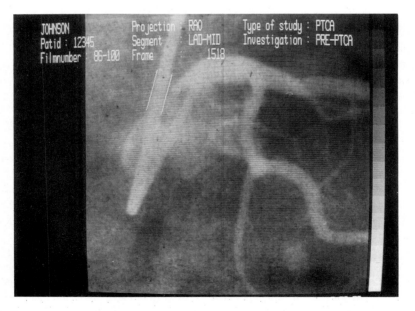

FIG. 2.   Example of automatically detected boundaries along shaft of coronary contrast catheter.

If biplane views are available, the calibration factor can be determined by measuring the distance of cardiomarker rings, which have been placed with 1 cm spacing on the tip portion of the catheter (third approach). Because of the fact that the length of this measuring device is roughly a factor of four greater than the diameter of the catheter, the precision of this calibration procedure is higher than by determining the size of the catheter; in addition, the positions of the rings are better defined than the boundaries of the catheter. The only requirement is that biplane views be available.

From the above it is clear that for the measurement of truly absolute sizes of coronary segments, two views, preferably but not necessarily orthogonal to each other, are required. If, however, one is interested only in the changes in sizes of coronary segments as a result of long- or short-term interventions, excellent results can be achieved from single-plane views. For these situations one must make sure that for the repeat angiogram the x-ray system is positioned in exactly the same geometry as during the first angiogram. This requires registration of the angles and height levels of the x-ray system, preferably on line with a microprocessor-based geometry read-out system.[32] Although the calibration factor used for a particular coronary arterial segment is then only an approximation of the true calibration factor, the same systematic error will be present for the first and repeat angiograms.

PINCUSHION DISTORTION AND CORRECTION

It is well-known that particularly the older types of image intensifiers introduce a geometric distortion, the so-called pincushion distortion. This results in selective magnification of an object near the edges of the image as compared to its size in the center of the field. These differences need to be corrected for, if absolute diameter measurements are to be derived from coronary angiograms. The standard procedure to assess the degree of distortion present is to film a cm-grid, which is positioned against the input screen of the image intensifier. This needs to be done only once for a given image intensifier tube at each of the available magnification modes.

A number of approaches to correct for pincushion distortion have been implemented. Theoretically, pincushion distortion is radially symmetric about the central x-ray beam, because of the rotational symmetry of the curved image intensifier input screen and its internal fields. The first approach, therefore, is based on the assumption that the distortion is indeed radially symmetric and that the relative magnification can be determined from the distance of the pixel under consideration from the center of the image intensifier. An empirically determined analytical function of the radius is then used to correct for the distortion.[31,34] The second method is also based on radial symmetry, but relative magnification factors for a single radial line are stored in the memory of the computer system. The relative magnification for each distance was obtained by averaging the four values measured in the four quadrants of the cm-grid image. Hence, no analytical function is employed.[25,35] The third method, which is in use in our center, makes no assumption about the geometrical distribution of the distortion and stores the relative magnifications of all the intersection points of the cm-grid.[36] We have developed a procedure that allows the fully automated detection of the wires and intersection points in the 1:1 projected cineframe (Fig. 3). For a given point in the image that does not coincide with one of the displayed intersection positions, the correction vector is determined by means of bilinear interpolation between the correction vectors of the four neighboring intersection points.

In their digital cardiac system, LeFree *et al.* have implemented a somewhat similar approach, except for the fact that they correct the entire image by piecewise linear warping and not only the contour positions of the catheter and arterial segment.[37] For these purposes a 1-cm spaced orthogonal array of bronze ball bearings is imaged at the image intensifier input screen.

CONTOUR DETECTION OF THE CORONARY ARTERIAL SEGMENT

For the computer-assisted definition of the boundaries of a selected coronary segment, in general, the following steps can be distinguished: (1) definition global centerline of coronary segment; (2) edge enhancement; and (3) contour definition. The different implementations of these steps will be discussed in some more detail in the following paragraphs.

1. Definition Global Centerline

Edge positions of coronary segments in the digitized images can best be detected along scanlines perpendicular to the local centerline direction of the segment. For

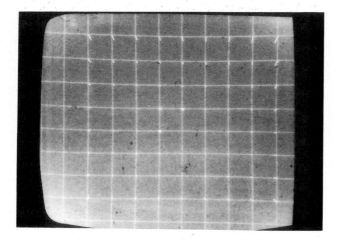

FIG. 3. Cm-grid with correction vectors computed from the automatically detected intersection positions.

these purposes the first step in the contour detection algorithm requires the definition of the global trajectory of the centerline.

In general, two approaches have been advocated:
(i) the user-definition of the global centerline, and
(ii) automated tracking of the centerline.

The user-interactive approach requires that the operator define a midline estimate for the arterial segment to be analyzed by indicating a few center points along the vessel by means of a sonic pen or writing tablet.[24,34,38–42] Figure 4 shows an example of a selected coronary arterial segment with the user-defined centerline. This centerline is then smoothed and defines the scanlines perpendicular to the local centerline directions for the computation of the edge positions. Several groups have advocated updating of this centerline by a new centerline computed from the contour positions once these have been detected and repeating the contour detection procedure.[24,40] By means of this iterative approach, the influence of the user definition of the center points on the detected contour positions can be minimized.

Barth *et al.* have developed an automated tracking procedure for the centerline; the user only indicates a starting position and a flow direction within the arterial segment of interest.[43,44]

LeFree *et al.* also have developed an automated procedure for the definition of the centerline applied to digital cardiac images.[37] A polar coordinate search algorithm is used to identify the centerline of the artery following operator assignment of the approximate center of the lesion and the length of the arterial segment to be evaluated.

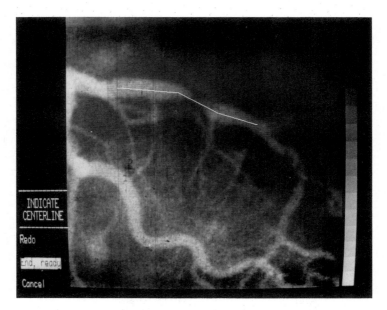

FIG. 4.   Example of magnified LAD mid-coronary segment with user-defined centerline.

2. Edge Enhancement

Edge enhancement of the digitized data is usually based on the application of first or second derivative functions or a combination of these two. In general, these derivative functions are applied to the individual scanlines perpendicular to the local centerline directions, and the edge positions are subsequently defined on the basis of a given contour-definition criterion. To simplify and speed up the edge-enhancement and contour-definition procedures, both Barth *et al.* and Kooijman *et al.* resample the digital data along the scanlines, resulting in a stretched version of the arterial segment.[24,36,43,44] In this resampled matrix the centerline has become a straight vertical line, whereas the scanlines are oriented horizontally. Edge enhancement can now easily be achieved by applying simple one-dimensional gradient functions along the horizontal lines. Second derivative values can be obtained by applying the gradient function to the first-derivative matrix.

3. Contour Definition

To date there does not seem to be a generally accepted contour detection technique; each research group has developed and used its own algorithm. Six different approaches can be distinguished. The edge definition is based on: (1) manual tracing of the boundaries;[31] (2) 1st derivative function applied along the scanlines perpendicular to the local centerline direction;[25,35,38–40,45] (3) 2nd derivative function;[46] (4) 1st and 2nd derivative functions;[24,36,37] (5) the use of correlation techniques;[34,41–45] and (6) the selection of a global threshold level following background subtraction.[47] Among these different techniques, one can further distinguish between local- and global-edge definition procedures. With the local procedure the edge points are defined on a scanline by scanline basis, possibly using expectation windows to limit the search regions. With the global procedures, all the intensity and/or derivative information along the arterial segment is taken into account in the definition of the arterial contour.[36]

In most publications no mention is made of particular procedures to eliminate extraneous detected positions. Experience from our earlier work made clear that certain precautions need to be taken if the contours are determined on a line-to-line basis (local edge definition procedure). That means that one should define, for example, an expectation window for a certain scanline based on the detected position(s) on the previous scanline(s).

Only Brown *et al.* and Kirkeeide *et al.* correct the defined edge positions for the line-spread function of the x-ray system.[31,34] This seems particularly of importance for the vessel dimensions below 1.0 mm.

Following contour definition, a smoothing procedure is usually applied to each of the detected contour paths, which may consist of a least-squares error first-degree polynomial fit through a number of nearest points on each side of the edge point under consideration. On the basis of these smoothed contours, quantitative data about the arterial dimensions can be obtained in the contour analysis phase.

CONTOUR ANALYSIS

From the contours of the analyzed arterial segment, following pincushion correction and calibration, a diameter function can be determined by computing the distance between the left and right edges. From these data a number of parameters may be calculated such as: (1) minimal obstruction diameter; (2) obstruction area (assuming circular or elliptical cross sections, or by applying the densitometric technique); (3) extent of the obstruction; (4) reference diameter (either user- or computer-defined); (5) percentage diameter stenosis; (6) percentage area stenosis (assuming circular or elliptical cross sections, or by applying the densitometric technique); (7) symmetry of the stenosis; (8) area of the artherosclerotic plaque in a particular angiographic view; (9) hemodynamic parameters of the obstruction;[21] and (10) mean diameter of a nonobstructive coronary segment.[24] Particularly the minimal obstruction area is of great importance as it is present to the inverse second power in the formulas describing the pressure loss over a coronary obstruction. Moreover, to determine the effect of interventions on the severity of coronary obstructions, one should compute the changes in minimal obstruction area (or diameter) and not those in percentage area (or diameter) narrowing, as the reference position in general will also be affected by the intervention.[48]

However, as cardiologists have been trained to express the severity and also the changes in severity of an obstruction in terms of percentage diameter narrowing, these values are mostly included in quantitative reports. The usual way to determine percentage diameter stenosis of a coronary obstruction requires the user to indicate a reference position. A reference diameter is then usually computed as the average value of a number of diameter values in a symmetric region with its center at the user-defined reference position. It is clear that this computed %-D narrowing of an obstruction depends heavily on the selected reference position. In arteries with a focal obstructive lesion and a clearly normal proximal arterial segment, the choice of the reference region is straightforward and simple. However, in cases where the proximal part of the arterial segment shows combinations of stenotic and ectatic areas, the choice may be very difficult. To minimize these variations, alternative methods have been developed which are not dependent on a user-defined reference region.[24,34,36,38,39] By these methods, an estimate of the normal or pre-disease arterial size and luminal wall location is obtained on the basis of the computed centerline and the 90th percentile of the diameter values[38,39] or on the basis of a first-degree polynomial computed through the diameter values of the proximal and distal centerline segments followed by a translation to the 80th percentile level (reference diameter function);[24,36] tapering of the vessel to account for a decrease in arterial caliber associated with branches is taken care of. The reference diameter is now taken as the value of the reference diameter function at the location of the minimal obstruction diameter. The interpolated or computer-defined percentage diameter stenosis is computed by comparing the minimal diameter value at the obstruction with the corresponding value of the reference diameter. An example of our technique is shown in Figure 5 for an obstruction in the mid-portion of the

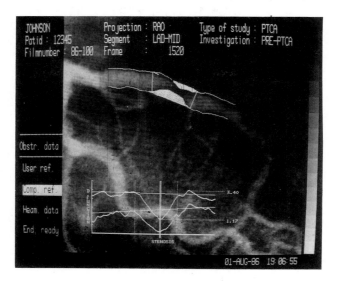

FIG. 5. Example of the automatically detected luminal boundaries of the mid-LAD segment and the estimated pre-disease dimensions of the vessel at the site of the obstruction (reference edges). The upper function is the diameter function, with the straight line through it being the reference diameter function; the lower function is the densitometric area function.

LAD in the RAO-projection. The actual contours of the arterial segment as well as the estimated pre-disease reference contours are superimposed in the image. The difference in area between the reference and the detected luminal contours is marked over the obstructive lesion; this area is a measure for the atherosclerotic plaque in this particular angiographic view. The upper function is the diameter function with the straight line being the reference diameter function; the lower function is the densitometric area function (see following section on Densitometry).

In addition, this interpolated or computer-defined reference diameter technique allows the assessment of the symmetry or asymmetry of the lesion in a given view with respect to a reconstructed centerline. Vessel midpoints for the proximal and distal "normal" portions are found by averaging the coordinates of the left and right contour points. However, for the obstructive region the vessel midpoints are obtained by interpolation between the proximal and distal vessel midpoints with a second degree polynomial. The symmetry measure is given as a value between 0 and 1, with 1 representing a concentric lesion and 0 the most severe case of asymmetry or eccentricity. The extent of the obstruction is determined from the diameter function on the basis of significant maxima in curvature using variable degrees of smoothing. In addition to the fact that the interpolated technique provides data about the area of the artherosclerotic plaque and the lesion's symmetry in a given view, there is another very practical advantage. By this technique, knowledge about the exact location of a reference, either proximal or distal to the stenosis, is not required for the analysis of repeated angiograms.

From the available morphological data of the obstruction, the Poisseuille and turbulent resistances at different flows and thus the resulting transstenotic pressure gradients can be computed on the basis of the well-known fluid-dynamic equations.[21,24]

For the example of Figure 5, the following quantitative measurements were obtained:

extent obstruction	7.51 mm
reference diameter	3.16 mm
obstruction diameter	1.17 mm
reference area (assuming circular cross sections)	7.86 mm^2
obstruction area (densitometric)	0.84 mm^2
area atherosclerotic plaque	9.90 mm^2
symmetry measure	0.53
diameter stenosis	63.1 %
area stenosis (densitometric)	89.4 %
transstenotic pressure gradient at mean flow of 1 ml/sec	3.04 mmHg

The mean diameter of a nonobstructive coronary segment can easily be determined from the diameter data by requesting the user to indicate with a writing tablet, lightpen or similar device the proximal and distal boundaries of the desired segment; the length of the segment in mm is usually also provided. For intervention studies coronary branch points may be used to define the boundaries of the segment, as these can be determined fairly reproducibly.

Information about the "roughness" of the arterial segment and thus about diffuse coronary artery disease may be obtained by subdividing the coronary segment into an integer number of subsegments with a length of about 5 mm and calculating for each subsegment the minimal, maximal, mean diameter, and the standard deviation of the diameter values. The standard deviation possibly is a measure for diffuse atherosclerosis; clinical validation procedures need to be carried out to determine the true value of this parameter. On the basis of the quotient of the standard deviation value and the difference between minimal and maximal diameters, it can be determined whether a subsegment is focally or diffusely diseased, or normal. Figure 6 shows the four subsegments for the example of Figure 5; the derived subsegmental data are given in Table I.

DENSITOMETRY

Since the luminal cross-section at a coronary obstruction is frequently irregular in shape, percentage diameter reduction measured in a single angiographic view is of limited diagnostic value. The hemodynamic resistance of an obstruction is deter-

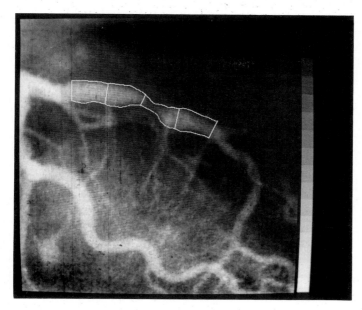

FIG. 6. To obtain information about the "roughness" (irregularities) of the arterial segment, the segment is subdivided into an integer number of subsegments with lengths of approximately 5 mm, and for each subsegment the standard deviation with respect to the mean value is computed. The subsegmental data for this example is presented in Table I.

mined to a great extent by the minimal cross-sectional area. Computation of this cross-sectional area reduction from the percentage diameter reduction measured in a single view requires the assumption of, e.g., circular cross-sections, an assumption which hardly ever holds. The resulting error may be reduced by incorporating two orthogonal projections and computing elliptical cross-sections. However, with the often occurring eccentric lesions even this last approach may yield inaccurate results.

The edge detection techniques described above, in general are based on the measurement of changes in the brightness profiles along scanlines perpendicular to local centerline segments. If, however, one could constitute the relationship between the path lengths of the x-rays through the artery and the absolute brightness values

TABLE I. *Subsegmental data for the example of Figure 6. Segment No. 1 is the most proximal segment*

Segment	1	2	3	4
Length (mm)	5.51	5.51	5.51	5.51
Minimal diameter (mm)	2.92	1.74	1.17	2.68
Maximal diameter (mm)	3.29	3.27	3.03	3.40
Mean diameter (mm)	3.04	2.85	2.02	2.99
Standard deviation (mm)	0.12	0.48	0.69	0.24
Focal or Diffuse Disease	No	Yes	Yes	No

in the digitized image, one would obtain the information required to compute the cross-sectional areas from a single view. It is clear that a homogeneous mixing of the contrast agent with the blood must be assumed for the measurement to have any meaning.

A simplified block diagram of a complete x-ray/cine acquisition and analysis system is shown in Figure 7. In a digital cardiac system the cinefilm components are absent and the video camera at the output screen of the image intensifier (not shown in Figure 7) is connected directly to the A/D-converter.

Constitution of the relationship between path length and brightness values requires detailed analysis of the complete imaging system. In a simplified approach, we are only interested in the static properties of the system. Analysis of the static transfer function of each link in the chain reveals that computation of the complete transfer function is very difficult. There is a large number of parameters involved, many of which are spatially variant.[24,49] A few different approaches towards densitometric analysis of selected coronary arterial segments have been published and will be described briefly in the following paragraphs.

Most authors assume that the x-ray absorption process, comprising the first part of the imaging chain from x-ray source to the image intensifier output screen, can be described by the Lambert-Beer law. Despite many potential sources of errors in the absorption process (for example, nonmonochromatic x-ray spectrum, beam hardening, scattering and veiling glare), it has indeed been demonstrated by Bürsch and Heintzen that by the use of appropriate filters and scatter grids the Lambert-Beer law is applicable for densitometric measurements in clinical studies with a sufficient degree of accuracy.[50,51]

On the other hand, Doriot *et al.* have indicated that the Lambert-Beer absorption law cannot account for the nonlinear relationship between densitometric signal and

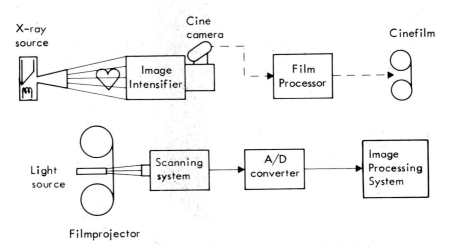

FIG. 7.   Block diagram of an x-ray/cine acquisition and analysis system.

logarithmic x-ray transmission through the lumen of an opacified coronary artery.[46,52] Therefore, they have developed a physical model that takes the polychromasia and scattered radiation into account and have shown that this relation can be approximated by a 2nd order polynomial. The coefficients of this polynomial depend primarily on the voltage applied to the x-ray tube and on the iodine concentration of the injected contrast medium. For a particular x-ray system the coefficients of the polynomial can be simply obtained by means of a linear wedge filled with contrast material.

Different approaches are being investigated to try to correct for the scattered radiation and the veiling glare in the image intensifier.[53,54]

In general, however, for the remaining subsystems of the cinefilm imaging chain, comprising the cinefilm exposure and development process, and the film-sampling process, which may be achieved via video and A/D conversion, with a CCD camera or other device, simplified formulas relating measured brightness levels with the irradiated object thicknesses are used, neglecting the influence of spatially non-homogeneous responses.[34,43,55] By this approach the response of film exposure, the density D versus log (exposure) curve, is being linearized (linear transfer function). Nichols *et al.* use a logarithmic transfer function.[56]

We have implemented a more complicated approach in an attempt to correct for the nonlinearities in the D versus log(E) plot and for the daily variations in the cinefilm processing.[24,49] For this purpose, a special sensitometer has been developed which allows 21 full cineframes covering the entire densitometric range of the film to be exposed on each film cassette before it is mounted on the image intensifier of the x-ray system. The color temperature of the light source is the same as the one from the output screen of the image intensifier. The analysis procedure of a coronary cineangiogram therefore starts with the digitization of these 21 sensitometric frames, allowing the assessment of a nonlinear transfer function.

By means of this calibration procedure many nonlinear, both temporally and spatially variant, effects in the film-processing and film-video or film-CCD camera system are taken into account. It has indeed been shown that this sensitometric approach improves the accuracy of cross-sectional area measurements as compared to the linear approach.[57]

In a digital cardiac system, the transfer function from the output of the image intensifier up to the digitized image can be assumed to be a linear function.[37,41,42,58]

In general, the basic steps in a densitometric procedure to compute percentage cross-sectional area reduction of a selected lesion can be summarized as follows (Fig. 8). The contours of a selected arterial segment are detected as described before. On each scanline perpendicular to the centerline, a profile of brightness values is measured. This profile is transformed into an absorption profile by means of the computed transfer functions (linear or nonlinear depending on the technique used). The background contribution is estimated by computing the linear regression line through the background points directly left and right of the detected contours. Subtraction of this background portion from the absorption profile within the arterial contours yields the net cross-sectional absorption profile. Integration of this function

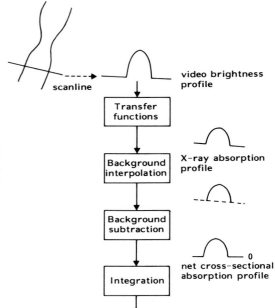

FIG. 8. Diagrammatic presentation of a densitometric analysis procedure to compute the cross-sectional area data from the brightness information within the arterial segment.

results in a measure for the cross-sectional area at the particular scanline. By repeating this procedure for all the scanlines, the cross-sectional area function A(i) is obtained. Percentage area reduction of an obstruction is determined by comparing the minimal area value at the obstruction with the mean value at a selected reference position. The earlier mentioned interpolated approach can also be applied for the estimation of the pre-disease area values. If we assume that the cross-section at the reference position is circular, absolute cross-sectional value (in mm²) for the arterial segments and thus for the minimal cross-section can be obtained.

The lower function in the example of Figure 5 is the densitometric area function for this segment. A percentage densitometric cross-sectional area reduction of 89.4% was found, indicating that the obstruction is slightly more severe than one would estimate by assuming circular cross-sections (86% area reduction).

It will be clear that the densitometric analysis of coronary arterial segments is difficult because of all the potential problems that may arise. In addition to all the possible error sources mentioned above, another important aspect is the orientation of the vessel of interest with respect to the x-ray beam.[59] In addition, sidebranches or branches lying very close to the arterial segment to be analyzed will cause errors in the background correction technique. One of the most essential requirements for a densitometric technique to meet is that the computed densitometric obstruction area values, assessed from different angiographic views, are equal within the variability range of the technique. Although various *in vitro* and *in vivo* phantom studies have been published on densitometric analysis of obstructions, until now not a single technique has proven to provide highly accurate and reproducible results in a well-designed *in vivo* study.

MEASUREMENT VARIABILITIES AND VALIDATION PROCEDURES

Although different approaches on the morphologic and densitometric analysis of coronary obstructions have been published in the literature, as described above, it is very difficult, if not impossible, at this point in time to compare these systems quantitatively, i.e., the question how well all these systems work with routinely obtained coronary angiograms cannot be answered. Data on the accuracy and precision of the edge detection and analysis procedures, the success scores under different image qualities and computation time, are usually not provided in the publications; if they are provided, different parameters to describe the validation results have been used, making comparisons very difficult. Recently, discussions among several groups active in this field have taken place in an attempt to define commonly acceptable validation procedures for the quantitative coronary angiography analysis systems and to use the same statistical techniques to present the results.[60]

In my opinion the following validation procedures should be carried out:

Assessment of Accuracy of Edge Detection and Densitometric Techniques

- Phantom studies of coronary obstructions with dimensions from 0.5 to 5.0 mm under different imaging conditions (various concentrations of the contrast agent, different kV-levels covering the routinely used range) and under static and dynamic flow conditions.
- *In vivo* animal studies with hollow plastic cylinders of various luminal shapes and sizes inserted in the coronary arteries.[58,61–63]

[Note that for densitometric studies the results should be independent of the angiographic views in which these studies were acquired.]

Reproducibility

- Repeated analysis of a set of clinical coronary angiograms of sufficient size obtained under various imaging conditions to assess inter- and intra-observer variabilities. At the present time, the variability of repeated cinefilm analysis in absolute dimensions is about 0.10 mm and in percentage diameter (%-D) stenosis 3%.

Parameters Describing the Validation Results

It has been suggested that the results from the validation studies should be described in terms of the mean differences (accuracy) and the standard deviations of the differences (precision) between the true and measured values or between the values from repeated measurements. Note that the differences should be calculated as (measurement 1 − measurement 2) or (measurement 2 − measurement 1); absolute differences should not be used.

APPROACHES TOWARDS STANDARDIZATION IN ANGIOGRAPHIC DATA ACQUISITION AND ANALYSIS

It has been shown that the variabilities in the arterial measurements can be decreased by standardizing of the angiographic data acquisition and analysis procedures.[32,64] In summary, the following measures have been proposed:

- Precise registration of the angulations of the x-ray system for the different angiographic views, so that the repeat angiographies can be performed in the same views.
- Administration of a vasodilator drug immediately prior to angiographic investigations.
- Use of modern isoviscous and iso-osmolar contrast agents.
- Administration of contrast medium preferably by ECG-triggered injector.
- Selection of a contrast catheter constructed of such material that a high-quality image results (high angiographic image contrast and edge gradient).
- Measurement of the actual size of the catheter with a micrometer following catheterization procedure.

REFERENCES

1. Zir LM, Miller SW, Dinsmore RE, Gilbert JP, Harthorne JW. Interobserver variability in coronary angiography. *Circulation* 1976; **53**:627–32.
2. Detre KM, Wright E, Murphy ML, Takaro T. Observer agreement in evaluating coronary angiograms. *Circulation* 1975; **52**:979–86.
3. DeRouen TA, Murray JA, Owen W. Variability in the analysis of coronary arteriograms. *Circulation* 1977; **55**:324–8.
4. Sanmarco ME, Brooks SH, Blankenhorn DH. Reproducibility of a consensus panel in the interpretation of coronary angiograms. *Am Heart J* 1978; **96**:430–7.
5. Shub C, Vlietstra RE, Smith HC, Fulton RE, Elveback LR. The impredictable progression of symptomatic coronary artery disease. A serial clinical-angiographic analysis. *Mayo Clin Proc* 1981; **56**:155–60.
6. Fisher LD, Judkins MP, Lespérance J, *et al.* Reproducibility of coronary arteriographic reading in the Coronary Artery Surgery Study (CASS). *Cathet Cardiovasc Diagn* 1982; **8**:565–75.
7. Meier B, Gruentzig AR, Goebel N, Pyle R, Von Gosslar W, Schlumpf M. Assessment of stenoses in coronary angioplasty. Inter- and intraobserver variability. *Int J Cardiol* 1983; **3**:159–69.
8. Cameron A, Kemp HG, Fisher LD, *et al.* Left main coronary artery stenosis: Angiographic determination. *Circulation* 1983; **68**:484–9.

9. Zir LM. Observer variability in coronary angiography (editorial note). *Int J Cardiol* 1983; **3**:171–3.

10. Serruys PW, Reiber JHC, Wijns W, *et al*. Assessment of percutaneous transluminal coronary angioplasty by quantitative coronary angiography: Diameter versus densitometric area measurements. *Am J Cardiol* 1984; **54**:482–8.

11. Serruys PW, Geuskens R, Feyter P de, *et al*. Incidence of restenosis 30 and 60 days after successful PTCA: A quantitative coronary angiography study in 200 consecutive patients. *Circulation* 1985; **72**(Suppl III):III–140 (abstract).

12. Serruys PW, Wijns W, Brand M van den, *et al*. Is transluminal coronary angioplasty mandatory after successful thrombolysis? A quantitative coronary angiographic study. *Br Heart J* 1983; **50**:257–65.

13. Serruys PW, Arnold AER, Brower RW, *et al*. Quantitative assessment of the effect of continued rt-PA infusion on the residual stenosis after initial recanalisation in acute myocardial infarction. *Circulation* 1986; **74**:II–368 (abstract).

14. Serruys PW, Arnold AER, Brower RW, *et al*. Effect of continued rt-PA administration on the residual stenosis after initially successful recanalization in acute myocardial infarction–a quantitative coronary angiography study of a randomized trial. *Eur Heart J* 1987; **8** (in press).

15. Sigwart U, Puel J, Mirkovitch V, Joffre F, Kappenberger L. Intravascular stents to prevent occlusion and restenosis after transluminal angioplasty. *N Engl J Med* 1987; **316**:701–6.

16. Isner JM, Clarke RH. Laser angioplasty: unraveling the Gordian Knot. *J Am Coll Cardiol* 1986; **7**:705–8.

17. Slager CJ, Essed CA, Schuurbiers JCH, Bom N, Serruys PW, Meester GT. Vaporization of atherosclerotic plaques by spark erosion. *J Am Coll Cardiol* 1985; **5**:1382–6.

18. Serruys PW, Lablanche JM, Reiber JHC, Bertrand ME, Hugenholtz PG. Contribution of dynamic vascular wall thickening to luminal narrowing during coronary arterial vasomotion. *Z Kardiol* 1983; **72**:116–23.

19. Serruys PW, Deckers JW, Luyten HE, *et al*. Long-acting coronary vasodilatory action of the molsidomine metabolite Sin 1: A quantitative angiographic study. *Eur Heart J* 1987; **8**:263–70.

20. Arntzenius AC, Kromhout D, Barth JD, *et al*. Diet, lipoproteins, and the progression of coronary atherosclerosis. The Leiden Intervention Trial. *N Engl J Med* 1985; **312**:805–11.

21. Gould KL, Kirkeeide RL. Assessment of stenosis severity. *In:* Reiber JHC, Serruys PW, eds. *State of the Art in Quantitative Coronary Arteriography*. Dordrecht/Boston/Lancaster, Martinus Nijhoff Publishers, 1986; 209–28.

22. Blankenhorn DH, Brooks SH. Angiographic trials of lipid-lowering therapy. *Arteriosclerosis* 1981; **1**:242–9.

23. Reiber JHC, Kooijman CJ, Slager CJ, *et al*. Computer-assisted analysis of the severity of obstructions from coronary cineangiograms: a methodological review. *Automedica* 1984; **5**:219–38.

24. Reiber JHC, Serruys PW, Slager CJ. *Quantitative Coronary and Left Ventricular Cineangiography; Methodology and Clinical Applications*. Boston/Dordrecht/Lancaster: Martinus Nijhoff Publishers, 1986.

25. Sanders WJ, Alderman EL, Harrison DC. Coronary artery quantitation using digital image processing techniques. *Comput Cardiol* 1979; 15–20.

26. Ellis S, Sanders W, Goulet C, *et al*. Optimal detection of the progression of coronary artery disease: comparison of methods suitable for risk factor intervention trials. *Circulation* 1986; **74**:1235–42.

27. Reiber JHC, Kooijman CJ, Slager CJ, *et al*. Taking a quantitative approach to cine-angiogram analysis. *Diagn Imaging* 1985; (April):87–9.

28. Selzer RH, Shircore A, Lee PL, Hemphill L, Blankenhorn DH. A second look at quantitative coronary angiography: some unexpected problems. *In:* Reiber JHC, Serruys PW, eds. *State of the Art in Quantitative Coronary Arteriography*. Dordrecht/Boston/Lancaster, Martinus Nijhoff Publishers, 1986; 125–43.

29. Kooijman CJ, Kalberg R, Slager CJ, Tijdens FO, Plas J van der, Reiber JHC. Densitometric analysis of coronary arteries. *In:* Young IT, Biemond J, Duin RPW, Gerbrands JJ, eds. *Signal Processing III: Theories and Applications*. North-Holland, Amsterdam/New York/Oxford/Tokyo, 1986; 1405–8.

30. Wollschlaeger H, Lee P, Zeiher A, Solzbach U, Bonzel T, Just H. Improvement of quantitative angiography by exact calculation of radiological magnification factors. *Comput Cardiol* 1985; 483–6.

31. Brown BG, Bolson E, Frimer M, Dodge HT. Quantitative coronary arteriography. Estimation of dimensions, hemodynamic resistance, and atheroma mass of coronary artery lesions using the arteriograms and digital computation. *Circulation* 1977; **55**:329–37.
32. Reiber JHC, Serruys PW, Kooijman CJ, Slager CJ, Schuurbiers JCH, Boer A den. Approaches towards standardization in acquisition and quantitation of arterial dimensions from cineangiograms. *In:* Reiber JHC, Serruys PW, eds. *State of the Art in Quantitative Coronary Arteriography.* Dordrecht/Boston/Lancaster, Martinus Nijhoff Publishers, 1986; 145–72.
33. Reiber JHC, Kooijman CJ, Boer A den, Serruys PW. Assessment of dimensions and image quality of coronary contrast catheters from cineangiograms. *Cathet Cardiovasc Diagn* 1985; **11**:521–31.
34. Wong W-H, Kirkeeide RL, Gould KL. Computer applications in angiography. *In:* Collins SM, Skorton DJ, eds. *Cardiac Imaging and Image Processing.* New York: McGraw-Hill, 1986; 206–38.
35. Alderman EL, Berte LE, Harrison DC, Sanders W. Quantitation of coronary artery dimensions using digital imaging processing. *In:* Brody WR, ed. *Digital Radiography.* SPIE 1982; **314**:273–8.
36. Kooijman CJ, Reiber JHC, Gerbrands JJ. *et al.* Computer-aided quantitation of the severity of coronary obstructions from single view cineangiograms. First IEEE Comp Soc Int Symp on Medical Imaging and Image Interpretation, IEEE Cat No 82 CH1804-4, 1982; 59–64.
37. LeFree M, Simon SB, Lewis RJ, Bates ER, Vogel RA. Digital radiographic coronary artery quantification. *Comput Cardiol* 1985; 99–102.
38. Selzer RH, Blankenhorn DH, Crawford DW, Brooks SH, Barndt R. Computer Analysis of Cardiovascular Imagery. Proceedings of the Caltech/JPL Conference on Image Processing Technology, Data Sources and Software for Commercial and Scientific Applications, Pasadena, 1976; 1–20.
39. Ledbetter DC, Selzer RH, Gordon RM, Blankenhorn DH, Sanmarco ME. Computer quantitation of coronary angiograms. *In:* Miller HA, Schmidt EV, Harrison DC, eds. *Noninvasive Cardiovascular Measurements,* SPIE 1978; **167**:17–20.
40. Siebes M, D'Argenio DZ, Selzer RH. Computer assessment of hemodynamic severity of coronary artery stenosis from angiograms. *Comput Methods Programs Biomed* 1985; **21**:143–52.
41. Parker DL, Pope DL, White KS, Tarbox LR, Marshall HW. Three-Dimensional Reconstruction of Vascular Beds. Proc Conf Inf Proces Med Imag, Georgetown, 1985; 415–30.
42. Parker DL, Pope DL, Van Bree R, Desai R. Three-dimensional reconstruction of vascular beds from digital angiographic projections. Int Workshop on Physics and Eng in Comput/Multi-dimensional Imag Processing, Newport Beach, 1986 (in press).
43. Barth K, Epple E, Irion KM, Faust U, Decker D. Quantifizierung von Stenosen der Herzkranzgefässe durch Digitale Bildauswertung. *Erg Bd Biomed Technik* 1981: 26.
44. Barth K, Faust U, Both A, Wedekind K. A critical examination of angiographic stenosis quantitation by digital image processing. First IEEE Comp Soc Int Symp on Medical Imaging and Image Interpretation, IEEE Cat No 82 CH1804-4, 1982; 71–6.
45. Kirkeeide RL, Fung P, Smalling RW, Gould KL. Automated evaluation of vessel diameter from arteriograms. *Comput Cardiol* 1982; 215–8.
46. Doriot PA. Non-linearity by densitometric measurements of coronary arteries. *In:* Heintzen PH, ed. *Progress in Digital Angiocardiography.* Dordrecht: Martinus Nijhoff Publishers, 1987 (in press).
47. Smith DN, Colfer H, Brymer JF, Pitt B, Kliman SH. A semiautomatic computer technique for processing coronary anoiograms. *Comput Cardiol* 1982; 325–8.
48. Beatt KJ, Luijten HE, Katen HJ ten, Reiber JHC, Serruys PW. Early regression and late progression of stenosis in the first four months following successful coronary angioplasty. *In:* Reiber JHC, Serruys PW, eds. *New Developments in Quantitative Coronary Arteriography.* Dordrecht: Martinus Nijhoff Publishers, 1988 (in press).
49. Reiber JHC, Slager CJ, Schuurbiers JCH, *et al.* Transfer functions of the X-ray-cine-video chain applied to digital processing of coronary cineangiograms. *In:* Heintzen PH, Brennecke R, eds. *Digital Imaging in Cardiovascular Radiology.* Stuttgart: Georg Thieme Verlag, 1983; 89–104.
50. Bürsch J, Johs R, Heintzen P. Validity of Lambert-Beer's law in roentgendensitometry of contrast material (Urografin) using continuous radiation. *In:* Heintzen PH, ed. *Roentgen-, Cine and Videodensitometry: Fundamentals and Applications for Blood Flow and Heart Volume Determinations.* Stuttgart: Georg Thieme Verlag, 1971; 81–4.
51. Heintzen P, Moldenhauer M. X-ray absorption by contrast material using pulsed radiation. *In:* Heintzen PH, ed. *Roentgen, Cine- and Videodensitometry: Fundamentals and Applications for Blood Flow and Heart Volume Determinations.* Stuttgart: Georg Thieme Verlag, 1971; 73–81.

52. Doriot P-A, Pochon Y, Rasoamanambelo L, Chatelain P, Welz R, Rutishauser W. Densitometry of coronary arteries—an improved physical model. *Comput Cardiol* 1985; 91–4.
53. Shaw CG, Ergun DI, Lysel MS van, *et al.* Quantitation techniques in digital subtraction video-angiography. *In:* Brody WR, ed. *Digital Radiography.* SPIE 1982; **314**:121–9.
54. Pfaff JM, Whiting JS, Eigler NE, Forrester JS. Increased accuracy of cross-sectional area calculations following correction for scatter and veiling glare. *In:* Reiber JHC, Serruys PW, eds. *New Developments in Quantitative Coronary Arteriography.* Dordrecht: Martinus Nijhoff Publishers, 1988 (in press).
55. Sandor T, Als AV, Paulin S. Cine-densitometric measurement of coronary arterial stenoses. *Cathet Cardiovasc Diagn* 1979; **5**:229–45.
56. Nichols AB, Gabrieli CFO, Fenoglio JJ, Esser PD. Quantification of relative coronary arterial stenosis by cine-videodensitometric analysis of coronary arteriograms. *Circulation* 1984; **69**:512–22.
57. Reiber JHC, Kooijman CJ, Slager CJ, Boer A den, Serruys PW. Improved densitometric assessment % area-stenosis from coronary cineangiograms. X World Congress of Cardiology, Washington, 1986; 39 (abstract).
58. Wiesel J, Grunwald AM, Tobiasz C, Robin B, Bodenheimer MM. Quantitation of absolute area of a coronary arterial stenosis: experimental validation with a preparation *in vivo. Circulation* 1986; **74**:1099–106.
59. Parker DL, Pope DL, Petersen JC, Clayton PD, Gustafson DE. Quantitation in cardiac video-densitometry. *Comput Cardiol* 1984; 119–22.
60. Herrington DM. Issues of validation in quantitative coronary angiography. *In:* Reiber JHC, Serruys PW, eds. *New Developments in Quantitative Coronary Arteriography.* Dordrecht. Martinus Nijhoff Publishers, 1988 (in press).
61. Block M, Bove AA, Ritman EL. Coronary angiographic examination with the dynamic spatial reconstructor. *Circulation* 1984; **70**:209–16.
62. Mancini CBJ, Simon SB, McGillem MJ, LeFree MT, Friedman HZ, Vogel RA. Automated quantitative coronary arteriography: morphologic and physiologic validation *in vivo* of a rapid digital angiographic method. *Circulation* 1987; **75**:452–60.
63. Reiber JHC, Serruys, PW, Mancini GBJ. Accuracy of coronary quantitation from cinefilm; *in-vivo* validation. Abstract submitted to AHA-scientific meeting, 1987.
64. Reiber JHC, Serruys PW, Kooijman CJ, *et al.* Assessment of short-, medium- and long-term variations in arterial dimensions from computer-assisted quantitation of coronary cineangiograms. *Circulation* 1985; **71**:280–8.

SUMMARY

There is an increasing demand for the objective and reproducible assessment of coronary arterial dimensions to study the efficacy of new recanalization techniques in the catheterization laboratory, to study new approaches to achieve regression or no-growth of coronary atherosclerosis, and also as a means for diagnostic and therapeutic decision-making during the cardiac catheterization procedure. This last application requires the use of digital cardiac imaging systems with the capability of storing the images on-line; at the present time, the other applications are usually evaluated off-line from 35mm cinefilm.

In this chapter an overview is presented on the different techniques that have been developed for the quantitative analysis of the size and shape of coronary arterial segments, and in particular of coronary obstructions. The first approaches have been directed towards the (semi)-automated boundary detection of the arterial segments and the subsequent computation of the relative and absolute length and width dimensions; more recent approaches have attempted to determine the cross-sectional narrowing of obstructions from a single angiographic view by densitometry. In general, the algorithms are applicable to both digitized cineframes and the on-line acquired digital images, possibly requiring slight modifications from the one medium to the other.

Finally, recommendations for the validation procedures of the techniques, as well as for standardized image acquisition and analysis, are provided.

RÉSUMÉ

Il y a une demande croissante d'évaluation objective et reproductible des dimensions coronariennes artérielles afin d'étudier l'efficacité des nouvelles techniques de recanalisation dans les laboratoire de cathétérisme, afin d'étudier les nouvelles approches permettant d'arriver à une régression ou à un arrêt de croissance de l'athérosclérose coronaire, et aussi comme moyen de décision dans le choix du diagnostique et de la thérapie au cours d'un cathétérisme cardiaque. Cette dernière application nécessite l'utilisation d'un appareil de systèmes d'images cardiaques digitales capable de stocker les images en direct; actuellement, les autres applications sont généralement évaluées indirectement sur des films de 35mm.

Dans ce chapitre on présentera une vue d'ensemble des différentes techniques développées pour l'analyse quantitative de la taille et de la forme des segments artériels coronaires et en particulier des obstructions coronaires. Les premières approches ont été dirigées vers la détection semi-automatique de délimitation des segments artériels et le calcul consécutif de la longueur et de la largeur relative et absolue; de plus récentes approches ont tenté de déterminer le rétrécissement en coupe des obstructions à partir d'une seule prise de vue angiographique, par densitométrie. En général, les algorithmes s'appliquent à la fois aux cadres codifiés en numérique et aux images digitales acquises de façon directe, exigeant parfois une légère modification lorsqu'on passe d'un milieu à un autre.

Pour terminer, on propose des recommandations pour les procédures de validation des techniques, ainsi que pour l'acquisition de l'image standardisée et l'analyse.

ZUSAMMENFASSUNG

Es existiert ein steigender Bedarf an objektiven und wiederholbaren Feststellungen der Dimensionen der Kranzarterien, um die Wirksamkeit der neuen Rekanalisationstechniken in dem Katheterisierungslabor zu studieren, und um neue Methoden zur Rückbildung oder "kein Wachsen" der koronaren Atherosklerose als Mittel zur diagnostischen und therapeutischen Entscheidungskraft während des kardialen Katheterisierungsverfahrens zu studieren. Diese letzte Anwendung benötigt den Gebrauch von digitalen kardialen Bildbearbeitungssystemen mit der Möglichkeit einer direkten Speicherung der Bilder; momentan werden die anderen Anwendungen normalerweise indirekt durch 35-mm Kinefilm ausgewertet.

In diesem Kapitel wird ein Überblick der verschiedenen Techniken vorgelegt, die für die Mengenbestimmung der Größe und Form der kranzarteriellen Segmente, und im besonderen der koronaren Verstopfungen entwickelt wurden. Die ersten Versuche sind auf die (halb) automatische Grenzlinien-Ermittlung der arteriellen Segmente und der folgenden Berechnung der relativen und absoluten Länge- und Breitedimensionen gerichtet; Methoden jüngeren Datums haben versucht, die Querschnittsverengung der Obstruktionen aus einer einzigen angiographischen Ansicht densitometrisch zu ermitteln. Im allgemeinen sind die Algorithmen sowohl auf digitalisierte Kinebilder als auch auf direkt erworbene digitale Bilder anwendbar, obwohl kleine Modifikationen von dem einem Medium zum anderen nötig sein können.

Zum Schluß sind Empfehlungen für die Verfahren zur Gültigkeitserklärungen der Techniken sowohl als auch für die standardisierte Erwerbung und Analyse von Bildern geliefert.

SOMMARIO

C'è una crescente richiesta per la valutazione oggettiva e riproducibile di dimensioni arteriali coronarie per studiare l'efficacia di nuove tecniche di ricanalizzazione nel laboratorio di cateterizzazione, lo studio di nuovi approcci per raggiungere regressione o almeno il non-progresso dell'aterosclerosi coronaria ed anche un metodo per arrivare alla diagnosi e alla decisione terapeutica durante il procedimento della cateterizzazione cardiaca. Quest'ultima applicazione richiede l'uso dei sistemi d'immagine cardiaca digitale con la capacità di memorizzare le immagini in linea; al momento le altre applicazioni sono solo valutate fuori-linea da un cinefilm di 35 mm. In questo capitolo verrà presentato un sommario delle varie tecniche che sono state sviluppate per le analisi quantitative delle misure e delle forme di sezioni arteriali coronarie, e in particolar modo delle ostruzioni coronarie. I primi approcci sono stati diretti verso le (semi) automizzate scoperte di limiti delle sezioni arteriali e della susseguente computazione delle dimensioni delle relative e assolute lunghezza e larghezza. Piú recentemente gli approcci han cercato di determinare la ristrettezza della sezione trasversale delle ostruzioni da una sola vista angiografica per densitometria. In generale, gli algoritmi sono applicabili sia per le digitizzate cine-cornici, sia per le acquistate immagini digitali e in-linea, richiedendo possibilmente delle piccole modifiche da un mezzo all'altro. Finalmente, vengono provviste delle raccomandazioni per il procedimento di convalida delle tecniche, come pure per l'acquisizione delle immagini standardizzate e delle analisi.

SUMÁRIO

Há uma procur cada vez maior para a avaliação objetiva e reproduzível das dimensões das artérias coronárias para estudar a eficácia de novas técnicas de recanalização no laboratório de cateterismo, para estudar novos métodos para conseguir a regressão ou nenhum-crescimento da aterosclerose coronária e também como um meio para a decisão diagnóstica e terapêutica durante o procedimento de cateterismo cardíaco. Esta última utilização requer o uso de sistemas digitais de imagens cardíacas com a capacidade de armazenar as imagens diretamente; atualmente, as outras utilizações são gèralmente avaliadas indiretamente com película de 35 mm.

Neste capítulo um sumário será apresentado sobre as técnicas diferentes que têm sido desenvolvidas para a análise quantitativa do tamanho e forma de segmentos arteriais coronários, e em particular de obstruções coronárias. As primeiras tentativas têm sido dirigidas à detecção semi-automática dos limites dos segmentos arteriais e o cálculo subseqüente das dimenções relativas e absolutas do comprimento e largura; tentativas mais recentes têm tëñtado calcular o estreitamento da secção transversāl de obstáculos com uma vista única angiográfica atrayés de densitômetria. Geralmente, os algoritmos são aplicáveis tanto às vistas cinematográficas digitalizadas como às imagens digitais obtidas diretamente, possivelmente precisando de modifições ligeiras dum méio para o outro.

Finalmente, as recomendações para os procedimentos de confirmação das técnicas, como também para a compra e análise de imagens estandardizadas são fornecidas.

RESUMEN

Cada vez hay una mayor demanda de evaluación objetiva y reproducible de las dimensiones de las arterias coronarias para estudiar la eficacia de nuevas técnicas de recanalización en el laboratorio de cateterización, con el fin de estudiar nuevos enfoques para obtener la regresión o detención de la expansión de la aterosclerosis coronaria y también como un medio para tomar decisiones diagnósticas y terapéuticas durante el procedimiento de cateterización cardíaca. Esta última aplicación requiere el uso de sistemas digitales de producción de imágenes cardiológicas, capaces de almacenar las imágenes directamente (en línea); en la actualidad las otras aplicaciones generalmente se evalúan indirectamente (fuera de línea) mediante películas de 35 mm.

Se presenta un panorama general de las diferentes técnicas que se han desarrollado para el análisis cuantitativo del tamaño y forma de los segmentos de las arterias coronarias, y en particular de obstrucciones coronarias. Los primeros enfoques se han dirigido hacia la detección (semi)automática de los límites entre segmentos arteriales y la consiguiente computación de las dimensiones absolutas y relativas del largo y-el ancho; un enfoque más reciente ha tratado de determinar el estrechamiento en sección transversal de las obstrucciones mediante una imagen angiográfica simple obtenida por densitometría. En general, los algoritmos pueden aplicarse tanto a las vistas cinematográficas digitalizadas como a las imágenes digitales obtenidas directamente, pero posiblemente se requiera una ligera modificación para cambiar de un medio a otro.

Finalmente, se proporcionan recomendaciones para los procedimientos de validación de las técnicas, así como para el análisis y la obtención de imágenes estándar.

The Role of Cholesterol in Atherosclerosis:
New Therapeutic Opportunities, edited by S. M. Grundy
and A. G. Bearn, Hanley & Belfus, Inc., Philadelphia.

Discussion

JULIAN: Dr. Reiber, you have been talking in terms of luminal diameter. Looked at from the point of view of myocardial infarction, we are more concerned about the constitution of the plaque. If we can convert all fatty plaques to fibrous plaques we might succeed in preventing infarction without affecting luminal diameter. Is there any way of looking at the constitution of plaques and their liability to rupture:

REIBER: Not that I know of by x-ray techniques, by which we can see only the lumen of the vessel that is still open. The plaque itself is not visible and therefore we cannot determine the type of plaque radiographically. Recently, high frequency intraoperative echocardiographic techniques have been developed by which the wall of the vessel can be imaged. Possibly, in the future, the content of the plaque may be determined by this approach.

POOLE-WILSON: I would like to comment on the methods of visual angiography, as I think Dr. Reiber is being a bit unfair to the radiologists. This particular technique is applied to proximal lesions. In the example you showed, there were two distal lesions and they would be very difficult to measure. If you have a 3 mm coronary artery, which has to be 80% occluded to affect flow, then the diameter of the artery will be down to about 0.4 mm; and the sensitivity is about 0.3 mm. The detection of a change in the size would be marginal.

REIBER: In the nifedipine trial, which we are now analyzing with Professor Lichtlen from Hannover, the entire coronary tree is quantitated in two angiographic projections, i.e., the distal, mid- and proximal segments are computer-processed. We can process vessels down to 0.7 mm–0.8 mm in size. We have performed phantom studies with diameters about 0.3 mm in size, but it is clear that imaging becomes impossible at such small sizes. Angiographically, only vessels with diameters of at least 0.5 mm in size are clearly visible. We are very close to measuring these small lesions with acceptable accuracy, so the technique is certainly not limited to the 2 or 3 mm obstructions in proximal vessels. Distal lesions can be quantitated, and it is generally agreed that a method should allow quantitation of vessel sizes of 0.5 mm and up with sufficient accuracy.

LEDINGHAM: Dr. Reiber, what do you feel about the last NHLBI publication on the rate of progress of coronary lesions in relation to treatment? It did not go into the complex computerized techniques that you have described. Were the conclusions acceptable in your view?

REIBER: I think if the changes in the size of the vessels are quite dramatic, then you can interpret such results visually with confidence. If, however, the expected changes in size are only of the order of a few tenths of a millimeter, you would need a very large number of patient studies to determine accurately by visual inspection whether any change has occurred or not. The quantitative techniques that I presented allow, in a limited group of patients, the assessment of small changes in size with sufficient accuracy. I believe that there is now a consensus in the cardiological community that intervention studies should be analyzed quantitatively with computer-based techniques.

JOHNSTON: Dr. Smith, the converse of the studies you cited on the degree of stenosis and the dramatic fall in blood flow is that, presumably, small regressions should lead to quite dramatic increases in blood flow. Do you think in the future it may be a very sensitive way of detecting changes in coronary luminal diameter by measuring changes in regional blood flow?

129

SMITH: I agree. It may not take a very dramatic macroscopic reduction in the degree of stenosis to improve clinical state. One hopes that the physiological information one can get from flow-imaging or other non-invasive tests such as exercise-tolerance testing may provide this important information.

REIBER: It is now possible to determine the coronary flow reserve from coronary angiograms by measuring the transit time of the contrast agent within the coronary vessels. From a coronary angiogram, therefore, you can now determine both the anatomy and the functional significance of stenoses; such approaches are now available for long-term studies.

NORRBY: Dr. Smith, when licensing a new lipid-lowering drug, do you think that one should request only that it lowers blood cholesterol, or should some documented evidence of clinical benefit be required?

SMITH: This is a difficult question. Asking pharmaceutical companies to fund large studies lasting long enough to provide clinical outcome data may not be realistic. But at the least one can and should ask for careful post-marketing surveillance studies to collect as much safety and efficacy data as possible.

LENFANT: It is interesting that the Federal Drug Administration (FDA) in the USA refused to approve the use of a tissue plasminogen activator because a beneficial effect on mortality had not been demonstrated. Many people thought this was not the purpose of the drug to start with. I think the question remains open.

DOLLERY: The WHO clofibrate trial, a multi-country, randomized, controlled trial with 15,000 patients, produced some alarming results. In the five-year-long trial, the total mortality in the treated group was higher after five years. They then continued follow-up but stopped treatment, and the total mortality in the treated group continued to diverge from that of the placebo group over the next five years. There was a small reduction in cholesterol (5 or 7%) and there was a small reduction in non-fatal myocardial infarction. The consistent increase in total mortality was very worrying.

JULIAN: The fact that the mortality was higher in treated than in untreated individuals would not have emerged if the clofibrate study had been smaller or less carefully conducted. Simply doing a post-marketing survey would not have shown up that evidence.

MONCLOA: We do have studies planned to attempt to answer the mortality question.

LEWIS: Could I express a little anxiety about attempts to draw conclusions on total mortality change from the published trials of lipid-lowering agents. The trials have been designed, and their statistical power has been worked out, in order to assess the change in coronary incidence and/or coronary mortality. To investigate rarer end-points, such as non-cardiovascular diseases, the trial would have to be considerably larger. Where there has been a gross change, as in the WHO clofibrate trial, clearly one must draw provisional conclusions, but I think it is dangerous to say, for example, that the cholestyramine study did or did not show a change in any disease other than coronary heart disease.

The Role of Cholesterol in Atherosclerosis:
New Therapeutic Opportunities, edited by S. M. Grundy
and A. G. Bearn, Hanley & Belfus, Inc., Philadelphia.

Physician Attitudes Toward Elevated Lipid Levels: An International Perspective

C. Boyd Clarke

The medical dimensions of the link between elevated levels of blood cholesterol and the increased risk of coronary artery disease have been described from a variety of perspectives. For example, the pathology, molecular biology, epidemiology and clinical manifestations of lipid-related disorders have been extensively discussed and debated, and the confluence of findings from these disciplines has served as the backbone of the now widely distributed "consensus" documents on the prevention of coronary disease.[1] The objective of this paper is to approach the issue of elevated blood cholesterol levels (and other lipid disorders) from a somewhat different perspective—how do practicing physicians perceive the problem of elevated cholesterol levels and how aggressive are they currently prepared to be in their approach to the problem.

THE "CONSENSUS" DOCUMENTS AND THE PREVALENCE OF CHOLESTEROL-RELATED DISEASES

The publication of the policy statement of the National Institutes of Health Consensus Development Conference represented a watershed in the treatment of cholesterol-related disorders.[2] From the perspective of the practicing clinician, perhaps two recommendations were central to the guidelines:

1. Americans over the age of 40 between the 75th percentile (240 mg/dl; 6.2 mmol/L) and 90th percentile (260 mg/dl; 6.7 mmol/L) of blood cholesterol levels were defined as being at "moderate risk." Consequently, they became candidates for dietary therapy to reduce their blood cholesterol.
2. Those in the upper decile of cholesterol values (over 260 mg/dl; 6.7 mmol/L) were defined as being at "high risk." The recommendation was that such people should be treated intensively by dietary means, under the supervision of a physician, and that if the response to the dietary prescription was inadequate, appropriate drugs should be added to the regimen.

The implication of such guidelines for clinicians in the United States was profound. Among the adult population, over 18 million Americans were classified as "high risk," becoming *potential* candidates for drug therapy, and many more were classified as moderate risk.

The implications of the NIH consensus document were at least as far-reaching in the European context. Shaper and Pocock noted that if the American consensus was implemented in Great Britian, approximately 49% of the British middle-aged male population would be intensively treated by diet, and an undetermined number by drug therapy.[4] Similarly, the PROCAM Study in Germany indicated that the upper decile of cholesterol values in the United States included 17.5% of their population.[5] However, when a Study Group of the European Atherosclerosis Society sought to develop a similar policy document, they argued that it was "not meaningful to regard a cholesterol level of, for example, 225 mg/dl (5.8 mmol/L) as normal in one country and pathological in another." Their policy document noted that there was no readily definable biological threshold over which intervention could be recommended, but nevertheless suggested that at levels in excess of 200 mg/dl (5.2 mmol/L), intervention could commence by giving nutritional advice and by correcting other risk factors if present, whereas at levels in excess of 250 mg/dl (6.5 mmol/L), a lipid-lowering diet should be commenced, and, if the response to diet was inadequate, cholesterol-reducing medications could be considered. A significant proportion of the European population was thus defined as potential candidates for drug therapy, and the limits of intervention were defined in a manner that was essentially consistent with that of the American consensus.

Given the essential harmony between recommendations to treat elevated serum cholesterol levels in both Europe and the United States, one can foresee two interlocking factors that might have an impact on the numbers of patients being diagnosed and treated for elevated blood lipid values within a particular country. First, the distribution of lipoprotein values within the population and presumably the prevalence of the coronary artery disease for which elevated cholesterol is a major risk factor would define in broad terms the potential "yield" of patients within the medical system. However, the "local medical culture" (e.g., the availability of and reimbursement for various medications, the attitudes of physicians toward preventive medicine generally, and toward cholesterol reduction specifically) would have a major impact on the extent to which the potential yield of patients predicted by the epidemiology and the consensus recommendations was actually realized. The remainder of this chapter addresses international variations in local medical cultures.

DIAGNOSIS AND TREATMENT OF HYPERLIPIDEMIA: A MULTI-NATIONAL COMPARISON

Diagnostic patterns for hyperlipidemia vary markedly from country to country and have no relationship to the known epidemiology of cholesterol-related disease. Table

I presents a multi-national comparison of the number of office visits in which hyperlipidemia was diagnosed or treated (with or without drugs) by the physician. When compared on the basis of annual visits per 100,000 population, it is clear that the countries divide into two tiers: in Northern Europe or North America such visits are relatively less frequent, and in Central or Southern Europe, physicians appear to be far more active in the diagnosis of and therapy for hyperlipidemia. This pattern is at variance with international patterns of ischemic heart disease mortality (Table II). In countries with high rates of mortality due to ischemic heart disease (i.e., Finland, the United Kingdom and the United States) the frequency with which physicians diagnose or treat hyperlipidemia is relatively low; in countries with relatively lower rates of mortality due to ischemic heart disease (i.e., Italy, France and Spain) the reverse is true. The prevalence of the disease therefore appears to have relatively little impact on the frequency of diagnosis and treatment of hyperlipidemia. Such comparisons of patient visits may be misleading. Such visits do not distinguish between diagnostic and return visits, so that the figures could simply reflect more intensive monitoring in treated patients in Southern Europe, perhaps related to the impact of the local medical and reimbursement system. Countries with medical systems that favor longer intervals between repeat visits and prescriptions then appear to be less active in the treatment of hyperlipidemia than countries favoring shorter intervals between repeat visits.

A comparison between physician activity in the treatment of hyperlipidemia and that involved in the treatment of hypertension then becomes instructive. As two of the major risk factors for coronary artery disease, hypertension and high cholesterol levels provide an interesting means to approach the current attitudes of physicians to the dimensions of preventive cardiology. Depending on the definition of what comprises ''high'' cholesterol or ''high'' blood pressure, the risk factors are not that dissimilar in terms of their prevalence or in terms of their predictive capacity for the future development of coronary artery disease.[3] Yet, throughout the world, the diagnosis and control of high blood pressure is a much more established part of the control of risk factors by physicians than is the control of elevated cholesterol.

TABLE I. *A multi-national comparison of office visits for hyperlipidemia (1986)**

Country	Annual office visits for hyperlipidemia (000's)	Visits per 100,000 of population
United Kingdom	452	800
Netherlands	133	900
Finland	63	1,300
United States	4,917	2,100
Germany	4,312	7,200
Portugal	814	8,600
Belgium	1,129	11,400
Italy	7,076	12,200
France	6,797	12,500
Spain	5,825	14,900

* Source: Merck & Co., Inc. (Rahway, N.J., U.S.A.) estimates based on IMS data.

TABLE II. *Hyperlipidemia and ischemic heart disease (IHD) mortality: A comparison of annual office visits per 100,000 of population (1986) and age-standardized mortality rate per 100,000 aged 40–69 (1980)*[7]

Country	Annual hyperlipidemia visits per 100,000 of population	IHD mortality per 100,000 of population
United Kingdom	800	482–630
Netherlands	900	323
Finland	1,300	599
United States	2,100	398
Germany	7,200	314
Belgium	11,400	264
Italy	12,200	212
France	12,500	137

Table III compares the annual number of visits per 1,000 population in which the physician either diagnoses or treats hyperlipidemia or diagnoses and treats hypertension. There is much less variability in international patterns of diagnosis and treatment of hypertension than there is in hyperlipidemia, suggesting an international consensus on therapy. Even in countries that appear to be relatively active in efforts to monitor and control hyperlipidemia, the level of such activity is still far lower than that predicted by their effort to control hypertension. Nevertheless the number of visits required remained greater in all South/Central European countries.

Such data say nothing about the intensity of the action the physician might take, including the prescription of a hypolipidemic medication. However, Table IV demonstrates that countries which have a low frequency of office visits for hyperlipidemia have a low frequency of prescription. Furthermore, compared to the willingness to prescribe a medication for hypertension, the willingness to prescribe drugs for

TABLE III. *A multi-national comparison of office visits for hypertension and hyperlipidemia (1986)**

Country	Hypertensive visits/1,000	Hyperlipidemic visits/1,000	Ratio of hypertensive to hyperlipidemic visits
United Kingdom	374	8	46
Holland	251	9	27
Finland	177	13	14
United States	292	21	14
Germany	375	72	5
Portugal	476	86	6
Belgium	400	114	3
Italy	536	112	4
France	486	125	4
Spain	401	149	3
Japan	1,463	466	3

* Source: Merck & Co., Inc. (Rahway, N.J., U.S.A.) estimates based on IMS data.

TABLE IV.   *The frequency of prescription for hyperlipidemia and hypertension (1986)**

Country	Ratio of hypertensive to hyperlipidemic prescriptions	Ratio of hypertensive to hyperlipidemic visits
United Kingdom	73	46
Netherlands	55	27
Finland	17	14
United States	29	14
Germany	5	5
Portugal	6	6
Belgium	4	3
Italy	4	4
France	6	4
Spain	3	3

* Source: Merck & Co., Inc. (Rahway, N.J., U.S.A.) estimates based on IMS data.

hyperlipidemia is very poorly developed in the United Kingdom, Finland, the Netherlands, and the United States.

PHYSICIAN ATTITUDES TOWARD THERAPY FOR HYPERLIPIDEMIA

The data presented suggest that physician concerns about hypercholestolemia as a cardiovascular risk factor are less highly developed than their concerns about elevated blood pressure. In addition, the data suggest that the therapeutic guidelines recommended in the various consensus documents represent a major educational challenge throughout the world, particularly in Northern Europe and North America. To amplify these findings Merck & Co., Inc. (Rahway, N.J., U.S.A.) has performed a series of surveys of the attitudes of physicians toward hypercholesterolemia.

Surveys conducted among representative samples of physicians in 1986 sought to determine the level at which various therapies for hypercholesterolemia were implemented (Table V).

The geographical distinctions seen previously in the more objective measures of actual prescribing habits and the frequency of office visits were less obvious. When physicians in the United States were asked to describe their therapeutic thresholds, the levels were more aggressive than might be predicted from their prescribing patterns. Table V demonstrates that physicians in "Northern" Europe (the United Kingdom, Finland and Norway) have therapeutic thresholds that are far higher than those generally in Southern or Central Europe (e.g., Spain, Italy and Germany). In addition there is a striking contrast between the stated mean therapeutic levels and the various consensus documents. If, as the European Policy Document recommends, physicians need to consider aggressive intervention to reduce serum cholesterol at levels over 250 mg/dl (6.5 mmol/L), it would seem there is an enormous educational task that needs addressing, even in those countries where physicians have demonstrated the greatest propensity to treat elevated cholesterol.

TABLE V. *Mean therapeutic thresholds for elevated serum cholesterol levels by country**

Country	Number of MD's	Commence dietary therapy[†]	Commence drug therapy[†]
United States (card.)	100	232	277
United States (GP)	100	241	294
United Kingdom	100	275	331
Finland (hosp.)	50	318	348
Norway (hosp.)	54	318	396
Germany (GP)	100	249	283
Spain (GP)	100	253	282
Argentina (GP)	102	257	281
Brazil (GP)	100	262	322
France (GP)	100	280	314
Belgium (GP)	79	263	313
Italy	100	267	291

* Source: Merck & Co., Inc. (Rahway, N.J., U.S.A.) surveys.
† 250 mg/dl = 6.5 mmol/L serum cholesterol.

Where, for example, Scandinavian physicians do not commence even dietary therapy until levels of cholesterol reach 320 mg/dl (8.3 mmol/L), the recommendations of the European Policy Document seem far distant.

The stated intervention levels in the surveys described may underestimate the extent of the task, because the describing of an intervention level is much easier than actually monitoring and treating the patient. In order to determine what physicians actually did in the diagnosis and treatment of hypercholesterolemia, a representative sample of physicians was asked to keep a diary on patients whose serum cholesterol levels were known to the physician. The basic instructions were that any time the physician consciously measured the cholesterol of a patient during a week, he or she was asked to record the actions taken thereafter. Data from five countries are presented in Table VI. It is curious that the mean values of intervention (except Norway), be they diet or drug, did not differ greatly from country to country, but in all countries the levels used as indicators are far in excess of the levels suggested by the various consensus documents. In both the United Kingdom and Norway a significant minority (15–21%) of patients were not treated by the phy-

TABLE VI. *International intervention levels: Results of one-week diary studies**

Country	Number of MD's	Patients screened weekly per MD	% patients no action (mean choles. value)	% patients dietary advice (mean value)	% patients drug added (mean value)
Norway (hosp.)	54	1.5	21 (251)	56 (373)	223 (464)
United Kingdom (GP)	100	1.3	15 (262)	62 (296)	23 (328)
Germany (GP)	100	9.5	5 (265)	41 (285)	52 (321)
Italy (GP)	100	7.1	4 (227)	35 (278)	61 (328)
Spain (GP)	100	7.3	4 (272)	33 (274)	63 (317)

* 250 mg/dl = 6.5 mmol/L serum cholesterol.

sician, although their cholesterol levels exceeded the guideline for "aggressive intervention." Finally, and perhaps most significantly, although the patterns of cholesterol intervention were not particularly different from country to country, the vigor with which physicians were willing to screen varied markedly. Slightly more than one patient per week was screened in the United Kingdom and Norway, whereas 7 to 10 were screened in Germany, Spain and Italy.

TRENDS IN THE TREATMENT OF HYPERCHOLESTEROLEMIA

Although there may be a gap between consensus levels for treatment and current actions, this does not tell us the extent to which attitudes might be changing. The publication in 1984 of the landmark Lipid Research Clinics Coronary Primary Prevention Trial (LRC-CPPT)[4] and the release of the NIH Consensus Guidelines provide both a rationale and the reference point for a more aggressive approach to hypercholesterolemia. There are two ways in which the response of physicians' attitudes to the momentum generated by these events may be measured. Table VII provides a measure of the attitudes of physicians toward treatment of elevated serum cholesterol levels. In most countries, and particularly in the United States, pre-scribing increased. Sequential attudinal surveys conducted in the United States (Table VIII) show that, since 1984, both general practitioners and cardiologists have lowered their therapeutic thresholds, although the levels remain higher than those suggested by the consensus documents.

CONCLUSIONS

A variety of data sources describe the international attitudes of physicians toward hyperlipidemia generally and hypercholesterolemia specifically. Physicians in Northern Europe and North America appear to be relatively less aggressive in their treatment of and screening for high blood cholesterol than their counterparts elsewhere in Europe. In all areas of Western Europe and North America, the levels of elevated cholesterol being treated by diet or drugs are considerably in excess of those sug-

TABLE VII.   *Global trends in total prescriptions for hyperlipidemia (000's)**

Country	1981	1982	1983	1984	1985	1986	Growth rate 86/81	Growth rate 86/83
United Kingdom	280	229	204	209	238	235	− 3%	+ 5%
United States	2569	2429	2411	2667	3199	4181	+ 10%	+ 20%
Holland	75	66	53	64	69	64	− 3%	+ 7%
France	5510	5254	5324	6045	6204	7632	+ 7%	+ 13%
Germany	3543	3660	3696	3634	3622	3903	+ 2%	+ 2%
Italy	6210	5595	5609	5890	6417	7146	+ 3%	+ 8%
Spain	2715	2686	2642	2607	2806	3089	+ 2%	+ 5%

* Source: IMS.

TABLE VIII. *Physician attitudes and behavior trends in drug intervention (United States)**

	mg/dl	
	Generalists	Cardiologists
1984	327	320
1985	323	292
1986	294	277

* Source: Merck & Co., Inc. (Rahway, N.J., U.S.A.) estimates based on IMS data.

gested by either the NIH Consensus Development Conference or the European Atherosclerosis Society. In spite of the magnitude of the educational challenge represented by the dissonance between existing physician attitudes and the recommendations of the consensus groups, there is some evidence that the trend is toward a more aggressive therapeutic resolve by physicians.

REFERENCES

1. See Consensus Conference: Lowering blood cholesterol to prevent heart disease. *JAMA* 1985; **253**:2080–2086. Also Study Group, European Atherosclerosis Society: Strategies for the prevention of coronary heart disease: A policy statement of the European Atherosclerosis Society. *Eur Heart J* 1987; **8**:77–88. A somewhat more conservative but directionally similar document may be found in *Report of the British Cardiac Society Working Group on Coronary Disease Prevention* (1987).
2. Consensus Conference: Lowering blood cholesterol to prevent heart disease. *JAMA* 1985; **253**:2080–2056.
3. See for example Oliver MF, Consensus or nonsensus conferences on coronary heart disease. *Lancet* 1985; 1087–1089. Also, Olsen RE, Mass intervention vs. screening and selective intervention for the prevention of coronary heart disease. *JAMA* 1986; **255**:2204–2207.
4. Shaper and Pocock. Blood cholesterol and the American consensus (correspondence). *Br Med J* 1985; 480–481.
5. Assmann G, Schulte G. *Prospective Cardiovascular Munster Trial (PROCAM)*. Zurich: Panscienta Verlag, 1987, 10.
6. Study Group, European Atherosclerosis Society, *op. cit.*, p. 81.
7. Simon L. Interrelations of lipids and lipoproteins with coronary artery disease mortality in 19 countries. *Am J Cardiol* 1986; **57**:5G–10G.
8. Danben TR. *The Framingham Study: The Epidemiology of Atherosclerotic Disease*. London: Harvard University Press, 1980, 91–120, 121–141. See also Assmann and Schulte, *op. cit.*, pp. 10ff.
9. Lipid Research Clinics Program. The Lipid Research Clinics Coronary Primary Prevention Trial Results. *JAMA* 1984; **251**:351–361.

SUMMARY

This paper considers the issue of elevated blood cholesterol levels from the viewpoint of the practicing physician. How do they perceive the problem of elevated cholesterol levels and how aggressive are they in their approach to the problem? A variety of data sources are examined, including the policy statement of the National Institute of Health Consensus Development Conference. Through an international comparison of the diagnosis and treatment of hypercholesterolemia, geographical differences emerge. For example, physicians in Northern Europe and North America appear to be less aggressive in their treatment of and screening for high blood cholesterol than their counterparts elsewhere in Europe. It was also noted that in all areas of Western Europe and North America the blood cholesterol levels at which diet or drug therapy is being implemented are considerably higher than those suggested by either the NIH Consensus Development Conference or the European Atherosclerosis Society. Despite the disparity between the present attitudes of physicians and the recommendations of the consensus groups, there is evidence, particularly in the United States, of a trend towards a more aggressive therapeutic resolve on the part of the physicians.

RÉSUMÉ

Cet article examine le point de vue des médecins traitants sur les problèmes de niveaux élevés de cholestérol dans le sang. Comment les médecins perçoivent-ils le problème des taux élevés de cholestérol? Abordent-ils le problème de façon agressive? De nombreuses sources de données sont étudiées y compris les recommandations du Rapport de la Conférence de Consensus des Instituts Nationaux de la Santé (NIH). Lorsque l'on compare les diagnostics et les traitements de l'hypercholestérolémie à l'échelle nationale, on note de profondes différences géographiques. Il semble, par exemple, que les médecins d'Europe du Nord et d'Amérique du Nord traitent moins agressivement leurs patients et soient moins stricts avec eux que leurs confrères d'autres pays d'Europe. On a aussi remarqué que dans toutes les régions de l'Europe de l'Ouest et de l'Amérique du Nord les niveaux de cholestérol des patients soumis à un traitement thérapeutique ou à un régime alimentaire étaient beaucoup plus élevés que ceux suggérés soit par la Conférence de Consensus des Instituts Nationaux de la Santé (NIH) soit par la Société Européenne d'Athérosclérose. En dépit de la grande différence d'écart qui existe entre les attitudes actuelles des médecins et les recommandations de ces deux groupes, il y a une tendance manifeste chez les médecins, en particulier aux Etats-Unis, à vouloir traiter les patients de façon plus agressive.

Pour terminer, on propose des recommandations pour les procédures de validation des techniques, ainsi que pour l'acquisition de l'image standardisée et l'analyse.

ZUSAMMENFASSUNG

Dieser Vortrag zieht das Problem des erhöhten Blut-Cholesterin-Spiegels vom Standpunkt des praktisierenden Arztes in Betracht. Wie verstehen sie das Problem von erhöhten Cholesterin-Spiegeln und wie aggressiv sind sie in der Handhabung dieses Problems? Eine Reihe von Datenquellen sind untersucht, einschließlich der Verfahrensdarlegung der Übereinstimmungschaffenden Konferenz der Nationalen Gesundheitsinstitute. Durch internationale Vergleiche der Diagnose und Behandlung von Hypercholesterinämie tauchen geographische Unterschiede auf. Zum Beispiel scheinen Ärzte in Nordeuropa und Nordamerika weniger aggressiv in ihrer Behandlung und Assuchen des hohen Blut-Cholesterins als ihre Kollegen anderswo in Europa zu sein. Es wurde auch bemerkt, daß in allen Gegenden Westeuropas und Nordamerikas die Blut-Cholesterin-Spiegel, bei denen Diät oder Drogen-Therapie eingesetzt wird, erheblich höher sind als jene empfohlen von entweder der Übereinstimmungschaffenden Konferenz der NIH oder der. Europäischen Atherosklerose-Gesellschaft. Trotz der Verschiedenheit zwischen den derzeitigen Einstellungen der Ärzte und den Empfehlungen der Übereinstimmungsgruppen, gibt es Beweise, besonders in den Vereinigten Staaten, einer Tendenz in Richtung auf eine aggressivere therapeutische Entschlossenheit von seiten der Ärzte.

SOMMARIO

Questo saggio discute il problema degli alti livelli del colesterolo nel sangue dal punto di vista di un medico che esercita la professione. Come vedono il problema degli alti livelli del colesterolo e in che modo riescono ad affrontare il problema? Una varietà di dati vengono esaminati, incluso l'esposizione di prassi dalla Conferenza di consenso promossa dall'Istituto Nazionale di Sanità. Attraverso un paragone internazionale delle diagnosi e delle cure per ipercolesterolemia, sorgono diversità geografiche. Per esempio i medici dell'America del Nord e dell'Europa del Nord sembrano meno aggressivi nelle loro cure ed esaminazioni per l'alto colesterolo nel sangue che i medici in altre parti d'Europa. È stato inoltre notato che in tutte le zone dell'Europa occidentale e dell'America del Nord i livelli del colesterolo nel sangue, per cui una terapia di droga o di dieta viene iniziata, sono considerabilmente piú alti di quelli suggeriti dalla INS Conferenza di Consenso o dalla Società Europea dell'Aterosclerosi. Nonostante la disparità fra gli attegiamenti attuali dei medici e la raccomandazioni dei gruppi di consenso c'è evidenza, particolarmente negli Stati Uniti, di una tendenza verso una terapia piú aggressiva da parte dei medici.

SUMÁRIO

Este papel consídera o assunto do nìveis elevados de colésterol no sangue do ponto de vista do médico praticante. Como é que êles encaram o problema do níveis elevados de colésterol e quão agressivos são êles no seu modo de tratar o problema? Uma variedade de fontes de informação são examinadas, incluindo a declaração de política da Conferência do Instituto Nacional para o Desenvolvimento dum Consenso de Saúde. Através duma comparação internacional da diagnose e do tratamento de hipercolesterolémia, diferenças geográficas emergem. Por exemplo, os médicos no Norte da Europa e na América do Norte aparecem ser menos agressivos no seu tratamento e na sua examinação para níveis elevados de colésterol no sangue do que os seus colegas nas outras partes da Europa. Foi também notado que em todas áreas do Oeste da Europa e da América do Norte, os níveis de colésterol no sangue aos quais um regime alimentar ou uma terapia farmacológica é executada são muito mais altos do que aquêles sugeridos pela Conferência *NIH* para o Desenvolvimento dum Consenso ou pela Sociedade de Aterosclerose da Europa. A pesar da disparidade entre as atitudes atuais dos médicos e as recomendações dos grupos de consenso, há uma evidência, especialmente nos Estados Unidos, duma tendência para uma determinação terapêutica mais agressiva da parte dos médicos.

RESUMEN

Se considera el tema de los niveles séricos elevados de colesterol desde el punto de vista del médico practico. ¿Cómo perciben ellos este problema y cuán vigorosas son sus estrategias para resolverlo? Se examinan datos procedentos de diversas fuentas, incluyendo la declaración de principios de la Conferencia Pro-consenso del National Institutes of Health—NIH— (Institutos Nacionales de Salud). Al hacer una comparación internacional del diagnóstico y tratamiento de la hipercolesterolemia emergen diferencias geográficas. Por ejemplo, los médicos de Norteamérica y del norte de Europa aparentemente emplean un enfoque menos vigoroso en el tratamiento y la identificación de los niveles séricos elevados de colesterol que los médicos del resto de Europa. También sobresale el hecho que en todas las áreas de Europa Occidental y Norteamérica los niveles séricos de colesterol a los que se empieza un tratamiento dietético o farmacológico son mucho más elevados que aquéllos sugeridos por la Conferencia Pro-consenso del NIH o la Sociedad Europea de Aterosclerosis. A pesar de la disparidad observada entre las actitudes actuales de los médicos y las recomendaciones de los grupos de consenso, existen evidencias, particularmente en los Estados Unidos, de una tendencia a un enfoque terapéutico más agresivo por parte de los médicos.

The Role of Cholesterol in Atherosclerosis:
New Therapeutic Opportunities, edited by S. M. Grundy
and A. G. Bearn, Hanley & Belfus, Inc., Philadelphia.

Coronary Heart Disease: Differences in the Occurrence Between Populations and Changing Trends Within Populations; Relationship to Serum Cholesterol Levels

Kalevi Pyörälä

It has long been known on the basis of international mortality statistics that there are striking differences in coronary heart disease (CHD) mortality between countries. Until the 1970s, CHD mortality appeared to be increasing in a number of "Western" countries. During the last 15 years, however, CHD mortality has markedly declined in several countries; at the same time some other countries have experienced a rise or no change. Great differences in CHD rates between populations and marked changes in these rates over relatively short periods of time indicate that the occurrence of CHD must be strongly influenced by environmental factors related to lifestyle.

Diet and its influence on blood lipids are known to have a central role among the factors contributing to the mass occurrence of CHD in populations. Differences between populations in the mean levels of serum total cholesterol—mainly reflecting low density lipoprotein (LDL) cholesterol levels—are determined by differences in the habitual diets of populations, and the dietary determinants of serum cholesterol include the intake of total and saturated fat, the ratio between polyunsaturated, monounsaturated and saturated fats, and the intake of cholesterol, fiber, and complex carbohydrates.

This review first examines the magnitude of differences between populations in the occurrence of CHD and recent international trends in CHD rates. The data available concerning interpopulation correlations between serum cholesterol and the occurrence of CHD will then be summarized. Some examples will be mentioned indicating that differences in the levels of other CHD risk factors may importantly modify the impact of serum cholesterol levels on the occurrence of CHD in populations. Scarce data available concerning time trends in population mean levels for serum cholesterol in relation to time trends in CHD rates within populations will be briefly discussed.

143

DIFFERENCES IN CHD RATES BETWEEN POPULATIONS AND CHANGES IN THESE RATES WITHIN POPULATIONS

The rank order of countries in the international CHD mortality statistics has undergone changes due to differences between countries in CHD mortality trends. Finland was long the leading country in the international CHD mortality statistics for middle-aged men, but due to a decline in CHD mortality in Finland it is now in third place, Northern Ireland and Scotland having the highest male CHD mortality rates (Fig. 1).[1,2] Male CHD mortality rates in the three leading countries—Northern

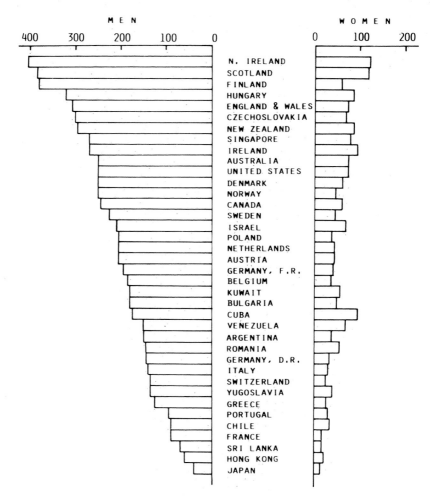

FIG. 1. Age standardized CHD mortality rates for men and women aged 35–64 in 38 countries in 1980–1982 (based on data obtained from WHO;[1] Pyörälä,[2] with permission).

Ireland, Scotland and Finland—are about five times higher than male CHD mortality rates in some southern European countries, such as Portugal and France, and about ten times higher than male CHD mortality rate in Japan. Differences between populations in female CHD mortality rates are of similar magnitude to those for men and, as for men, Northern Ireland and Scotland show the highest CHD mortality rates for women. Finnish women have a more favorable position in these international comparisons, being in fifteenth place.

A myocardial infarction register study, carried out in 1971 in 21 towns from 16 countries under the coordination of the World Health Organization,[3] confirmed that the official international mortality statistics had given a true picture of the magnitude of differences between populations in the occurrence of CHD, and this study also showed that differences between the study populations in the incidence of acute myocardial infarction paralleled national CHD mortality rates. Likewise, the Seven Countries Study,[4,5] a prospective study of 16 cohorts of middle-aged men in seven countries, demonstrated marked differences between study cohorts in CHD mortality and in the incidence of non-fatal CHD events. As shown in Table I, the differences between study cohorts in CHD mortality were actually much larger than those shown by international mortality statistics given for whole countries. Thus, men living in East Finland, having the highest CHD mortality rate among the study cohorts, had a 20–30 times higher CHD mortality rate than men living in Velika Krsna, Yugoslavia, or in Crete, Greece. This amplification of differences between populations in CHD mortality rates is due to the existence of marked regional differences in CHD mortality within some countries, including Finland, Yugoslavia and Greece. East Finland men showed a 1.6-times higher CHD mortality rate than West Finland men, in accordance with regional mortality statistics and findings from other prospective population studies carried out in Finland.[6,7] Regional dif-

TABLE I. *Seven Countries Study: Deaths from coronary heart disease in 15 years in 15 cohorts of men aged 40–59 at entry; age-standardized rates per 10,000 (Keys et al.[5])*

Cohort	Rate
East Finland	1202
U.S. Railroad	773
West Finland	741
Zutphen, Netherlands	637
Rome Railroad, Italy	516
Montegiorgio, Italy	447
Crevalcore, Italy	425
Slavonia, Yugoslavia	389
Zrenjanin, Yugoslavia	298
Dalmatia, Yugoslavia	216
Corfu, Greece	202
Tanushimaru, Japan	144
Ushibuka, Japan	128
Velika Krsna, Yugoslavia	67
Crete, Greece	38

ferences in the occurrence of CHD are also known to exist in some other European countries[8] and in the United States.[9]

A declining trend in CHD mortality started in the United States around 1970 or a little earlier.[10,11] About the same time a declining CHD mortality became evident in a number of other countries, although in most instances this was of a lesser degree than that occurring in the United States. In most of the remaining countries CHD mortality either was still increasing or showed no change.[12,13] Figures 2 and 3 show the percentage change in age-standardized CHD mortality rates for middle-aged men and women in 26 countries during a 10-year period from the beginning of the 1970s until the beginning of the 1980s.[14] The United States and Australia showed the most marked decreases in both male and female CHD mortality. It is worth noting that declining CHD mortality trends were not confined to countries with exceptionally high CHD mortality rates; substantial decreases also occurred in several countries in the middle of the rank order of the international CHD mortality

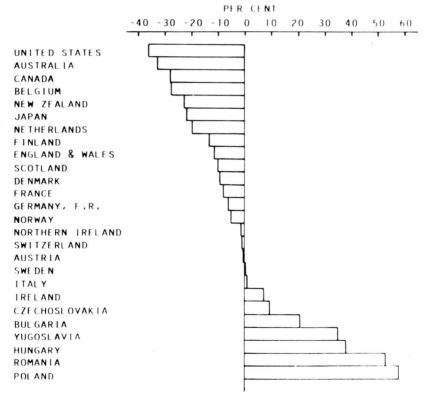

FIG. 2. Percentage change in age-standardized CHD mortality rate in men aged 40–69 in 26 countries during a 10-year period from 1970–1973 until 1980–1983 (based on data from Uemura and Pisa,[14] with permission).

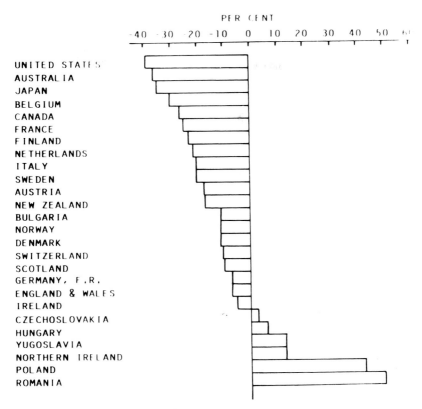

FIG. 3. Percentage change in age-standardized CHD mortality rate in women aged 40–69 in 26 countries during a 10-year period from 1970–1973 until 1980–1983 (based on data from Uemura and Pisa,[14] with permission).

statistics, such as Belgium and the Netherlands, and also in some countries with initially low CHD mortality rates, for example France and Japan. At the same time, a marked increase in CHD mortality occurred in several countries, whereas in a few countries very little change took place. It is of interest that in most of the countries showing declining CHD mortality trends, the decline was somewhat greater in women than in men and, similarly, in the countries showing increasing CHD mortality trends, the increase in women was, with few exceptions, less marked than in men or there was no increasing CHD trend in women.

Very few data are so far available concerning time trends in the incidence of non-fatal CHD events in countries showing changing trends in CHD mortality. Some data, however, have been published from the United States[15,16] and Finland[7,17,18] indicating that decreases in hospitalization rates for an acute myocardial infarction accompany the decline in CHD mortality rate in these countries.

Information about time trends in CHD mortality from countries showing regional differences in CHD rates is scarce. In Finland, the decline in CHD mortality began at the end of the 1960s in the central, eastern, and northern parts of the country with the highest CHD mortality rates, and in the western and southern parts with the lowest CHD mortality rates, the percentage decline until the beginning of the 1980s being almost similar in all parts of the country.[7] Thus, the regional differences in the occurrence of CHD within Finland have so far remained unchanged.

In many industrialized countries, in addition to regional differences in CHD mortality there are marked differences in CHD mortality rates between social classes, low social classes nowadays usually having the highest rates. Time trends in CHD mortality rates may show differences between social classes, as indicated in a recent report from Great Britain by Marmot and McDowall[19] demonstrating that in both sexes CHD mortality rates were declining among people in non-manual occupations, but remained unchanged among people in manual occupations; thus, the difference between social classes in CHD mortality actually increased.

INTERPOPULATION CORRELATIONS BETWEEN SERUM CHOLESTEROL LEVELS AND THE OCCURRENCE OF CHD

In the Seven Countries Study[4,5] all the methods, including biochemical methods for serum cholesterol determination, were carefully standardized. At the baseline examination a strong relationship was observed between the amount and proportions of saturated and polyunsaturated dietary fats in the habitual diets of the 16 study cohorts and their median serum cholesterol levels.[4] The population median of the serum total cholesterol levels at the baseline examination ranged from about 160 mg/dl (4.1 mmol/L) to above 250 mg/dl (6.5 mmol/L). As shown in Figure 4, a strong positive relationship was observed between the population median serum total cholesterol and 10-year CHD mortality ($r = 0.80$). The relationship between the population median serum total cholesterol level and the 10-year incidence of "hard" CHD (a definite myocardial infarction or CHD death) was essentially similar.

Rose[20] has used the Seven Countries Study data for the assessment of the issue of the "incubation period" of the CHD, i.e., the interval between the exposure of a population to a high serum cholesterol level and the occurrence of its clinical effects. As shown in Figure 5, the correlation between the mean serum cholesterol levels at the start of the study and the contemporary national mortality rates was strong ($r = 0.86$), but the USA rate was too high and the Greece rate too low. Over the next 15 years those deviating from the mean came progressively into line, and ultimately the original mean serum cholesterol levels gave an almost perfect prediction of the national CHD mortality 15 years later ($r = 0.96$).

Knuiman *et al.*[21,22] studied serum total cholesterol levels by carefully standardized methods in 26 schoolboy populations aged 7–8 years and in 14 adult male populations (age groups 33–38 years and 43–48 years) in 13 countries. There was a

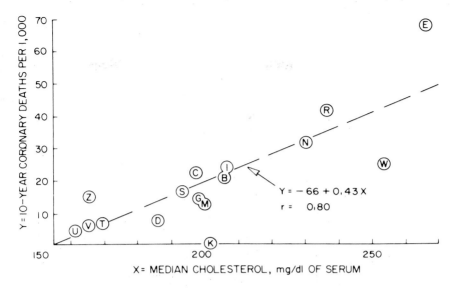

FIG. 4. The relationship of the median serum total cholesterol level to 10-year CHD mortality in the 16 male cohorts of the Seven Countries Study (Keys,[4] with permission). B = Belgrade; C = Crevalcore; D = Dalmatia; E = East Finland; G = Corfu; I = Italian Railroad; K = Crete; M = Montegiorgio; N = Zutphen; R = American Railroad; S = Slavonia; T = Tanushimaru; U = Ushibuka; V = Velika Krsna; W = West Finland; Z = Zrenjanin.

wide range in the population mean serum total cholesterol levels both among the schoolboy and adult male populations. Mean serum total cholesterol levels for adult men were low in populations from Africa (116–166 mg/dl; 3.0–4.3 mmol/L), intermediate in populations from Pakistan, the Philippines, Surinam, Hungary, Poland and the Mediterranean countries (170–213 mg/dl; 4.4–5.5 mmol/L), and high in populations from the Netherlands and Finland (217–248 mg/dl; 5.6–6.4 mmol/L). There was also about a twofold range in the population mean HDL cholesterol levels both among the schoolboy and adult male populations. Mean serum HDL cholesterol levels for adult men tended to be lower in populations from Africa, Asia and Surinam (27–50 mg/dl; 0.7–1.3 mmol/L) than in populations from Europe (43–58 mg/dl; 1.1–1.5 mmol/L). A strong positive correlation between population mean levels for serum total cholesterol and HDL cholesterol was observed both in schoolboys (r = 0.90) and adult men (r = 0.57–0.64). Knuiman et al.[22] calculated correlations between the mean serum total and HDL cholesterol levels in eight populations and corresponding national CHD mortality rates. A strong positive correlation was observed between serum total cholesterol and CHD mortality (r = 0.86), and the correlation between serum HDL cholesterol and CHD mortality was also positive (r = 0.57).

Simons[23] analyzed correlations between population mean levels for serum lipids and lipoproteins and corresponding national CHD mortality rates, and used for these

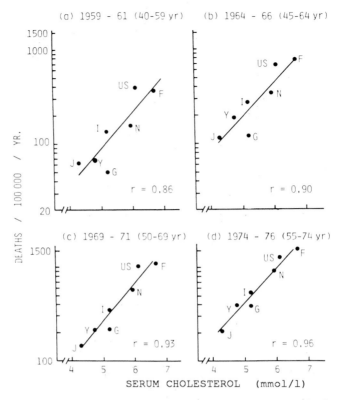

FIG. 5.   The relationship of the mean entry values for serum cholesterol in the Seven Countries Study national cohorts to corresponding national CHD mortality rates (a) at the time of the initial examination, (b) 5 years later, (c) 10 years later, and (d) 15 years later (Rose,[19] with permission). G = Greece; F = Finland; I = Italy; J = Japan; N = The Netherlands; US = United States; Y = Yugoslavia.

analyses serum lipid and lipoprotein data obtained from investigators in 19 of the 27 countries included in the report on cardiovascular mortality trends by Uemura and Pisa.[14] These data on serum lipids and lipoproteins were based on different types of population studies carried out in the 1970s, and the study populations were not necessarily representative of the whole nation. Furthermore, diverse biochemical methods had been used by different centers for serum lipid and lipoprotein measurements, and there had been no standardization and comparison of the levels of measurements between the centers. National CHD mortality data for the year 1980 were used in these analyses, and the data were age-standardized within the 40–64-year age group. As shown in Figure 6, population mean levels for serum total cholesterol ranged from about 200 mg/dl to about 270 mg/dl (5.2–7.0 mmol/L), and there was a strong positive correlation between the mean serum total cholesterol level and CHD mortality in men ($r = 0.67$; $p < 0.001$), whereas no statistically

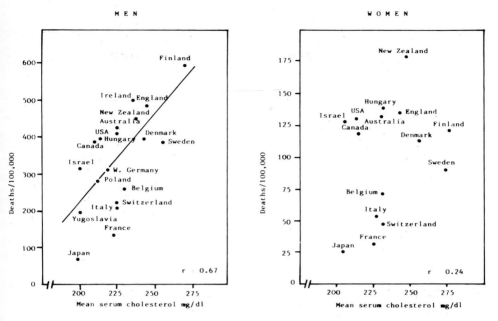

FIG. 6. The relationship of the mean serum total cholesterol to CHD mortality in men in 19 countries and in women in 15 countries (Simons,[23] with permission).

significant correlation between the mean serum total cholesterol and CHD mortality was observed in women. Serum HDL cholesterol data were available for men from 14 countries and for women from 11 countries. Population mean levels for serum HDL cholesterol ranged from 40 mg/dl to 55 mg/dl (1–1.4 mmol/L) in men and from 50 mg/dl to 65 mg/dl in women (1.3–1.7 mmol/L) (Fig. 7). There was an inverse correlation between the mean serum HDL cholesterol and CHD mortality in men ($r = -0.57$; $p < 0.02$), but no statistically significant correlation between the mean serum HDL cholesterol and CHD mortality was observed in women. As shown in Figure 8, the mean serum total cholesterol/HDL cholesterol ratio showed a strong positive correlation to CHD mortality in both sexes (mean: $r = 0.74$, $p < 0.002$; women: $r = 0.56$, $p < 0.04$). The mean serum triglyceride level did not show any correlation to CHD mortality both in men and women.

Kesteloot et al.[24] analyzed interpopulation correlations between serum total cholesterol and all causes and CHD mortality within Belgium, using as a starting point a study on serum lipids and lipoproteins in candidates for the military officers' academy of the Belgian army. The study comprised 1319 men from different Belgian provinces with a mean age of 20 years. Men from the four northern Dutch-speaking provinces—Limburg, Oost-Vlaanderen, Antwerpen and West-Vlaanderen—showed lower mean serum total cholesterol levels (184–190 mg/dl; 4.7–4.9 mmol/L) than men from the four southern French-speaking provinces (191–203 mg/dl; 5.0–5.2

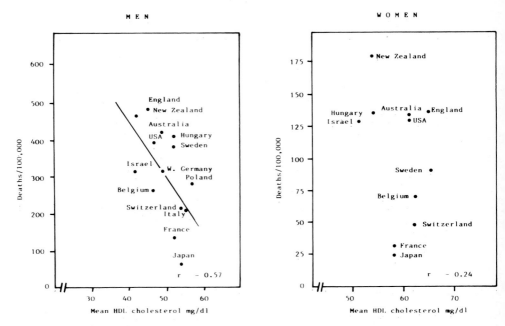

FIG. 7. The relationship of the mean serum HDL cholesterol level to CHD mortality in men in 14 countries and in women in 11 countries (Simons,[23] with permission).

mmol/L). Men from the bilingual province of Brabant, which includes the capital city Brussels, had a mean serum cholesterol level of 186 mg/dl (4.8 mmol/L), resembling those for men from the northern Dutch-speaking provinces. As to the mean levels for HDL cholesterol, there were no significant differences between men from Dutch-speaking and French-speaking provinces (Kesteloot, personal communication).

There are substantial regional differences within Belgium in butter and saturated fat consumption, and these differences correlate with regional differences in CHD mortality.[25,26] Saturated fat consumption is higher in the southern French-speaking provinces, mainly due to a higher butter consumption, than in the northern Dutch-speaking provinces, and CHD mortality is higher in the south than in the north. The mean provincial serum total cholesterol level in young Belgian military officer candidates showed a statistically significant positive correlation with provincial butter consumption and an inverse correlation with provincial margarine consumption.[24] A statistically significant positive correlation was observed between the mean provincial serum total cholesterol and provincial mortality from all causes and CHD, and it was estimated that a difference of 20 mg/dl (0.5 mmol/L) in the serum total cholesterol level at the age of 20 years would correspond with a difference of 20% in mortality from all causes and of 21% in mortality from CHD In the 45–64 year age group.

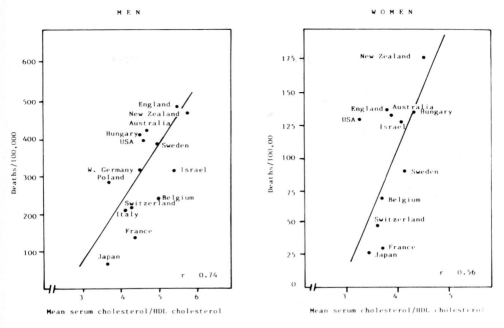

FIG. 8.   The relationship of the mean serum cholesterol/HDL cholesterol ratio to CHD mortality in men in 14 countries and in women in 11 countries (Simons,[23] with permission).

Looking at Figures 4 and 6, showing the relationship between the population mean serum total cholesterol and CHD mortality from two different types of epidemiological analyses, it becomes immediately apparent that despite the strong overall relationship between serum total cholesterol and CHD mortality, there are many examples of marked disparities in CHD mortality rates between populations with similar or almost similar mean levels for serum total cholesterol. An example of such a disparity studied in much detail is the marked difference in CHD mortality between East and West Finns (about 1.6-fold), although their mean total cholesterol levels show a difference of only about 20 mg/dl (0.5 mmol/L).[6,7] Applying epidemiological predictions from other studies such as the Framingham Study,[27] this difference in serum total cholesterol mean levels would explain no more than a 15% difference in CHD mortality. Hypertension is more common in East Finland, and formerly East Finland men were more often smokers and smoked more heavily than West Finland men, although this difference has now disappeared.[6,7] These differences in other major risk factors factors evidently contribute in part to the notable disparity in the CHD mortality experience between East and West Finns, but do not explain it completely.

Another example of an even greater disparity in CHD mortality experience between populations, despite almost similar mean levels for serum total cholesterol, is given by the carefully standardized study on CHD risk factors in men aged 40 in Edinburgh and Stockholm,[28] Edinburgh having about a three times higher male CHD mortality than Stockholm. Mean value for total serum cholesterol was 214 mg/dl (5.54 mmol/L) in Edinburgh men and 208 mg/dl (5.39 mmol/L) in Stockholm men. Edinburgh men were shorter and fatter, had higher systolic and diastolic blood pressures, drank more alcohol, and smoked more cigarettes, although the proportion of cigarette smokers in both groups was similar. Edinburgh men had higher mean levels for serum total, VLDL, LDL and HDL triglycerides and VLDL cholesterol, and a lower mean level for serum HDL cholesterol. The relative linoleic acid content of plasma triglycerides and cholesterol esters was lower in Edinburgh men, and their subcutaneous adipose tissue glycerides had a lower polyunsaturated/saturated fatty acid ratio and a markedly lower relative linoleic acid content. Edinburgh men also had a greater plasma insulin response in an oral glucose tolerance test, although the glucose response was the same in both groups. This study points out that a number of lifestyle factors and metabolic factors, which in turn may be related to diet and other lifestyles, may explain deviations from the overall interpopulation correlation between serum cholesterol and the occurrence of CHD.

TIME TRENDS IN POPULATION MEAN SERUM CHOLESTEROL LEVELS VERSUS TIME TRENDS IN THE OCCURRENCE OF CHD

There is paucity of well-standardized longitudinal studies on time trends in population mean serum cholesterol levels from countries undergoing marked changes in CHD rates. A recent report on trends in serum cholesterol levels among the adult population of the United States, based on data from National Health and Nutrition Examination Surveys (NHANES), showed that between the 1960–1962 and the 1976–1980 surveys the mean serum cholesterol level had decreased among white men from 218 mg/dl (5.6 mmol/L) to 211 mg/dl (5.5 mmol/L) and among white women from 224 mg/dl (5.8 mmol/L) to 215 mg/dl (5.6 mmol/L) (Table II).[29] Among black men and women no definite change in mean serum cholesterol took

TABLE II. *Changes in age-adjusted mean serum cholesterol levels of adults aged 20–74 years in the United States, by sex and race. Data from NHANES surveys, 1960 to 1980 (National Center for Health Statistics–National Heart, Lung, and Blood Institute Collaborative Lipid Group[29])*

	Mean serum cholesterol, mg/dl			Change, %	
	1960–1962	1971–1974	1976–1980	1960–1962 to 1971–1974	1960–1962 to 1976–1980
White men	218	214	211	−2	−3
White women	224	216	215	−4	−4
Black men	221	213	209	+1	−1
Black women	216	218	214	+1	−1

Conversion factor: 1 mg/dl = 0.0258 mmol/L

place. These trends in serum cholesterol levels in the United States white population are compatible with information available concerning dietary changes from the 1960s until the 1980s, although it is not possible to assess the possible contributions of changes in the use of individual nutrients. Using logistic regression coefficients from the Framingham Study data,[27] the NHANES investigators concluded that the 3–4% decline in mean serum cholesterol level would translate into a 6–8% reduction in CHD mortality. As shown above, there has been in the United States since the beginning of the 1970s until the beginning of the 1980s an almost 40% reduction in the CHD mortality of men and women, and thus only about one fifth of this would be explained by the decline in serum cholesterol.

Data based on the 5-year follow-up examinations of the East and West Finland cohorts of the Seven Countries Study[30] showed that the mean serum cholesterol levels in both areas peaked between 1964 and 1969, and then started to decline, as could be predicted on the basis of changes in the habitual diet of the Finnish population since the beginning of the 1960s.[7] Puska et al.[31] have reported changes in the mean serum cholesterol levels among men and women from two provinces in East Finland, North Karelia and Kuopio, during a 10-year period 1972–1982. In North Karelia a comprehensive community program to control cardiovascular diseases, the so-called North Karelia project, was started in 1972 with an intensive health education programme in 1972–1977, and Kuopio province served as a reference area to reflect ongoing national trends. As shown in Table III, a decline in mean serum cholesterol levels occurred from 1972 until 1982 in both provinces in both sexes, and these changes were more marked in North Karelia during the first 5-year period. The serum cholesterol data given in Table III have not been adjusted for the effect of a change in the biochemical methods used for serum cholesterol measurements in different surveys, but even allowing for that, a substantial reduction in the mean serum cholesterol level by about 6–7% has occurred in these two East Finland populations during the period 1972–1982. According to epidemiological

TABLE III. *Changes in mean serum cholesterol levels in North Karelia and Kuopio provinces, East Finland, based on surveys of random samples of men and women aged 30–59 years, 1972–1982 (Puska et al.[31])*

	Mean serum cholesterol, mmol/L			Change, %	
	1972	1977	1982	1972–1977	1972–1982
North Karelia					
Men	7.1	6.7	6.3	−6	−11
Women	7.0	6.6	6.2	−6	−11
Kuopio					
Men	6.9	6.8	6.3	−1	−9
Women	6.8	6.5	6.0	−4	−12

Conversion factor: 1 mmol/L = 38.7 mg/dl

predictions mentioned above, this change would translate into a 12–14% decline in CHD mortality. Tuomilehto *et al.*[32] have calculated linear trends for CHD mortality in the population aged 35–64 years in North Karelia and the rest of Finland for the period from 1969–1982. Using the average figures for the annual decline in CHD mortality obtained from these calculations, the male CHD mortality declined during the 10-year period preceding 1982 by 29% in North Karelia and by 20% in the rest of Finland. The female CHD mortality declined during the 10-year period by 49% in North Karelia and by 30% in the rest of Finland. Thus, it appears that the decline in population mean serum cholesterol level may have been greater in Finland than in the United States and in Finland contributed more to the decline in CHD mortality.

CONCLUSIONS

Interpopulation correlations between serum total cholesterol and CHD mortality from epidemiological studies using different approaches are strong and consistent. In univariate analyses, correlation coefficients ranged from 0.67 to 0.86, which means that from 45%–74% of the variation in CHD mortality between populations would be explained by differences in the population mean cholesterol levels. Since the habitual diet of the population is the strongest determinant of the position and central tendency of its serum cholesterol distribution, these observations emphasize the powerful impact of dietary factors on the occurrence of CHD and the key importance of appropriate dietary changes in the prevention of CHD in populations with high population mean levels for serum cholesterol and high CHD rates.

Data from the Seven Countries Study[4] on the serum cholesterol-CHD mortality relationship across populations indicate that the occurrence of CHD in populations begins to increase with increasing population median serum total cholesterol at levels even below 200 mg/dl (5.2 mmol/L). This is in accordance with data on the serum cholesterol-CHD mortality relationship from a six-year follow-up of 361,662 Multiple Risk Factor Intervention Trial screenees.[33,34] Within this large group of men living in cities of the United States, a curvilinear relationship was observed between the serum total cholesterol level and their six-year risk of CHD, and the risk started to increase at levels below 200 mg/dl (5.2 mmol/L). The Seven Countries Study included only few cohorts with median serum total cholesterol levels around or above 250 mg/dl (6.5 mmol/L). Thus, the question remains open as to whether the serum cholesterol-CHD mortality relationship between populations actually would be curvilinear rather than linear, as seen in within-population analyses.

Marked deviations from the overall interpopulation correlation between serum total cholesterol and the occurrence of CHD were observed both in the Seven Countries Study data and in the analyses carried out by Simons using serum cholesterol mean values from population studies among men and national male CHD mortality rates from 19 countries. Differences in other major CHD risk factors, like blood pressure and smoking, independent of serum cholesterol levels, may explain in part disparities in the occurrence of CHD between populations with rather similar mean serum cholesterol levels. Observations from the Edinburgh-Stockholm study,[28] however, emphasize that more complex cluster of metabolic and other factors may be involved in such disparities. The observation concerning a low relative linoleic acid content of plasma and adipose tissue lipids in Edinburgh men with a high CHD rate as compared with that observed in Stockholm men with a low CHD rate is of great interest. Later studies both across populations and within populations suggest in accordance with the Edinburgh-Stockholm study that fatty acid composition of plasma and tissue lipids may have links with the development of CHD through several mechanisms, for example, effects on thrombogenesis and blood pressure level.[35–39] These findings again emphasize the importance of dietary factors as determinants of the occurrence of CHD, but through mechanisms other than the cholesterol-atherosclerosis relationship.

The only information available concerning the serum cholesterol-CHD relationship in women is the report by Simons[23] showing no statistically significant correlation between the mean serum cholesterol levels from population studies among women and national female CHD mortality rates from 15 countries. The possibility has to be taken into account, however, that the serum cholesterol data for women available for these analyses were not representative of the national averages, and thus a correlation that may exist would not have become evident. It is also possible, and even likely, that differences between nationalities with respect to other CHD risk factors, such as cigarette smoking, which do not always run parallel in both sexes for cultural reasons, could explain the disparity between data for men and women concerning the serum cholesterol-CHD relationship.

Data for interpopulation correlations between serum HDL cholesterol and CHD mortality are available only from two analyses and their results are diametrically opposite, Knuiman et al.[22] reporting a positive correlation and Simons[23] an inverse correlation between serum HDL cholesterol and CHD mortality in male populations. Thus, the possible contribution of differences in the population distributions of serum HDL cholesterol to the between-population variation in the occurrence of CHD so far remains an unsolved issue needing for its clarification new studies using well-standardized methods for HDL cholesterol measurement.

Data from the United States[15,29] and Finland[7,30,31] indicate that recent declining trends in CHD mortality and morbidity in these countries have been preceded and paralleled by changes in the habitual diets of the countries and declining population mean levels for serum cholesterol. Well-standardized data on serum lipids and lipoproteins and other CHD risk factors, based on repeated random sample surveys of adult populations, and CHD mortality and morbidity data on the same populations are currently being collected in 26 countries in the WHO-coordinated MONICA project (Multinational Monitoring of the Trends and Determinants in Cardiovascular Disease).[40] Therefore, it may be expected that important new information will be forthcoming from MONICA Project about cross-sectional interpopulation correlations between serum lipids and lipoproteins and other risk factors and the occurrence of CHD, as well as about time trends in the levels of serum lipids and lipoproteins and other risk factors in relation to time trends in the occurrence of CHD.

REFERENCES

1. World Health Statistics Annual. Geneva: WHO, 1984–85.
2. Pyörälä K. Interpopulation correlations between serum cholesterol level and the occurrence of coronary heart disease. *Eur Heart J* 1987; **8**(Suppl E):23–30.
3. World Health Organization. Myocardial infarction community registers. Public Health in Europe 5. Copenhagen: Regional Office for Europe, 1976.
4. Keys A. Seven countries. A multivariate analysis of death and coronary heart disease. Cambridge, Massachusetts: Harvard University Press, 1980.
5. Keys A, Menotti A, Aravanis C, *et al.* The seven countries study: 2,289 deaths in 15 years. *Prev Med* 1984; **13**:141–154.
6. Pyörälä K, Valkonen T. The high ischaemic heart disease mortality in Finland. International comparisons, regional differences, trends and possible causes. Skandia International Symposia. Medical Aspects of Mortality Statistics. Stockholm: Almquist & Wicksell International, 1981, 37–57.
7. Pyörälä K, Salonen JT, Valkonen T. Trends in coronary heart disease mortality and morbidity and related factors in Finland. *Cardiology* 1985; **72**:35–51.
8. Smith WC, Tunstall Pedoe H. European regional variation in cardiovascular mortality. *Br Med Bull* 1984; **40**:374–379.
9. Working Group on Arteriosclerosis of the National Heart, Lung, and Blood Institute. *Arteriosclerosis 1981.* Vol. 2. Report of the Working Group on Arteriosclerosis of the National Heart, Lung, and Blood Institute. U.S. Department of Health and Human Services, NIH Publication No. 82-2035. Bethesda, Md.: US Public Health Service, 1981.
10. Walker WJ. Coronary mortality: What is going on? *JAMA* 1974; **227**:1045–1046.
11. Gordon T, Thom T. The recent decrease in CHD mortality. *Prev Med* 1975; **4**:115–125.
12. Epstein FH, Pisa Z. International comparisons in ischaemic heart disease mortality. *In*: Havlik R, Feinleib M. (eds.). *Proceedings of the Conference on the Decline in Coronary Heart Disease Mortality.* US Department of Health, Education, and Welfare, Public Health Service, National Institutes of Health. NIH Publication No. 79-1610. Washington: DHEW, 1979, 55–58.
13. Pisa Z, Uemura K. Trends of mortality from ischaemic heart disease and other cardiovascular diseases in 27 countries, 1968–1977. *World Health Stat Q* 1982; **35**:11–47.
14. Uemura K, Pisa Z. Recent trends in cardiovascular mortality in 27 industrialized countries. *World Health Stat Q* 1985; **38**:142–162.
15. Stamler J. The marked decline in coronary heart disease mortality rates in the United States, 1968–1981; summary of findings and possible explanations. *Cardiology* 1985; **72**:11–22.
16. Pell S, Fayerweather WE. Trends in the incidence of myocardial infarction and in associated mortality and morbidity in a large employed population, 1957–1983. *N Engl J Med* 1985; **312**:1005–1011.
17. Koskenvuo M, Kaprio J, Langinvainio H, *et al.* Changes in incidence and prognosis of ischaemic heart disease in Finland: a record linkage for 1972 and 1981. *Br Med J* 1985; **290**:1773–1775.
18. Pohjola-Sintonen S, Siltanen P, Haapakoski J, *et al.* The declining trends in the incidence of acute myocardial infarction in Finland. The results of Helsinki Coronary Register during 1970–1977. *Eur Heart J* 1985; **6**:834–839.
19. Marmot M, McDowall ME. Mortality decline and widening social inequalities. *Lancet* 1986; **2**:274–276.
20. Rose G. Incubation period of coronary heart disease. *Br Med J* 1982; **284**:1600–1601.
21. Knuiman JT, Hermus RJJ, Hautwast JGAJ. Serum total and high density lipoprotein (HDL) cholesterol concentrations in rural and urban boys from 16 countries. *Atherosclerosis* 1980; **36**:529–537.
22. Knuiman JT, West CE, Burema J. Serum total and high density lipoprotein cholesterol concentrations and body mass index in adult men from 13 countries. *Am J Epidemiol* 1982; **116**:631–642.
23. Simons LA. Interrelations of lipids and lipoproteins with coronary artery disease in 19 countries. *Am J Cardiol* 1986; **57**:5G–10G.

24. Kesteloot H, Bandle J, Pille J *et al*. Serum lipid distribution and mortality in Belgium. *Eur Heart J* 1984; **5**:778–783.
25. Joossens JV. Epidemiology of coronary heart disease. Lessons from North and South Belgium. *Postgrad Med J* 1980; **56**:548–556.
26. Joossens JV, Brems-Heynes E, Claes JH *et al*. The pattern of food and mortality in Belgium. *Lancet* 1977; **1**:1069–1072.
27. Shurtleff D. Some characteristics related to the incidence of cardiovascular disease and health: The Framingham Study. US Department of Health, Education, and Welfare, Public Health Service, National Institutes of Health. NIH Publication No. 74-599. Washington: DHEW, 1974, Section 30, Table 6-3.
28. Logan RL, Riemersma RA, Thomson M, *et al*. Risk factors for ischaemic heart-disease in normal men aged 40. Edinburgh-Stockholm study. *Lancet* 1978; **1**:949–954.
29. National Centre for Health Statistics—National Heart, Lung and Blod Institute Collaborative Lipid Group. Trends in serum cholesterol levels among US adults aged 20 to 74 years. Data from the National Health and Nutrition Examination Surveys, 1960 to 1980. *JAMA* 1987; **257**:937–942.
30. Pekkanen J. Coronary heart disease during a 25-year follow-up. Risk factors and their secular trends in the Finnish cohorts of the Seven Countries Study. Academic Dissertation. Helsinki: University of Helsinki, 1987.
31. Puska P, Salonen JT, Nissinen A, *et al*. Changes in risk factors for coronary heart disease during 10 years of a community intervention programme (North Karelia project). *Br Med J* 1983; **287**:1840–1844.
32. Tuomilehto J, Geboers J, Salonen JT, *et al*. Decline in cardiovascular mortality in North Karelia and other parts of Finland. *Br Med J* 1986; **293**:1068–1071.
33. Martin MJ, Hulley SB, Browner WS, *et al*. Serum cholesterol, blood pressure, and mortality: implications from a cohort of 361,622 men. *Lancet* 1986; **2**:933–936.
34. Stamler J, Wentworth D, Neaton J. Is the relationship between serum cholesterol and the risk for death from coronary heart disease continuous and graded? Findings on the 356,222 primary screenees of the Multiple Risk Factor Intervention Trial (MRFIT). *JAMA* 1986; **256**:2833–2828.
35. Puska P, Iacono JM, Nissinen, *et al*. Controlled, randomized trial of the effect of dietary fat on blood pressure. *Lancet* 1983; **1**:1–5.
36. Miettinen TA, Naukkarinen V, Huttunen JK, *et al*. Fatty acid composition of serum lipids predict myocardial infarction. *Br Med J* 1982; **285**:933–936.
37. Wood DA, Butler S, Riemersma RA, *et al*. Adipose tissue and platelet fatty acids and coronary heart disease. *Lancet* 1984; **2**:117–121.
38. Riemersma RA, Wood DA, Butler S, *et al*. Linoleic acid content in adipose tissue and coronary heart disease. *Br Med J* 1986; **292**:1423–1427.
39. Wood DA, Riemersma RA, Butler S, *et al*. Linoleic acid eicosapentaenoic acids in adipose tissue and platelets and risk of coronary heart disease. *Lancet* 1987; **1**:177–182.
40. Pisa A. The MONICA project for cardiovascular diseases. *World Health Forum* 1982; **3**:336–337.

SUMMARY

International mortality statistics indicate striking differences in mortality from coronary heart disease (CHD) between countries. The increase in mortality seen during the 1970s in some ''Western'' countries now appears to be declining, whilst in other countries it is still on the increase. It is clear that diet, in particular a high intake of total and saturated fats, has considerable influence on blood lipid levels, notably low density lipoprotein cholesterol and this in turn is a vital contributing factor in the occurrence of CHD in populations. This review examines the magnitude of the differences between populations in the occurrence of CHD and recent international trends in CHD rates. Current data on interpopulation correlations between serum cholesterol and the occurrence of CHD are summarized. Examples are given indicating that differences in the levels of risk factors other than serum cholesterol also have an important influence on the occurrence of CHD in populations. Data available from the United States and Finland concerning time trends in population mean levels for serum cholesterol in relationship to time trends in CHD mortality rates in these countries are discussed.

RÉSUMÉ

Les statistiques internationales de mortalité montrent des différences frappantes entre les pays en ce qui concerne la mortalité à la suite de maladies coronariennes. L'accroissement des mortalités dans les années 70 dans certains pays de l'Ouest semble maintenant en régression, alors que dans d'autres pays l'accroissement persiste. Il est évident que le régime alimentaire, notamment la forte comsommation de graisses saturées entières, a une influence considérable sur les niveaux de lipides dans le sang, surtout du cholestérol des lipoprotéines de faible densité, et ceci à son tour est un facteur vital déterminant des maladies coronariennes parmi les populations. Cet article examine l'ampleur des différences qui existent entre les populations frappées de maladies coronariennes et les récentes tendances internationales des taux de maladies coronariennes. On récapitule les données actuelles sur les rapports qui existent entre les niveaux élevés de cholestérol et les incidences de maladies coronariennes dans divers pays. On donne aussi des exemples de facteurs de risques autres que le cholestérol qui jouent un rôle important dans le développement des maladies coronariennes dans les populations. A partir de données des Etats-Unis et de Finlande on discute les tendances actuelles en oe qui concerne les niveaux moyens de cholestérol dans la population par rapport aux tendances actuelles des taux de mortalité dans ces pays à la suite de maladies coronariennes.

ZUSAMMENFASSUNG

Internationale Sterblichkeitsstatistiken deuten auf schlagende Unterschiede in der Sterblichkeitsrate durch koronare Herzkrankheit (CHD) zwischen verschiedenen Ländern. Der Anstieg der Sterblichkeitsrate in einigen "westlichen Ländern," wie man ihn in den 1970 ziger Jahren gesehen hat, scheint jetzt abzunehmen, während er in anderen Ländern immer noch am Anstieg ist. Es ist klar, daß Diät, im besonderen hohe Einnahme von Gesamt und gesättigten Fetten, einen erheblichen Einfluß auf Blut-Lipid-Spiegel und besonders auf niedrigdichtes Lipoprotein-Cholesterin hat. Dies ist wiederum ein wichtiger, beitragender Faktor in dem Auftreten von CHD in Bevölkerungen. Diese Revision prüft die Größe der Unterschiede zwischen Bevölkerungen beim Auftreten des CHD und unlängste internationale Tendenzen in CHD-Raten. Gegenwärtige Daten betreffend Zwischen-Bevölkerungs-Wechselbeziehungen zwischen Serum-Cholesterin und dem Auftreten von CHD sind zusammengefaßt. Beispiele sind gegeben, die besagen, daß Unterschiede in den Spiegeln von Risikofaktoren anderer als Serum-Cholesterin ebenfalls einen wichtigen Einfluß auf das Auftreten von CHD in Bevölkerungen hat. Daten von den Vereinigten Staaten und Finland betreffend Zeitten-

denzen in mittleren Bevölkerungsspiegelwerten für Serum-Cholesterin in Verhältnis zu Zeit-
tendenzen der CHD-Sterblichkeitsrate in diesen Ländern sind erörtert.

SOMMARIO

Statistiche internazionali sulla mortalità indicano estreme differenze nella morte causata dalla
malattia coronaria del cuore (MCC) da una nazione all'altra. L'aumento dei morti visto negli
anni 70 in alcuni paesi dell' ''Ouest'' sembra adesso in declino, mentre in altre nazioni è
ancora in aumento. E'chiaro che la dieta, in particolar modo un alto consumo di grassi totali
e saturati ha un'influenza considerevole nel livello lipide del sangue, notevolmente colesterolo
di lipoproteina con bassa densità, e questo è a sua volta un fattore vitale che contribuisce
alla MCC delle popolazioni. Questa recensione esamina la magnitudine delle differenze fra
le popolazioni quando occorre la MCC e nelle tendenze internazionali delle rate della MCC.
Dati correnti sulle correlazioni delle interpopolazioni fra il colesterolo del siero e l'occorrenza
della MCC vengono riassunti. Vengono dati degli esempi che indicano che le differenze nei
livelli dei fattori rischio, oltre al colesterolo del siero, hanno anche un'influsso importante
nell'occorrenza della MCC nei popoli. Vengono discussi dati disponibili dagli Stati Uniti e
dalla Finlandia riguardanti le tendenze di tempo verso i livelli del colesterolo nel siero delle
popolazioni in relazione all'tasso di mortalità causato dalla MCC.

SUMÁRIO

Os dados estatísticos internacionais de mortalidade indicam diferenças notáveis em mortalidade de cardiopátia coronária (CHD) entre os países. O aumento em mortalidade visto
durante a década de 1970 em alguns países ''do Ocidente'' agora aparece estar em declínio,
enquanto em outros países ainda está aumentando. É claro que o regime alimentar, em
particular um consumo alto de gorduras totais e saturadas, tem influência considerável sobre
os níveis de lípidos no sangue, notávelmente o colesterol de lipoproteína de baixa densidade
e isto em sua vez é um fator vital contribuindo para a ocorrência de CHD nas populações.
Esta revista examina a magnitude das diferenças entre populações na ocorrência de CHD e
as tendências internacionais recentes nas taxas de CHD. Os dados atuais sobre as correlações
interpopulações entre níveis de colesterol no soro e a ocorrência de CHD são sumariados.
Exemplos são dados indicando que as diferenças no níveis dos fatores de risco além de
colesterol no soro tambem têm uma influência sobre a ocorrência de CHD nas populações.
Os dados disponíveis dos Estados Unidos e da Finlândia no que respeito às tendências de
tempo nos niveis médios de colesterol no soro das populações em relação às tendências de
tempo nas taxas de mortalidade em CHD nestes países são discutidos.

RESUMEN

Las estadísticas internacionales de mortalidad dan a entender que hay grandes diferencias
en los índices de mortalidad de cardiopatía coronaria (CHD) entre países. Actualmente parece

que el incremento en la mortalidad visto durante la década del setenta en algunos países "occidentales" está declinando, mientras que en otros países continúa en aumento. Es claro que la dieta, en particular una ingesta elevada de grasas tanto saturadas como total, ejerce una influencia considerable en los niveles séricos de lípidos, en particular el colesterol de lipoproteínas de baja densidad, y esto a su vez es un importantísimo factor en la ocurencia de CHD entre la población. Aquí se analiza la magnitud de las diferencias entre las poblaciones en cuanto a los índices de CHD, y las tendencias internacionales recientes en los índices de CHD. Se resumen los datos actuales en cuanto a las correlaciones interpoblación entre los niveles séricos de colesterol y la ocurencia de CHD. Se dan ejemplos que indican que las diferencias en los niveles de otros factores de riesgo aparte del colesterol sérico también tienen un papel importante en la aparición de CHD entre poblaciones. Se examinan los datos disponibles obtenidos en los Estados Unidos y en Finlandia con respecto a las tendencias en el tiempo en los niveles séricos medios de colesterol de la población en relación con las tendencias en el tiempo en los índices de mortalidad por CHD en estos países.

The Role of Cholesterol in Atherosclerosis:
New Therapeutic Opportunities, edited by S. M. Grundy
and A. G. Bearn, Hanley & Belfus, Inc., Philadelphia.

Desirable Plasma Lipid and Lipoprotein Levels in Adults

Barry Lewis

The concept of desirable levels of plasma lipids is based ultimately on epidemiologic relationships; it derives from longitudinal studies indicating a range of levels associated with minimum risk of coronary heart disease. Implicit in the concept is the recognition that abnormal lipid levels are of causal significance in relation to disease.

ETIOLOGIC RELATIONSHIPS BETWEEN LIPID DISORDERS AND COMMON DISEASES

The direct relations between coronary heart disease and plasma levels of cholesterol, and of low density lipoprotein (LDL) cholesterol have all the characteristics of a causal association.[1] This conclusion is justified by concordant evidence from epidemiology, controlled trials, studies of hyperlipidemic laboratory animals,[2,3] and cell-biologic studies of interactions between lipoproteins and the cellular elements of atherosclerotic plaque.

Very low levels of plasma cholesterol (39–58 mg/dl; 1–1.5 mmol/L) are seen in the genetic disorder abetalipoproteinemia, and are clearly associated with pathologic consequences in the CNS, retina and red cells; these abnormalities appear to reflect impaired transport of fat-soluble vitamins. Abetalipoproteinemia is a rare disorder. A few years ago, however, several sets of epidemiologic studies suggested that men with plasma cholesterol levels in the lowest quintile of the distribution were at increased risk for cancer, particularly carcinoma of the colon. In contrast to the direct relationship of plasma cholesterol to coronary heart disease, however, the inverse association between cholesterol and cancer lacks characteristics suggesting that hypocholesterolemia causes cancer.[4–7] The longitudinal epidemiologic studies are inconsistent and even in those in which an association is demonstrated, no "dose-response" relationship is present. Further, such studies within populations are inconsistent with observations in cross-cultural epidemiologic studies; in the latter a direct relation is evident between fat consumption (and by inference mean plasma cholesterol) and mortality from cancers of the breast, colon, lung, kidney, and pancreas. The temporal sequence lends credence to the view that low cholesterol levels may be a consequence of, rather than an antecedent to, undiagnosed cancer. Furthermore, no plausible mechanism has been put forward to explain a causal role of hypocholesterolemia.[8]

The evidence relating other plasma lipid and lipoprotein fractions to disease processes is suggestive but incomplete. Clinical observation and the effects of lipid-lowering therapy leave no doubt that marked hypertriglyceridemia (>885 mg/dl; 10 mmol/L) is a cause of acute pancreatitis. A positive association is evident between plasma triglyceride and the incidence of coronary heart disease on univariate analysis, but has been shown by multivariate analysis to be dependent on mutual associations with obesity and with low levels of high density lipoprotein (HDL) cholesterol. Recently the alternative statistical procedure, projected slope analysis, has been employed, reaffirming that triglyceride levels are independently predictive of coronary heart disease incidence in persons with low levels of HDL cholesterol. Nevertheless, evidence from other sources (clinical trials, animal models) has not as yet been forthcoming to confirm the causal nature of this association, plausible though this interpretation appears to be.

There is a strong, independent and relatively consistent negative association between HDL cholesterol and the incidence of coronary heart disease.[1] However the evidence that this reflects a causal relationship is far from compelling at the present time. High density lipoprotein undoubtedly plays a central role in the reverse transport of cholesterol. The cholesterol in this lipoprotein class, and some of the apolipoproteins too, are derived from multiple sources;[9] the absence of an independent correlation between levels of HDL components and the mass of cholesterol in tissue pools[10] argues against the hypothesis that plasma levels of this lipoprotein determine the rate of reverse transport of cholesterol. In addition, controlled trial evidence is as yet lacking that the risk of coronary heart disease is altered as a result of manipulations of HDL levels, although a recent study of gemfibrozil has been interpreted as suggesting this conclusion.[19a] Thus measurement of this lipoprotein class is of value in helping to assess the risk of coronary heart disease; but in the absence of cogent evidence of a directly protective role, it is not appropriate to assign "desirable levels" of high density lipoprotein cholesterol at the present time.

DESIRABLE AND NORMAL LEVELS AND ACTION LIMITS

Cholesterol

With the apparent exception of diabetes mellitus and impaired glucose tolerance, the major risk factors for coronary heart disease are continuous graded characteristics. In most large longitudinal studies no threshold is evident in the relation between plasma cholesterol and coronary heart disease. These conclusions derive particularly from a uniquely large longitudinal study of 361,000 men who underwent risk factor screening for inclusion in the Multiple Risk Factor Intervention Trial (MRFIT) (Fig. 1).[11] In

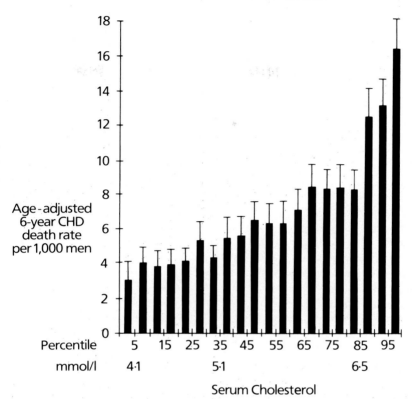

FIG. 1. Relation between serum cholesterol and six-year mortality from coronary heart disease in 361,662 men screened for entry into Multiple Risk Factor Intervention Trial. (Reproduced with permission from Martin MJ, *et al.* Serum cholesterol, blood pressure, and mortality: Implications from a cohort of 361,662 men. *Lancet* 1986; **2**:933–36.)

this, as in the longitudinal phase of the Seven Countries Study,[12] there was a steady increase in the incidence of coronary heart disease as serum cholesterol levels increased from 155–175 mg/dl (4–4.5 mmol/L) to 230–250 mg/dl (6–6.5 mmol/L). The incidence of coronary heart disease increased more steeply in relation to cholesterol levels in the range 250–300 mg/dl (6.5–7.8 mmol/L).

Outside the limits illuminated by these surveys, other sources of information must be invoked. In heterozygous familial hypercholesterolemia, in which cholesterol levels are elevated from birth (most adults having levels in the range of 350–540 mg/dl, 9–14 mmol/L), affected men have a coronary heart disease risk 8–10 fold greater than unaffected men. Clearly the increase in incidence in the highest reaches of the distribution is very steep indeed. There is a dearth of hard epidemiologic data on populations such as those in rural China, where mean cholesterol levels in the range of 97–155 mg/dl (2.5–4 mmol/L) are common; clinical observation suggests that coronary heart disease is strikingly uncommon in such communities.

The definition of desirable levels as those associated with minimum risk of coronary heart disease was pioneered by the American Health Foundation[13] and extended by a National Institutes of Health Consensus Development Panel.[14] Most recently this approach has been systematized by a Study Group of the European Atherosclerosis Society.[15] The basis is analogous to that underlying current definitions of desirable body weight or of diabetes mellitus. Given the continuous, graded nature of the plasma cholesterol–coronary heart disease relationship over so extensive a range of levels, it is somewhat arbitrary to select any values as an upper limit of ''desirable plasma cholesterol level.'' For didactic purposes, nevertheless, it is useful to set a series of action limits. Provided that these are flexibly employed, in conjunction with other clinical findings, they are of value in selecting the extent to which lipid-lowering therapy should be pursued. Such action limits are concordant with the study of men screened for the MRFIT study (Fig. 1) They are shown in Table I, which is based on the therapeutic categories proposed by the European Atherosclerosis Society (EAS).[15]

The EAS recommends that cholesterol levels exceeding about 200 mg/dl (5.2 mmol/L) deserve consideration for therapy, particularly in young adults. This is justified by the 2-fold greater risk of coronary disease shown in the MRFIT study in men with a serum cholesterol of 250 mg/dl (6.5 mmol/L), compared with those with levels of 200 mg/dl (5.2 mmol/L). The EAS stresses that for the majority of individuals with cholesterol levels in the range 200–250 mg/dl (5.2–6.5 mmol/L), management will comprise counseling designed to reinforce health recommendations made to the population as a whole (Table I). Such recommendations include moderate dietary change, weight control, avoidance of smoking, and the practice of suitable regular physical exercise. Only in exceptional circumstances, such as the presence of multiple risk factors conferring high overall risk or a strong family history of premature coronary disease, would individuals with levels in this range be considered for more aggressive treatment. Another category justifying more active management would be patients who have undergone coronary artery bypass grafting, endarterectomy, or other revascularization procedures.

The EAS regards the presence of plasma cholesterol levels greater than 250 mg/dl (6.5 mmol/L) due to an increase in low density lipoprotein as an indication for individual therapy, in conformity with the marked increase in risk conferred by such levels (Table I).[4] Among individuals with plasma cholesterol levels greater than 310 mg/dl (8 mmol/L), a substantial proportion will have major genetic disorders of lipoprotein metabolism, notably familial hypercholesterolemia and remnant (Type III) hyperlipoproteinemia. Most patients with such disorders will require lipid-lowering drug therapy in addition to diet therapy; hence a precise metabolic diagnosis is important in defining optimal therapy.

To minimize the risk of coronary heart disease, the goal of treatment is agreed, by the NIH Consensus Development Panel[14] as well as the EAS Study Group, to be to achieve a cholesterol level as close to 200 mg/dl (5.2 mmol/L) as possible in adults (the former body sets an even lower target of 180 mg/dl (4.7 mmol/L) for those between 20–29 years of age).

TABLE I. Graded management of hyperlipidemia*

Lipid levels	mmol/L	mg/dl	Investigation and assessment	Management
I. Cholesterol	5.2–6.5	200–250	Take into account age, family history of CHD, blood pressure, smoking, HDL cholesterol <1 mmol/L	Emphasize general dietary guidelines for serum lipid reduction. Deal with associated risk factors and overweight.
Glyceride	<2.3	<200		
II. Cholesterol	6.5–7.8	250–300	As in I	1. prescribe lipid-lowering diet, reduce energy intake if overweight. 2. monitor response; promote compliance. 3. consider lipid-lowering drug if cholesterol is persistently high.
Glyceride	<2.3	<200		
III. Cholesterol	<5.2	<200	Identify possible causes of hypertriglyceridemia: alcohol abuse, obesity, diabetes, use of diuretics, oestrogens, retinoids	Restrict food energy if overweight, emphasize general dietary guidelines for lipid reduction. Deal with causes if possible.
Glyceride	2.3–5.6	200–500		
IV. Cholesterol	5.2–7.8	200–300	As in I and II	As in II and III
Glyceride	2.3–5.6	200–500		
V. Cholesterol and/or	>7.8	>300	Assess cardiovascular status and investigate fully for causes of secondary hyperlipidemia	Proceed as under II and III or on referral to specialized lipid class. Therapy with appropriate drug(s) commonly necessary.
glyceride	>5.6	>500		

* Modified from European Atherosclerosis Society policy statement.[15]

There is no evidence that low plasma cholesterol (i.e., the lowest levels that can be achieved by presently available therapy in hyperlipidemic patients) is causally related to disease; hence it is inappropriate to designate a *lower* limit to desirable plasma cholesterol levels.

Triglyceride

The relation of hypertriglyceridemia to major diseases including pancreatitis was mentioned in an earlier section. The EAS Study Group took the view that elevated plasma triglyceride has yet to be shown to be a cause of atherosclerosis. Nevertheless there is some clinical and experimental support for the view that a specific class of triglyceride-rich lipoproteins (intermediate density lipoprotein and the denser subclass of very low density lipoprotein) play a role in atherogenesis. Pending a securer basis for therapeutic policy, the EAS, like the NIH Consensus report on treatment of hypertriglyceridemia,[16] regarded levels exceeding 530 mg/dl (6 mmol/L) as justifying vigorous therapy, including drug treatment if necessary. Similarly, when triglyceride levels are elevated as a manifestation of remnant hyperlipoproteinemia, dietary and drug therapy are usually appropriate.

The clinical approach to persons with triglyceride levels in the range of 180–530 mg/dl (2–6 mmol/L) is made easier by the fact that in many such individuals, hypertriglyceridemia results from underlying causes that justify correction in their own right, namely obesity, overuse of alcohol, and uncontrolled diabetes. In others it may result from medication (thiazides, estrogen-containing oral contraceptives, isotretinoin) for which alternatives are available. Further, moderate hypertriglyceridemia decreases in response to diets in which saturated fatty acids are partly substituted by polyunsaturated fatty acids of n-6 and n-3 series. Overall, therefore, the common abnormality of mildly elevated triglyceride levels can usually be dealt with by simple measures, and this approach is advocated by the EAS.

High Density Lipoprotein Cholesterol

Measurement of this lipoprotein is justified to improve the assessment of coronary heart disease risk, and also to recognize the small number of individuals, commonly women, in whom mildly elevated cholesterol levels are due to a marked increase in high density lipoprotein; such persons do not require lipid-lowering therapy. No sound basis exists for defined desirable levels at present. The EAS has suggested as a provisional guideline that levels of HDL cholesterol <35 mg/dl (0.9 mmol/L) should be included among indices of high risk for coronary heart disease. Like elevated triglyceride levels, low levels of HDL cholesterol often reflect remediable underlying causes, in this instance obesity, cigarette smoking, and thiazide and beta-blocker medication.

BIOMETRIC VARIABLES AND THE DEFINITION OF DESIRABLE LEVELS OF CHOLESTEROL

Plasma and LDL cholesterol levels are influenced by age, increasing in early life from low neonatal levels, and increasing again at the onset of puberty. In Western, coronary-disease-prone populations, levels increase again during adult life, reaching a maximum in the sixth decade[17,18] and subsequently declining.[17] Since this rise and fall during adult life are absent in several healthy populations studied in Africa and the Far East,[19] however, these trends in Western adults appear not to be physiological. They are best regarded as reflecting increasing prevalence of hyperlipidemia in middle age. It is therefore inappropriate to adjust desirable levels of plasma cholesterol or LDL cholesterol for adult age. Similar considerations probably apply to plasma triglyceride levels, although fewer studies have been performed.

To express desirable levels in terms of percentiles of the distribution among healthy persons would result in differing action limits in different populations. The EAS expressed the view that the varying distributions of lipids and lipoproteins in different countries do not influence their biological significance with respect to effects on the arterial wall. The EAS therefore recommended basing limits upon absolute levels.

FACTORS AFFECTING THE CHOICE OF THERAPY

As indicated in Table I, therapeutic decisions are influenced not only by the lipid action limits shown but also by the patient's age and overall risk for coronary heart disease. Introduction of treatment at as early an age as possible is presumed to offer the best chance of minimizing the development of atherosclerosis. Conversely, it would be arbitrary to assign an upper age beyond which all treatment should be withheld; however, in older persons, less-intensive therapy may be appropriate.

In reaching therapeutic decisions, the overall risk for coronary heart disease or its progression modulate the level of therapy. Overall risk is assessed on the basis of cholesterol level, family history, duration and extent of smoking, blood pressure, presence of diabetes or obesity, HDL level, and sex. The therapeutic level indicated in Table I for a given plasma lipid concentration may become appropriate for a patient with lower lipid concentrations if his or her overall risk is judged to be high.

PREVALENCE OF LIPID RISK FACTORS

The action limits chosen will define large segments of some populations as having undesirable or high levels of plasma cholesterol. In the United Kingdom, 65% of men and women aged 25–59 years currently have cholesterol levels greater than

200 mg/dl (5.2 mmol/L), and 25% at present have levels greater than 250 mg/dl (6.5 mmol/L).[20] Nevertheless these action limits are objectively based. Fortunately the prevalence of hyperlipidemia may be expected to decline as a result of the introduction of effective population strategies for coronary heart disease prevention, and the magnitude of this change in prevalence has been estimated.[21] The secular decrease in mean plasma cholesterol levels in the United States has recently been quantified.[22] Hence these considerations serve to underline the interdependence of population strategy and individual strategy, which require simultaneous vigorous application.

REFERENCES

1. Lewis B. The lipoproteins: predictors, protectors and pathogens. *Br Med J* 1983; **287**:1161–64.
2. La Ville A, Turner PR, Pittilo M, *et al*. Hereditary hyperlipidemia and atherosclerosis in the rabbit due to an overproduction of lipoprotein. I. Biochemical studies. *Arteriosclerosis* 1987; **7**:105–12.
3. Seddon A, Woolf N, La Ville A, *et al*. Hereditary hyperlipidemia in the rabbit. II. A preliminary report of the arterial pathology. *Arteriosclerosis* 1987; **7**:113–24.
4. Sherwin RW, Wentworth DN, Cutler JA, Hulley SB, Kuller L, Stamler J. Serum cholesterol levels and cancer mortality in 361,662 men screened for the Multiple Risk Factor Intervention Trial. *JAMA* 1987; **257**:943–48.
5. International Collaborative Group. Circulating cholesterol level and risk of death from cancer in men aged 40–69 years. *JAMA* 1982; **248**:2853–59.
6. Lewis B, Mancini M (chairmen). Hypocholesterolaemia: a risk factor? *In:* Schettler G, Gotto AM, Middelhof G, Habenicht A, Jurutha KR, eds. *Atherosclerosis VI.* Berlin: Springer-Verlag, 1984; 839–72.
7. Tornberg SA, Holm L-E, Carlensen JM, Eklund JA. Risks of cancer of the colon and rectum in relation to serum cholesterol and beta-lipoprotein. *N Engl J Med* 1986; **315**:1629–33.
8. Marenah CB, Hassall D, La Ville A, *et al*. Hypocholesterolaemia and non-cardiovascular disease: metabolic studies on subjects with low plasma cholesterol. *Br Med J* 1983; **286**:1603–6.
9. Eisenberg S. High density lipoprotein metabolism. *J Lipid Res* 1985; **25**:1017–28.
10. Blum CB, Dell RB, Palmer RH, Ramakrishnan R, Seplowitz AH, Goodman DS. Relationship of the parameters of body cholesterol metabolism with plasma levels of HDL cholesterol and the major HDL apoproteins. *J Lipid Res* 1985; **26**:1079–88.
10a. Frick MH, Elo O, Haapa K, *et al*. Helsinki Heart Study: Primary-prevention trial with gemfibrozil in middle-aged men with dyslipidemia: Safety of treatment, changes in risk factors, and incidence of coronary heart disease. *N Engl J Med* 1987; **317**:1237–1245.
11. Martin MJ, Hulley SB, Browner WS, Kuller LH, Wentworth D. Serum cholesterol, blood pressure, and mortality: implications from a cohort of 361,662 men. *Lancet* 1986; **2**:933–36.
12. Keys A. Seven Countries. Cambridge: Harvard University Press, 1981.
13. Blackburn HL, Lewis B, Wissler RW, Wynder EL. Health effects of blood lipids: optimal distribution for populations. *Prev Med* 1979; **8**:609–732.
14. NIH Consensus Development Panel (Steinberg D, chairman). Lowering blood cholesterol to prevent heart disease. NIH Consensus Development Conference Statement 1985; **5**:no 7, Bethesda, US Department of Health.
15. Assmann G, Lewis B, Mancini M, Paoletti R, Schettler G. Strategies for the prevention of coronary heart disease: a policy statement of the European Atherosclerosis Society. *Eur J Cardiol* 1987; **8**:77–88.
16. Grundy SM (chairman). Consensus conference: treatment of hypertriglyceridemia. *JAMA* 1984; **251**:1196–1200.
17. Lewis B, Chait A, Wootton IDP, *et al*. Frequency of risk factors for ischaemic heart disease in a healthy British population, with particular reference to serum lipoprotein levels. *Lancet* 1974; **1**:141–46.
18. David CE, Frantz ID, Heiss G. Lipoprotein-cholesterol distributions in selected North American populations: The Lipid Research Clinics Program Prevalence Study. *Circulation* 1980; **62**:302–15.

19. Rossouw JE, van Staden DA, Benade AJS, Jooste PL, Rossouw LJ, Steyn K, Langenhoven ML. Is it normal for serum cholesterol to rise with age? *In:* Fidge NM, Nestel PJ, eds. *Atherosclerosis VII.* Amsterdam: Elsevier, 1986; 37–40.
20. Lewis B, Mann JI, Shepherd J, Winder AF. UK Risk Factor Prevalence Study. In preparation.
21. Lewis B. Mann JI, Mancini M. Reducing the risks of coronary heart disease in individuals and in the population. *Lancet* 1986; **1**:956–59.
22. National Center for Health Statistics—NHLBI Collaborative Lipid Group. Trends in serum cholesterol levels among US adults aged 20 to 74 years. *JAMA* 1987; **257**:937–42.

SUMMARY

The concept of desirable levels of plasma lipids is based ultimately on epidemiologic relationships; it derives from longitudinal studies indicating a range of levels associated with the minimum risk of coronary heart disease. This concept has recently been utilized by the Study Group of the European Atherosclerosis Society (EAS). While recognizing that the selection of any values as "desirable plasma cholesterol levels" is somewhat arbitrary, the EAS sets out to provide certain action limits as guidelines. Recommendations, starting at a lower limit of 200 mg/dl (5.2 mmol/ L), include dietary change and weight control, leading to more aggressive treatment in patients with multiple risk factors and higher plasma cholesterol levels (250 mg/ dl, 6.5 mmol/L). Less is known about the role of raised plasma triglyceride in coronary heart disease: the EAS advocates attention to underlying causes and dietary measures for most patients, reserving drug therapy for those at high risk only. As yet there is insufficient evidence of a directly protective role of high density lipoprotein (HDL) cholesterol in coronary heart disease; hence, it is inappropriate at present to assign "desirable levels" of HDL cholesterol; but provisionally, levels below 35 mg/dl (0.9 mmol/L) are suggested by EAS to indicate high risk and thus to justify more vigorous therapy. The choice of therapy and the prevalence of lipid risk factors are also discussed, and a set of guidelines is provided for the investigation and management of hyperlipidemia of different grades of severity.

RÉSUMÉ

Le concept des niveaux souhaitables de lipides plasmatiques est fondamentalement basé sur des rapports épidémiologiques; il dérive d'études longitudinales qui indiquent un éventail de niveaux associés aux risques minimum de maladies coronariennes. Le Groupe d'Etudes de la Société Européenne d'Athérosclérose a récemment utilisé ce concept. Tout en admettant que le choix de valeurs de "niveaux souhaitables de cholestérol dans le plasma" demeure en quelque sorte arbitraire, la Société Européenne d'Athérosclérose a essayé d'etablir certaines règles d'action de conduite. Les recommandations, avec au départ une limite inférieure à 200 mg/dl (5,2 mmol/l) comprennent une modification du régime alimentaire, la régulation du poids corporel, et vont jusqu'à des traitements d'attaque chez les patients à risques multiples et à niveaux de cholestérol plus élevés (250 mg/dl, 6,5 mmol/l). Nos connaissances sont plus limitées en ce qui concerne le niveau élevé de triglycérides dans le plasma dans les maladies coronariennes: La Société Européenne d'Athérosclérose préconcise, pour la plupart des patients, de prêter attention aux causes sous-jacentes et de suivre un régime alimentaire approprié et de réserver le traitement thérapeutique pour les patients à très haut risque. Jusqu'à présent il n'y a encore que peu de preuves en ce qui concerne le rôle directement protecteur du cholestérol des lipoprotéines de forte densité dans les maladies coronariennes: il ne convient donc pas actuellement de déterminer "les niveaux souhaitables" du cholestérol des lipoproteínes de forte densité; mais, dans l'intérim, la Société Européenne d'Athérosclérose a tendance à croire que des niveaux inférieurs à 35mg/dl (0,9 mmol/l) sont indicateurs de hauts risques et justifient d'un traitement plus vigoureux. On discute ici du choix du traitement thérapeutique à suivre et de la prédominance des facteurs de risques lipidiques, et on donne un programme de démarches à suivre pour les recherches et le traitement de l'hyperlipidémie à différents stades de gravité.

ZUSAMMENFASSUNG

Das Konzept wünschenswerter Plasma-Lipid-Spiegel basiert letzten Endes auf epidemiologischen Verhältnissen; es stammt von longitudinalen Studien, die eine Reihe von Spiegeln erfordern, die mit dem minimalen Risiko der koronaren Herzkrankheit verbunden sind. Dies Konzept ist in letzter Zeit von der Studiengruppe der "Europäischen Atherosklerose-Gesellschaft" (EAS) benutzt worden. Während man erkannte, daß die Auswahl ewaiger Werte als "wünschenswerte Plasma-Cholesterin-Spiegel" etwas willkürlich ist, legt die EAS bestimmte Handlungsgrenzen als Richtlinien fest. Ihre Empfehlungen beginnen mit einem unteren Grenzwert von 200 mg/dl (5,2 mmol/l), einschließlich Diätswechsel und Gewichtskontrolle, und führen auf aggressive Behandlungen bei Patienten mit multipelen Risikofaktoren und höheren Plasma-Cholesterin-Spiegeln (250 mg/dl, 6,5 mmol/l). Weniger ist bekannt über die Rolle von erhöhtem Plasma-Triglyzerid bei koronarer Herzkrankheit—die EAS befürwortet Beachtung zugrundeliegender Ursachen und diätische Maßnahmen für die meisten Patienten, und die Rückstellung der Drogen-Therapie für nur jene Patienten, die ein hohes Risiko darstellen. Bislang ergab sich nur unvollständiger Beweis der "direkten Schutzrolle" von hochdichtem Lipoprotein-(HDL)-Cholesterin bei koronarer Herzkrankheit; daher scheint es im Moment nicht angemessen zu sein, "wünschenswerte Spiegel" des HDL-Cholesterins zuzuteilen; jedoch sind vorläufig Spiegel unter 35 mg/dl (0,9 mmol/l) von der EAS vorgeschlagen, um auf ein hohes Risiko hinzuweisen und um dadurch energischere Therapie zu rechtfertigen. Die Wahl der Therapie und das Überhandnehmen von Lipid Risikofaktoren ist auch diskutiert und eine Liste von Richtlinien ist für die Prüfung und Handhabung von verschiedenen Schweregraden der Hyperlipämie aufgestellt.

SOMMARIO

Il concetto di livelli desiderabili dei lipidi di plasma è basato, in fin dei conti, su relazioni epidemiologiche; deriva da studi longitudinali che indicano una serie di livelli associati con un rischio minimo di malattia coronaria del cuore. Questo concetto è stato recentemente utilizzato da un Gruppo di Studio della Societá Europea dell'Aterosclerosi (SEA). Pur realizzando che la selezione di alcuni valore come "livelli desiderabili del colesterolo" nel plasma sia [una selezione] piuttosto arbitraria, la SEA si prepara a provvedere alcuni limiti di azione come informazioni-guida. Le raccomandazioni, iniziando con un limite basso di 200 mg/dl (5.2 mmol/l) includono un cambiamento di dieta ed un controllo di peso, recandosi verso una cura piú aggressiva per pazienti con multipli fattori a rischio e con piu' alti livelli di colesterolo nel plasma (250 mg/dl, 6.5 mmol/l). C'è una minore conoscenza sul ruolo di aumento del trigliceride nel plasma in malattia coronaria del cuore. La SEA suggerisce attenzione alle cause sottostanti e a misure dietarie, per la maggior parte dei pazienti, riservando l'uso di medicine solo per quelli ad alto rischio. Per ora non c'è sufficiente evidenza di un ruolo diretto-protettivo di colesterolo con lipoproteina ad alta densita ''LAD'' verso la malattia coronaria del cuore; non è quindi appropriato, per il momento, assegnare ''livelli desiderabili'' di colesterolo LAD. Ma provvisoriamente la SEA suggerisce che i livelli sotto i 35/mg/dl (0.9 mmol/l) indicano un rischio alto e quindi una terapia vigorosa verrebbe giustificata. La scelta di cura e la prevalenza di fattori a rischio lipide vengono anche discussi, e viene fornita una serie di informazioni-guida per l'investigazione e l'amministrazione dell'iperlipidemia in gradi diversi di severità.

SUMÁRIO

O conceito de niveis desejáveis de lípidos plasmáticos é baseado em última análise sobre as relações epidemiológicas; é derivado de estudos longitudinais indicando um alcance de níveis associado com o risco mínimo de cardiopátia coronária. Este conceito tem sido utilizado recentemente pelo Grupo de Estudo da Sociedade Européia de Aterosclerose (EAS). Enquanto reconhece que a seleção de quaisquer valores como ''níveis desejáveis de colesterol plasmático'' é um pouco arbitrário, a EAS tenta fornecer certos limites de ação como guia. As recomendações, começando com um limite mais baixo de 200 mg/dl (5,2 mmol/l) abrangem uma mudança de regime alimentar e o contrôle de pêso, levando a tratamento mais agressivo com pacientes que têm fatores múltiplos de risco e níveis de colesterol plasmático mais altos (250 mg/dl. 6,5 mmol/l). Menos sabe-se sobre o papel de níveis elevados de triglicéridos plasmáticos em cardiopátia coronária; a EAS defende prestar atenção às causas latentes, e ao regime alimentar para a maioria dos pacientes, reservando a terapia de remédios para aquêles de alto risco somente. Por enquanto, há evidência insuficiente dum papel diretamente protetor do colesterol de lipoproteína de alta densidade (HDL) em cardiopátia coronária; assim é impróprio atualmente designar ''níveis desejáveis'' de colesterol-HDL; mas provisionalmente, os niveis abaixo de 35 mg/dl (0,9 mmol) são propostos pela EAS para indicar alto risco e assim para justificar uma terapia mais vigorosa. A escolha de terapia e a prevalência de fatores de risco de lípidos são também tratadas, e uma coleção de recomendações é fornecida para a investigação e o contrôle da hiperlipidemia em graus diferentes de severidade.

RESUMEN

El concepto de niveles deseables de lípidos plasmáticos se basa en ciertas relaciones epidemiológicas; se deriva de estudios longitudinales que indican que existe una gama de niveles asociados con el mínimo riesgo de cardiopatía coronaria. Este concepto ha sido empleado recientemente por parte del Grupo de Estudio de la European Atherosclerosis Society—EAS—(Sociedad Europea de Aterosclerosis). Aunque se reconoce que la selección de ciertos valores como "niveles deseables de colesterol plasmático" es algo arbitraria, la EAS desea proporcionar ciertos límites que sirvan de guía. Las recomendaciones—empezando con un límite inferior a 200 mg/dl (5,2 mmol/l)—incluyen cambios en la dieta y control del peso, hasta llegar a un tratamiento más vigoroso en pacientes con múltiples factores de riesgo y niveles más elevados de colesterol en el plasma (250 mg/dl, 6,5 mmol/l). Se sabe menos acerca del papel de los niveles plasmáticos elevados de triglicéridos en el desarrollo de cardiopatía coronaria: la EAS sugiere que se preste atención a las causas subyacentes y cambios en la dieta para la mayoría de pacientes, reservando la farmacoterapia solamente para aquellos que presentan riesgo elevado. Por ahora no existen evidencias suficientes de que el colesterol-HDL ejerza un papel directamente protector en cuanto a la cardiopatía coronaria; de modo que, por ahora no es apropiado asignar "niveles deseables" de colesterol HDL, pero provisionalmente, la EAS sugiere valores debajo de 35 mg/dl (0,9 mmol/l) para indicar un riesgo elevado y justificar así un tratamiento más vigoroso. También se discuten las opciones terapéuticas y la prevalencia de factores lípidos de riesgo, proporcionándose varias guías para la investigación y el manejo de la hiperlipidemia de diversos grados de severidad.

The Role of Cholesterol in Atherosclerosis: New Therapeutic Opportunities, edited by S. M. Grundy and A. G. Bearn, Hanley & Belfus, Inc., Philadelphia.

The 1984 National Institutes of Health Consensus Report on Cholesterol in Light of the Understanding of Lipoproteins and Coronary Heart Disease in 1987

Robert W. Mahley

In 1984, the National Institutes of Health (NIH) sponsored a Consensus Conference on Lowering Blood Cholesterol to Prevent Heart Disease. The 14-member panel, including experts ranging from a public interest attorney to a cardiologist and an experimental pathologist, was asked to hear testimony from a series of speakers versed in various aspects of the lipid-heart disease hypothesis, to review published data, and to prepare a statement on the basis of a series of questions presented to the panel. The major conclusions of the conference are presented below, followed by a consideration of possible modifications of the panel's recommendations on the basis of new insights into the relationship between lipoprotein metabolism and atherogenesis.

The major conclusions and recommendations, and the questions that prompted them, were as follows (for a complete discussion of the panel's report, see reference 1):

1. *Is there a causal relationship between blood cholesterol and coronary heart disease?* The evidence supporting a causal relationship between blood cholesterol levels and coronary heart disease (CHD) comes from a wealth of congruent results from genetic, experimental pathologic, epidemiologic, and intervention studies. The evidence was deemed to be overwhelming.

2. *Can cholesterol reduction prevent or retard coronary heart disease?* Data from a number of studies indicated that a reduction in blood cholesterol levels by various means could retard CHD. The recently completed Coronary Primary Prevention Trial indicated that for each 1% reduction in blood cholesterol levels there was an approximately 2% reduction in CHD.[2,3]

3. *Who should be treated and how?* Blood cholesterol levels above 200 to 230 mg/dl (5.2–6.0 mmol/L) are associated with an increased risk of developing premature CHD. The panel was impressed by the fact that about 50% of the adult population of the United States has these elevated cholesterol levels. It is clear from

various data, including population studies, that a more beneficial blood cholesterol level would be less than 200 mg/dl (5.2 mmol/L). However, it was also evident that realistic normal values, ones that could be attained by most individuals, had to be established.

As shown in Table I, the panel used two sets of values to define those at moderate and high risk. Moderate risk was defined as having blood cholesterol levels greater than 240 mg/dl (6.2 mmol/L) (the 75th percentile) at age 40, whereas high risk was defined as having levels greater than 260 mg/dl or 6.7 mmol/L (the 90th percentile) at that age. It was recommended that individuals with moderate-risk blood cholesterol levels be treated *intensively* by dietary means. Only when there is an inadequate response to an extended period of dietary therapy should drugs be added to the treatment regimen. Individuals with high-risk blood cholesterol levels should also be treated by dietary means, and by drug therapy if the response to diet is inadequate.

The panel stressed that dietary treatment was the first step in lowering blood cholesterol levels for all persons at risk. The guidelines recommended were consistent with recommendations of the American Heart Association and the Atherosclerosis Study Group of the Inter-Society Commission for Heart Disease Resources. The approach should be to lower the consumption of total fat, saturated fat, and cholesterol. In fact, it was stressed that everyone in the United States should be encouraged to consume a diet in which no more than 30% of the caloric intake is from fat and in which cholesterol is limited to 250 to 300 mg per day. An essential consideration was a reduction of saturated fat to 10% or less of total calories.

In my opinion, one of the most important recommendations of the NIH Consensus panel was to encourage the establishment of a National Cholesterol Education Program to educate physicians, other health professionals, and the public concerning cholesterol and heart disease. Under the leadership and direction of the National Heart, Lung and Blood Institute, more than a dozen nonprofit national organizations with interests in cholesterol and heart disease have provided the framework for this program, and various subcommittees are preparing the first phase of the program (see the report by Dr. Claude Lenfant, p. 213). Education at all levels of society is essential if we are to have the impact necessary to modify lifestyle and reduce CHD risk factors.

TABLE I. *Plasma cholesterol levels used in defining adults at moderate and high risk of developing premature coronary heart disease*

Age	Moderage risk	High risk
20–29	>200 mg/dl (5.2 mmol/L)	>220 mg/dl (5.7 mmol/L)
30–39	>220 mg/dl (5.7 mmol/L)	>240 mg/dl (6.2 mmol/L)
40 and over	>240 mg/dl (6.2 mmol/L)	>260 mg/dl (6.7 mmol/L)

Obviously, details of any recommendations require modification as new knowledge and understanding evolve. However, the major conclusions drawn by the panel have been strengthened by new findings since the Consensus Report was written two and a half years ago. At the same time, some modifications of the recommendations should be considered. These modifications include

(1) the inclusion of additional biochemical measurements for assigning CHD risk,

(2) a re-evaluation of lipid values considered to be normal, and

(3) the possible inclusion of genetic indicators for CHD risk.

The 1984 Consensus Panel used the measurement of total plasma cholesterol as the primary indicator of CHD risk. The usefulness of a measurement of high density lipoprotein (HDL) cholesterol was mentioned in the report; however, in 1984 there was concern about the reliability of this biochemical measurement and about its power to indicate risk. Although methodology and standardization of results remain a problem (and a challenge), the predictive value of HDL cholesterol as an independent risk factor has been established, necessitating its inclusion in plasma lipid evaluations for defining CHD risk. Furthermore, there continue to be reasons to lower the values for the upper limit of ''normal'' and to adopt the goal of reducing the plasma cholesterol level for the entire population to the more ideal value of around 180 mg/dl (4.7 mmol/L).

The panel's adoption of moderate- and high-risk cholesterol levels contributed to adjusting the thinking of physicians and scientists and to lowering the upper limits of acceptable plasma cholesterol levels. However, we are now beyond that phase; clearly, the moderate-risk cholesterol levels should be adopted as the upper limit of normal. I would suggest, therefore, that values greater than 240 mg/dl (6.2 mmol/L) at age 40 be considered as placing the individual at high risk and be considered as a level requiring dietary and perhaps drug treatment. Table II lists useful biochemical parameters and general values considered to be the upper limits of normal. These should be used as guidelines, in the clear recognition that other risk factors need to be considered. Physicians and scientists must continue to stress that the primary mode of therapy is diet and that long-term drug treatment should only be used after an ''honest'' attempt to normalize plasma cholesterol by dietary treatment.

Considerable attention is being focused on establishing genetic markers or indicators of CHD risk. Recently, several reports using restriction fragment length polymorphisms (RFLP) have described variations in DNA structure in and around important genes that govern lipoprotein metabolism and that appear to be associated

TABLE II. *Biochemical parameters used in defining adults at risk of developing premature coronary heart disease*

Plasma total cholesterol	>240 mg/dl (6.2 mmol/L)
High density lipoprotein cholesterol	< 35 mg/dl (0.9 mmol/L)
Low density lipoprotein cholesterol	>160 mg/dl (4.1 mmol/L)

with CHD risk.[4-7] These results are exciting; however, they need to be confirmed and extended to larger populations before their value as generalized indicators of CHD risk can be ascertained. In all likelihood, genetic markers, as determined by RFLP, will prove useful in assigning risk.

At the present time, one of the apolipoproteins, apo-E, displays a polymorphism that does correlate with low density lipoprotein (LDL) cholesterol levels and possibly with CHD. Apolipoprotein E occurs in one of three major forms (isoforms E2, E3, or E4) (for review, see refs. 8 and 9). Because the isoforms are the products of alleles of a single gene, there are three homozygous phenotypes (E2/2, E3/3, and E4/4) and three heterozygous phenotypes (E3/2, E4/3, and E4/2). Apolipoprotein E3 is the most common isoform. Apolipoprotein E2 is associated with the lipid disorder type III hyperlipoproteinemia, and this form of apo-E is defective in binding to the apo-B,E(LDL) receptor. However, only a small percentage of individuals with the apo-E2 allele actually develop gross hyperlipidemia, because an additional precipitatory factor other than being homozygous for apo-E2 is necessary. In fact, as will be discussed, individuals with apo-E2 are usually hypolipidemic.[10]

Apolipoproteins E2 and E4 differ from apo-E3 by single amino acid substitutions. The most common form of apo-E2 differs from apo-E3 at amino acid residue 158, where cysteine substitutes for the normally occurring arginine. Apolipoprotein E4 differs from apo-E3 at amino acid residue 112, where arginine substitutes for the normally occurring cysteine. These single substitutions have a profound effect on lipoprotein metabolism. For the present discussion, we will focus our attention on the impact of apo-E polymorphisms on plasma cholesterol and LDL levels.

Several studies have now shown that the apo-E2 allele is associated with low levels of both plasma cholesterol and LDL.[11,12] This is true for apo-E2/2 homozygotes and apo-E3/2 heterozygotes. On the other hand, the apo-E4 allele (apo-E4/4 or apo-E4/3) is associated with higher levels of plasma cholesterol and LDL. Therefore, the apo-E4 allele should be considered a genetic marker associated with increased CHD risk.

Several studies have determined the distribution of the various apo-E phenotypes within the populations of the United States and Europe (for review, see reference 10). As summarized in Table III, the apo-E4/3 and apo-E4/4 phenotypes are present in about 20% and 2% of the population, respectively. Therefore, this mutation,

TABLE III.   *Distribution of apolipoprotein E phenotypes in the population**

Phenotype	%
Apo-E3/3	60%
Apo-E4/3	20%
Apo-E3/2	15%
Apo-E4/4	2%
Apo-E2/2	1%
Apo-E4/2	2%

* Compiled from values reported in Mahley RW, Angelin B.[10]

which is associated with elevated plasma cholesterol and LDL levels, is quite common.

Furthermore, Assmann and associates[13] have studied 570 individuals presenting with a myocardial infarction and demonstrating one- to three-vessel disease by coronary angiography. A subset of these patients was separated into two groups on the basis of apo-E phenotype—those with the apo-E4 allele (E4/4, E4/3) and those with the apo-E2 allele (E2/2, E3/2). As expected, individuals with the apo-E4 allele had plasma cholesterol and LDL cholesterol levels that were respectively 23.6 and 22.2 mg/dl (0.61 and 0.58 mmol/L) higher than those in individuals with the apo-E2 allele. Very interestingly, patients with the apo-E4 allele had their myocardial infarction 4.3 years earlier than did those possessing the apo-E2 allele.

Individuals with the apo-E4 allele are, therefore, at increased risk, should be followed more carefully clinically, and should be instructed to eliminate other CHD risk factors.

In summary, I would conclude that while the conclusions of the 1984 Consensus Report have been further validated by new knowledge, it may be appropriate to modify some of the recommendations. Routine biochemical measurements should be expanded to include HDL cholesterol in order to define the lipid parameters of CHD risk. In addition, I believe that 240 mg/dl (6.2 mmol/L) at age 40 should now be used as the upper limit of normal for plasma cholesterol levels. Furthermore, I would suggest that apo-E phenotyping should be added to biochemical screens predicting CHD risk and that a routine methodology should be developed to accomplish this in clinical laboratories.

REFERENCES

1. Consensus Conference. Lowering blood cholesterol to prevent heart disease. *JAMA* 1985; **253**:2080–2086.
2. Lipid Research Clinics Program. The Lipid Research Clinics Coronary Primary Prevention Trial results. I. Reduction in incidence of coronary heart disease. *JAMA* 1984; **251**:351–364.
3. Lipid Research Clinics Program. The Lipid Research Clinics Coronary Primary Prevention Trial results. II. The relationship of reduction in incidence of coronary heart disease to cholesterol lowering. *JAMA* 1984; **251**:365–374.
4. Law A, Powell LM, Brunt H, *et al*. Common DNA polymorphism within coding sequence of apolipoprotein B gene associated with altered lipid levels. *Lancet* 1986; **1**:1301–1303.
5. Hegele RA, Huang L-S, Herbert PN, *et al*. Apolipoprotein B-gene DNA polymorphisms associated with myocardial infarction. *N Engl J Med* 1986; **315**:1509–1515.
6. Ordovas JM, Schaefer EJ, Salem D, *et al*. Apolipoprotein A-I gene polymorphism associated with premature coronary artery disease and familial hypoalphalipoproteinemia. *N Engl J Med* 1986; **314**:671–677.
7. Talmud PJ, Barni N, Kessling AM, *et al*. Apolipoprotein B gene variants are involved in the determination of serum cholesterol levels: a study in normo- and hyperlipidaemic individuals. *Atherosclerosis* 1987; **67**:81–89.
8. Mahley RW, Innerarity TL, Rall SC Jr, Weisgraber KH. Plasma lipoproteins: apolipoprotein structure and function. *J Lipid Res* 1984; **25**:1277–1294.
9. Mahley RW, Innerarity TL. Lipoprotein receptors and cholesterol homeostasis. *Biochim Biophys Acta* 1983; **737**:197–222.
10. Mahley RW, Angelin B. Type III hyperlipoproteinemia: recent insights into the genetic defect of familial dysbetalipoproteinemia. *Adv Intern Med* 1984; **29**:385–411.

11. Sing CF, Davignon J. Role of the apolipoprotein E polymorphism in determining normal plasma lipid and lipoprotein variation. *Am J Hum Genet* 1985; **37**:268–285.
12. Utermann G, Kindermann I, Kaffarnik H, Steinmetz A. Apolipoprotein E phenotypes and hyperlipidemia. *Hum Genet* 1984; **65**:232–236.
13. Lenzen HJ, Assmann G, Buchwalsky R, Schulte H. Association of apolipoprotein E polymorphism, low-density lipoprotein cholesterol, and coronary artery disease. *Clin Chem* 1986; **32**:778–781.

SUMMARY

In 1984, the National Institutes of Health (NIH) sponsored a Consensus Conference on 'Lowering Blood Cholesterol to Prevent Heart Disease.' This chapter examines the major conclusions and recommendations of the Consensus Report and assesses whether, in 1987, their findings are refuted or validated by recent research. The Consensus Report concludes that: 1) there is overwhelming evidence of a causal relationship between blood cholesterol levels and coronary heart disease (CHD); 2) for every 1% reduction in blood cholesterol levels there is an approximately 2% reduction in CHD; and 3) blood cholesterol levels above 200–230 mg/dl (5.2–6.0 mmol/L) are associated with an increased risk of developing premature CHD. It was recommended that individuals with moderate-risk blood cholesterol levels (greater than 240 mg/dl or 6.2 mmol/L) should be treated intensively by dietary means. Those in the high-risk group (blood cholesterol greater than 260 mg/dl or 6.7 mmol/L) should also be treated by dietary means, and by drug therapy if response to diet is inadequate. One of the most important recommendations was to encourage the establishment of a National Cholesterol Education Program to educate physicians, other health professionals, and the public about cholesterol and heart disease. Since 1984, the major conclusions of the panel have been validated, but some modifications of their recommendations should be considered, namely: the inclusion of additional biochemical measurements for assigning CHD risk (e.g., HDL cholesterol), re-evaluation of lipid values considered to be normal, and the possible inclusion of genetic indicators for CHD risk. The chapter looks at some recent reports using restriction fragment length polymorphisms (RFLP) to describe variations in DNA structure in genes governing lipoprotein metabolism that appear to be associated with CHD risk. The finding that the apo-E4 allele (apo-E4/4 homozygotes or apo-E4/3 heterozygotes) is associated with higher levels of plasma cholesterol and LDL than the apo-E2 allele (apo-E2/2 homozygotes and apo-E3/2 heterozygotes) is also discussed.

RÉSUMÉ

En 1984, l'Institut National de la Santé à Washington (NIH) a sponsorisé une Conférence de Consensus intitulée ''Comment abaisser le taux de cholestérol afin d'éviter les maladies coronariennes.'' Dans ce chapitre on examine les principales conclusions et recommandations du rapport du Consensus et on évalue si, en 1987, leurs découvertes sont réfutées ou confirmées par les derniers travaux de recherche. Le rapport du Consensus conclut: 1) qu'il est absolument incontestable qu'il y a un rapport causal entre les niveaux de cholestérol dans le sang et les maladies coronariennes; 2) que pour une réduction de 1% du niveau de cholestérol dans le sang il y a une réduction d'environ 2% des maladies coronariennes; 3) et que les niveaux de cholestérol supérieurs à 200–230 mg/dl (5,2–6 mmol/l) sont liés à des risques accrus d'un développement prématuré de maladie coronarienne. Il a donc été recommandé que les personnes ayant un taux de cholestérol modérément élevé (supérieur à 240 mg/dl ou 6,2 mmol/l) soient soumises à un régime alimentaire approprié. Les patients faisant partie du groupe à haut risque (niveau de cholestérol supérieur à 260 mg/dl ou 6,7 mmol/l) devraient aussi suivre un régime alimentaire et si cette mesure s'avère insuffisante être alors soumis à un traitement thérapeutique. Une recommandation qui était très importante était d'encourager la création d'un programme national de formation et d'enseignement sur le cholestérol et les maladies cardiaques afin d'instruire les médecins, les professionnels de la santé et le public. Depuis 1984 les principales conclusions de ce Consensus ont été confirmées, mais il faudrait envisager quelques modifications à leurs recommandations, à savoir: l'inclusion d'autres paramètres biochimiques pour déterminer les risques de maladies coronariennes (par exemple le cholestérol des lipoprotéines de forte densité), la réévaluation du taux de normalisation des lipides, et peut-être aussi l'inclusion des facteurs génétiques qui entrent en cause dans le développement des maladies coronariennes. Ce chapitre examine quelques études récentes utilisant des polymorphismes de la longueur des fragments de restriction pour décrire les variations dans la structure du DNA des gènes régissant le métabolisme des lipoprotéines qui semble être lié aux risques de maladies coronariennes. On discute aussi la découverte que l'apo-E4 allele (apo-E4/4 homozygotes ou apo-E4/3 hétérozygotes) est lié à des niveaux plus élevés de cholestérol dans le plasma et de lipoprotéines de faible densité que l'apo-E2 allele (apo-E2/2 homozygotes et apo-E3/2 hétérozygotes).

ZUSAMMENFASSUNG

Im Jahre 1984 veranstalteten die ''Nationalen Gesundheits-Institute'' (National Institutes of Health) (NIH) eine Übereinstimmungskonferenz mit dem Thema ''Erniedrigung des Blut-Cholesterins zur Verhinderung von Herzkrankheiten.'' Dieses Kapitel überprüft die Hauptschlußfolgerung und Empfehlungen der Übereinstimmungskonferenz und überprüft, ob im Jahre 1987 ihre Befunde durch die Forschung jüngeren Datums zurückgewiesen oder bestätigt werden. Der Übereinstimmungsbericht beschloß, daß (1) es gibt überwältige Beweise der ursächlichen Beziehungen zwischen Blut-Cholesterin-Spiegeln und CHD; (2) für jede 1%ige Erniedrigung der Blut-Cholesterin-Spiegeln ergab sich eine ungefähr 2%ige Erniedrigung der CHD; und (3) Blut-Cholesterin-Spiegel über 200–230 mg/dl (5,2–6,0 mmol/l) sind mit einem erhöhtem Risiko für die vorzeitige Entwicklung von CHD verbunden. Es wurde vorgeschlagen, daß Personen, die ein mäßiges Risiko in Bezug auf Blut-Cholesterin-Spiegel (größer als 240 mg/dl oder 6,2 mmol/l) haben, intensiv durch diätetische Mittel behandelt werden sollen. Jene in der hohen Risikogruppe (Blut-Cholesterin mehr als 260 mg/dl oder 6,7 mmol/l) sollen ebenfalls durch diätetische Maßnahmen behandelt werden, und durch Drogentherapie falls die Reaktionen auf Diät unzureichend ist. Die wichtigste Empfehlung war die Ermutigung zur Gründung eines ''Nationalen Cholesterin-Ausbildungsprogrammes'' zur Unterrichtung der Ärzte oder anderer Fachkräfte des Gesundheitswesens und der Öffentlichkeit über Cholesterin und Herzkrankheiten. Seit 1984 sind die Hauptbeschlüsse des Ausschußes als gültig erklärt worden, aber einige Modifikationen ihrer Empfehlungen sollten in Erwägung bezogen werden, im besonderen die Einbeziehung von weiteren biochemischen Maßstaben zur Zuteilung des CHD-Risikos (z. B., HDL-Cholesterin), nochmalige Untersuchung der Lipidwerte, die als normal angesehen werden, und die mögliche Einschließung von genetischen Indikatoren für CHD-Risiken. Das Kapitel überprüft einige neuerliche Berichte, die Polymorphismen der Länge der Einschränkungsfragmente (RFLP) benutzen, um Variationen in der DNA-Struktur von Lipoproteinstoffwechsel-regulierenden Genen, die mit dem CHD-Risiko verbunden zu sein scheinen, zu beschreiben. Die Entdeckung, daß das Apo-E4 Allel (Apo-E4/4 Homozygoten oder Apo-E4/3 Heterozygoten) mit höheren Spiegeln des Plasma-Cholesterins und LDL als das Apo-E2 Allel (Apo-E2/2 Homozygoten und Apo-E3/2 Heterozygoten) verbunden ist, ist auch erörtert.

SOMMARIO

Nel 1984, l'Istituto Nazionale della Sanità (INS) patrocinò una Conferenza di Consenso: ''Abbassare il livello del colesterolo nel sangue per prevenire la malattia del cuore.'' Questo capitolo esamina le conclusioni piú importanti e le raccomandazioni del Rapporto del Consenso e valuta se, nel 1987, le loro scoperte siano rifiutate o validate da ricerche recenti. Il Rapporto Consenso conclude che (1) c'è enorme evidenza di una relazione causale fra i livelli del colesterolo nel sangue e la Malattia Coronaria del Cuore (MCC); (2) per la riduzione di 1% nei livelli del colesterolo nel sangue c'era approssimativamente una riduzione del 2% nella MCC; e (3) i livelli del colesterolo nel sangue sopra 200–230 mg/dl (5.2–6.0 mml/l) sono associate con maggiore rischio per lo sviluppo di prematura MCC. È stato raccomandato che quegli individui con livelli di colesterolo nel sangue a rischio moderato, (piú di 240 mg/dl o 6.2 mmol/l) debbano essere intensamente curati con mezzi dietetici. Coloro i quali appartengono al gruppo di alto rischio (con colesterolo nel sangue piú di 260 mg/dl o 6.7 mmol/l dovrebbero) essere anche curati con mezzi dietetici, e con medicine se i risultati della dieta siano inadequati. Le raccomandazioni piú importanti sono state quelle di incoraggiare la fondazione del Programma Nazionale d'Istruzione sul Colesterolo (PNIC), d'istruire medici, altri professionisti e il pubblico in quanto al colesterolo e alla Malattia del Cuore. Dal 1984, le maggiori conclusioni dei partecipanti sono state validate, ma bisogna considerare alcune modifiche sulle loro raccomandazioni, in altre parole: l'aggiunta di altre misure biochimicha per l'assegnazione del rischio della MCC (per esempio il colesterolo LAD), rievalutazione dei valori del lipide anteriormente considerati normali, e la possibile aggiunta d'indici genetici per il rischio della MCC. Il capitolo studia alcuni rapporti recenti che usano polimorfismi della lunghezza dei frammenti de restrizione (PLFR) per descrivere cambiamenti nella struttura DNA nei geni che controllano il metabolismo della lipoproteina che sembrano essere in associazione con il rischio della MCC. La scoperta che l'Apo-E 4 allele (apo-E 4/4 omozigoti o apo-E 4/3 eterozigoti) è associato con livelli piú alti di colesterolo nel plasma e di LBD che l'apo-E 2 allele (apo-E 2/2 omozigoti e apo-E 3/2 eterozigoti) viene anche discussa.

SUMÁRIO

Em 1984, os "National Institutes of Health (NIH)" (os Institutos Nacionais de Saude) patrocinaram uma Conferência de Consenso sobre "Baixar o colesterol no sangue para evitar doença do coração." Este capítulo examina as principais conclusões e recomendações do Relatório de Consenso, e avalia se, em 1987, os seus descobrimentos são refutados ou confirmados por pesquisa recente. O Relatório de Consenso determina que (1) há evidência esmagadora duma relação causal entre níveis de colesterol no sangue e cardiopátia coronária (CHD); (2) por cada redução de 1% nos níveis de colesterol no sangue havia uma redução de aproximadamente 2% em CHD; e (3) os níveis de colesterol no sangue acima de 200–230 mg/dl (5,2–6,0 mmol/l) são associados com um risco aumentado de contrair CHD prematura. Foi recomendado que as pessoas com níveis de colesterol no sangue de risco moderado (mais do que 240 mg/dl ou 6,2 mmol/l) deviam ser tratadas intensivamente com um regime alimentar. Aquêles no grupo de alto risco (colesterol no sangue maior do que 260 mg/dl ou 6,7 mmol/l) deviam também ser tratados com um regime alimentar e com uma terapia farmacológica se a reação ao regime alimentar é inadequada. A recomendação mais importante foi de encorajar o estabelecimento dum Programa Nacional de Instrução sobre Colesterol para instruir os médicos, outros profissionais da saúde e o público sobre o colesterol e doença cardíaca. Desde 1984, as conclusões principais deste concelho têm sido confirmadas, mas algumas modificações das suas recomendações devem ser consideradas, isto é: a inclusão de mais medição bioquímica para avaliar o risco de CHD (e.g., colesterol HDL), uma re-avaliação de valôres de lípidos considerados a serem normais, e a possível inclusão de indicadores genéticos para o risco de CHD. O capítulo examina alguns relatórios recentes usando polimorfismos do comprimento dos fragmentos de restrição (RFLP) para descrever as variações na estrutura de DNA nos genes que governam o metabolismo das lipoproteínas que parece ser associado com risco de CHD. A descoberta que o allele Apo-E4 (apo-E4/4 homocigotos ou apo-E4/3 heterocigotos) é associado com níveis mais altos de colesterol plasmático e LDL do que o allele Apo-E2 (homocigotos apo E2/2 e heterocigotos apo E3/2) é também discutido.

RESUMEN

En 1984 el National Institutes of Health—NIH—(Institutos Nacionales de Salud) auspició una conferencia de consenso con el tema "Disminución de los niveles de colesterol para prevenir las enfermedades del corazón." Se examinan las conclusiones y recomendaciones más importantes del informe de la conferencia y se evalúa si, en 1987, sus conclusiones han sido desmentidas o confirmadas por las investigaciones más recientes. El informe de la conferencia concluye que: (1) existen evidencias sustanciales de una relación causal entre los niveles séricos de colesterol y CHD; (2) para cada reducción de 1% en los niveles de colesterol sérico había una reducción de aproximadamente 2% en CHD; y (3) niveles de colesterol sérico superiores a 200–230 mg/dl (5,2–6,0 mmol/l) se hallan asociados con un incremento en el riesgo de desarrollo prematuro de CHD. Se recomendó que los individuos con niveles séricos moderados de colesterol (superiores a 240 mg/dl o 6,2 mmol/l) deben recibir un tratamiento dietético intensivo. Aquéllos que se hallan en el grupo de alto riesgo (niveles séricos de colesterol superiores a 260 mg/dl o 6,7 mmol/l) también deben recibir un tratamiento dietético, y recibir tratamiento farmacológico si la respuesta al tratamiento dietético no es satisfactoria. La recomendación más importante fue apoyar el establecimiento de un ''Programa nacional de educación sobre el colesterol'' para informar a los médicos, otros profesionales de la salud y el público acerca del colesterol y las cardiopatías. Desde 1984 las conclusiones más importantes del panel han sido corroboradas, pero deben considerarse algunas modificaciones a sus recomendaciones: la inclusión de medidas bioquímicas adicionales para asignar el riesgo de CHD (por ejemplo, colesterol HDL), reevaluación de los valores lípidos considerados normales y la posible inclusión de indicadores genéticos del riesgo de CHD. Se examinan estudios recientes en que se emplearon polimorfismos de restricción de longitud fraccionaria (RFLP) para describir variaciones estructurales del DNA en los genes que controlan el metabolismo de las lipoproteínas y que parecen estar asociados con el riesgo de CHD. El descubrimiento de que el alelo apo-E4 (apo-E4/4 homocigotos o apo-E4/3 heterocigotos) se halla asociado con niveles más altos de colesterol sérico y LDL que el alelo apo-E2 (apo-E2/2 homocigotos y apo-E3/2 heterocigotos) también se discute.

The Role of Cholesterol in Atherosclerosis:
New Therapeutic Opportunities, edited by S. M. Grundy
and A. G. Bearn, Hanley & Belfus, Inc., Philadelphia.

Atherosclerosis and Lipid Metabolism in the Japanese

Hiroo Imura and Kinsuke Tsuda

The role and importance of various risk factors in the pathogenesis of atherosclerosis are not fully understood and so studies on the geographic differences in atherosclerotic diseases are of importance. It is well-known that coronary heart disease is much less common in Japan than in North American and European countries. Since atherosclerosis is the major pathogenetic factor in coronary heart disease, it is of interest to compare differences in atherogenic factors, in particular, lipid metabolism, in Japan and Western countries. The aim of this chapter is to review some characteristic features and changes of atherosclerosis in Japan in relation to lipid metabolism.

CHANGING PATTERNS OF ATHEROSCLEROTIC VASCULAR DISEASES IN JAPAN

Evaluation of the presence and severity of atherosclerosis by non-invasive methods is difficult, but changing patterns of diseases mainly due to atherosclerotic lesions can be assessed by the mortality due to vascular diseases. Figure 1 depicts changes in mortality rates of various heart diseases, based on the report of the Ministry of Health and Welfare in Japan. Although the death rate from rheumatic heart disease has gradually decreased, the death rate from ischemic heart disease has increased considerably over the past 35 years.[1] An increase in population age might contribute to this trend, but the age-adjusted death rate also shows an increase. Some types of coronary heart disease should probably be included with other heart diseases in Figure 1, due to uncertainty of diagnosis. Even when this is taken into account, however, it is evident that the death rate from ischemic heart disease is much less in Japan than in Western countries, indicating differences in risk factors for coronary heart disease.

Atherosclerotic lesions also cause cerebrovascular disease. Figure 2 illustrates changes in mortality from cerebrovascular disease during the past 30 years in Japan. The number of deaths from cerebral hemorrhage has decreased considerably in both males and females, whereas the death rate of cerebral infarction has been considerably increased.[2] Differential diagnosis between hemorrhage and infarction is no

185

IMURA ET AL.

CHANGES OF DEATH RATES OF VARIOUS HEART
DISEASES IN JAPAN

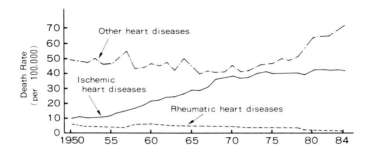

DEATH RATES OF VARIOUS HEART DISEASES
IN DIFFERENT COUNTRIES

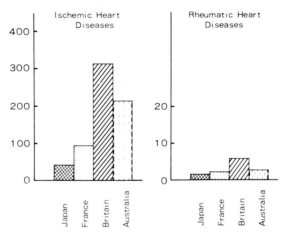

FIG. 1. Changes of death rates of various heart diseases in the past 30 years in Japan (upper panel: reference 1) and comparison of mortalities from ischemic and rheumatic heart diseases in different countries (lower panel: World Health Statistics Annual 1984–1985).

longer difficult, and this trend is evident following the introduction of computer-assisted tomography and in autopsy cases. Despite the decrease in mortality from cerebral hemorrhage, the total death rate of cerebrovascular diseases corrected for background population is, though significantly decreased, still higher in Japan than in Western countries.[2]

Murai et al.[3] reported that there are differences between the two types of cerebral infarction. The infarction of perforating arteries occurs in elderly individuals, is not related to altered lipid metabolism, and is caused by arteriosclerosis of small arteries. Infarction of cortical arteries, on the other hand, occurs in relatively young people who have high levels of low density lipoprotein (LDL) cholesterol and/or

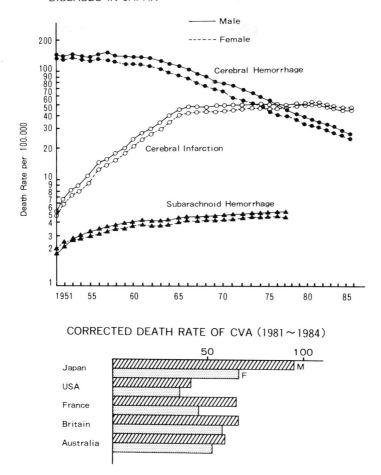

CHANGES OF DEATH RATES OF CEREBRAL VASCULAR DISEASES IN JAPAN

CORRECTED DEATH RATE OF CVA (1981~1984)

FIG. 2.   Changes of death rate of cerebrovascular diseases in approximately 30 years in Japan (upper panel: reference 1) and comparison of age-adjusted death rates of cerebrovascular diseases in some countries (lower panel: World Health Statistics Annual 1979–1980).

low levels of high density lipoprotein (HDL) cholesterol and is caused by atherosclerosis of moderate-size vessels. These findings suggest atherosclerotic lesions in the cerebral arteries are of importance in at least some patients with cerebral infarction.

CHANGES OF SERUM LIPIDS IN JAPAN

The remarkable changes in the mortality rates of coronary heart disease and cerebral infarction that have occurred in Japan in the past 30 years indicate altered risk factors for these diseases. Although several environmental factors are implicated in the development of atherosclerosis, altered lipid metabolism is considered to have contributed significantly to the development of atherosclerotic lesions.

A multi-institutional study was performed in Japan to determine normal serum cholesterol levels in 1960, 1970 and 1980.[4] As shown in Figure 3, the 1980 study showed that serum total cholesterol levels increased with age except during the first decade, reaching the peak in the seventh decade.[4] The mean serum cholesterol level in each generation was 10–15 mg/dl (0.2–0.4 mmol/L) higher than in the 1970 study. Serum triglyceride levels also increased with age and reached the maximum at the seventh decade. Although serum triglyceride was measured for the first time

Changes in serum total cholesterol levels of Japanese in the past 20 years.

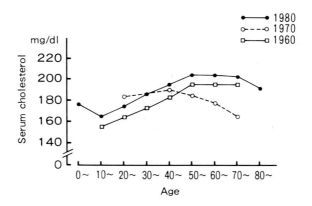

Changes in serum triglyceride levels of Japanese in the past 10 years.

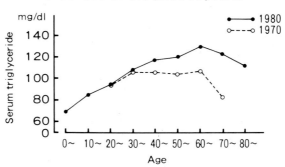

FIG. 3. Changes in serum total cholesterol and triglyceride levels of Japanese in the past 20 and 10 years, respectively. (Redrawn with permission from Sekimoto *et al. Jap Circ J* 1983; **47**:1351–8.[4])

in the 1970 study, the values in 1980 were 10–20 mg/dl (0.3–0.5 mmol/L) higher than those in 1970 in subjects after the fifth decade.[4] These results indicate that serum lipid levels have changed considerably in the Japanese during the past 20–30 years.

In 1960 serum cholesterol levels in Japanese were significantly lower than those of Western people over the corresponding period.[5,6] During the past 20 years, however, serum cholesterol levels have decreased in the United States,[7] whereas they have increased in Japan and are now approaching the present levels in Western countries. Such a change in plasma cholesterol is in agreement with the increase in death rates from atherosclerotic vascular diseases.

Recent advances in our understanding of lipoprotein metabolism have enabled us to study lipoproteins in serum and their relationship to the development of atherosclerosis. In Japanese studies, lipoprotein-cholesterol contents were also shown to change with age.[8] LDL-cholesterol increases gradually from the fourth decade in both sexes, but nevertheless the levels were lower than those in the United States.[9] On the other hand, HDL-cholesterol decreases after the sixth decade in both sexes in Japan, whereas it is almost unchanged with age in the United States.[9] The reason for this decrease in HDL-cholesterol in aged Japanese is still unknown. Low incidence of coronary heart disease in this generation in Japan as compared with Western countries may be explained by lower LDL-cholesterol.

The relationship between atherosclerosis and altered lipid metabolism has been studied also in Japan. Low HDL-cholesterol, especially low HDL_2-cholesterol, in association with high LDL-cholesterol was reported to be present more frequently in patients with coronary heart disease than in control subjects,[10] as in Western countries.[11] The atherogenic index is, therefore, high in these patients. A similarly high atherogenic index was found also in patients with infarction of cortical arteries in the brain.[3] Elevated serum levels of Lp(a), a lipoprotein fraction identified by an immunoprecipitation method, was found more frequently in coronary heart disease and cerebral infarction,[12] as in Western people.[13] These results suggest that altered lipid metabolism associated with atherosclerotic diseases is not fundamentally different in Japanese from that in Caucasians.

DISCUSSION

Several factors have been implicated in the development of atherosclerosis.[14] Some factors, such as heredity, aging and sex cannot be corrected, but most of them are correctable. Among these correctable factors, the importance of altered lipid metabolism has been pointed out by many clinical, epidemiological and experimental studies. Japanese experience with an increase of coronary heart disease and cerebral infarction in parallel with an increase in serum cholesterol is concordant with the concept that altered lipid metabolism plays an important pathogenetic role in atherosclerosis.

The major factor that has caused an increase of serum cholesterol in Japan in the past 20 to 30 years is considered to be a change in diet. Figure 4 shows changes of intake of total fat and animal fat in Japanese according to the study of the Ministry of Health and Welfare in Japan. Although total caloric intake increased about 10% in the past 20 years, an increase in fat intake was more than doubled. In particular, the increase in animal fat rich in saturated fatty acids was very remarkable. Such a change in diet seems to be responsible for the increase of serum cholesterol in Japanese.

Even though serum cholesterol levels in Japanese have now approached those in Americans, the incidence of coronary heart diseases is still considerably lower. This can be explained by several possibilities:

(1) Factors other than serum cholesterol play roles in the development of coronary heart disease—for example, hypertension, smoking and life style.
(2) It is possible that the development of diseases due to atherosclerosis requires a long latent period after the elevation of serum cholesterol. It is known that mild change in blood vessels, such as fatty streak and fibrous plaque, begin in early life, and this suggests gradual development of atherosclerotic changes that lead to clinical manifestations.

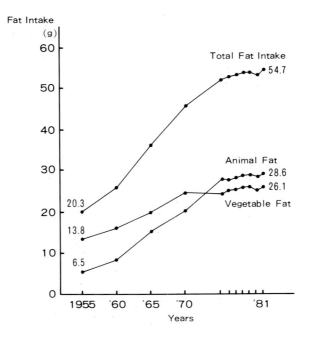

FIG. 4. Changes of fat intake of Japanese during the 25 years period, as expressed per person per day (report on nutrition of Japanese, Ministry of Health and Welfare).

(3) Genetic differences must be considered also. Several genetic markers have been reported recently that are involved in coronary heart disease or hyperlipidemia. Restriction fragment length polymorphisms (RFLPs) of the insulin gene, apolipoprotein AI-CIII gene, A-II gene, B gene and E gene are reported to be associated with hyperlipidemia or coronary heart diseases. Racial differences were found in RFLPs of the insulin gene and apolipoprotein AI-CIII gene.[15,16] An association of certain phenotypes of apolipoprotein E (E4/E4) with hyperlipidemia was also found and possible racial differences were also noted.[17,18] Polymorphisms in apolipoprotein genes or apolipoprotein phenotypes may cause differences in lipoprotein metabolism.

CONCLUSIONS

Genetic disposition may be an important factor in hyperlipidemia and coronary heart disease. However, the striking changes in serum cholesterol levels and mortality from atherosclerotic diseases observed in Japan in the past 30 years indicate the importance of environmental factors, especially diet, in the pathogenesis of atherosclerosis.

REFERENCES

1. Ministry of Health and Welfare. *Vital Statistics 1985, Japan.* 1985; 264–267.
2. Hirota Y. Epidemiology of stroke. *Brain Nerve* 1982; **34**:437–92.
3. Murai A, Tanaka T, Miyahara T, Kameyama M. Lipoprotein abnormalities in the pathogenesis of cerebral infarction and transient ischemic attacks. *Stroke* 1981; **12**:167–72.
4. Sekimoto H, Goto Y, Naito C, *et al.* Changes of serum total cholesterol and triglyceride levels in normal subjects in Japan in the past twenty years. *Jap Circ J* 1983; **47**:1351–8.
5. Keys A, Mickelsen O, Miller EO, Hayes ER, Todd RL. The concentration of cholesterol in the blood serum of normal man and its relation to age. *J Clin Invest* 1950; **29**:1347–53.
6. Lund E, Geill T, Andresen PH. Serum-cholesterol in normal subjects in Denmark. *Lancet* 1961; **2**:1383–5.
7. The Lipid Research Clinics Program Epidemiology Committee: Plasma lipid distributions in selected North American populations: The Lipid Research Clinics Program Prevalance Study. *Circulation* 1979; **60**:427–39.
8. Itakura H. Lipoprotein and its fractions. *Jap J Clin Med* 1985; **43**(**Suppl.**):333–9.
9. Heiss G, Johnson NJ, Reiland S, Davis CE, Tyroler HA. The epidemiology of plasma high-density lipoprotein cholesterol levels. The Lipid Research Clinics Program Prevalence Study. *Circulation* 1980; **62**(Suppl.IV):116–36.
10. Itakura H. Lipid metabolism and coronary sclerosis. Diagnosis and treatment. 1986; **74**:1557–62.
11. Miller NE. Association of high-density lipoprotein subclasses and apolipoproteins with ischemic heart disease and coronary atherosclerosis. *Am Heart J* 1987; **113**:589–97.
12. Murai A, Miyahara T, Fujimoto N, Matsuda M, Kameyama M. Lp(a) lipoprotein as a risk factor for coronary heart disease and cerebral infarction. *Atherosclerosis* 1986; **59**:197–204.
13. Frick MH, Dahlen G, Bergt K, Valle M, Hekali P. Serum lipids in angiographically assessed coronary atherosclerosis. *Chest* 1978; **73**:62–5.
14. Pollak OJ. Risk factors for atherosclerosis in proper perspective. *Atherosclerosis* 1987; **63**:257–62.
15. Takeda J, Seino Y, Fukumoto H, *et al.* The polymorphism linked to the human insulin gene: its lack of association with either IDDM or NIDDM in Japanese. *Acta Endocrinol* 1986; **113**:268–71.

16. Rees A, Stocks J, Paul H, Ohbuchi Y, Galton D. Haplotypes identified by DNA polymorphisms at the apolipoprotein A-I and C-III loci and hypertriglyceridemia. A study in a Japanese population. *Hum Genet* 1986; **72**:168–71.
17. Utermann G, Pruin N, Steinmetz A. Polymorphism of apolipoprotein E. III. Effect of a single polymorphic gene locus on plasma lipid levels in man. *Clin Genet* 1979; **15**:63–72.
18. Eto M, Watanabe K, Ishii K. A racial difference in apolipoprotein E allele frequencies between the Japanese and Caucasian populations. *Clin Genet* 1986; **30**:422–7.

SUMMARY

Coronary heart disease (CHD) is much less common in Japan than in North America and European countries. Since atherosclerosis is the major pathogenetic factor in coronary heart disease, it is of value to compare differences in atherogenic factors, in particular lipid metabolism, between Japan and Western countries. This chapter reviews some of the characteristic features and changes of atherosclerosis in Japan over the last 35 years in relation to lipid metabolism. A study of the mortality rates from various heart diseases in Japan shows that the rate from ischemic heart disease has increased over the past 35 years, but it is still much less than in Western countries. By contrast, the total death rate from cerebrovascular disease in Japan has significantly decreased over the same period, but the figure is still higher than in Western countries. Altered lipid metabolism has probably contributed significantly to the development of atherosclerotic lesions and hence to the mortality rates from CHD. Since 1960 in Japan, there have been increases in serum total cholesterol and triglyceride levels, and serum cholesterol levels are now approaching those seen in the United States. A change in diet among the Japanese is thought to be a major factor contributing to the increase in serum cholesterol. Their consumption of fat has more than doubled over the past 20 years, with a particularly marked increase in saturated animal fats. Reasons why the incidence of CHD is still considerably lower in Japan than in the United States, even though the serum cholesterol levels are now quite similar, are examined. Other risk factors, such as life-style, hypertension and cigarette smoking, may be relevant. A latent period may be required before the development of atherosclerosis. Genetic differences, with particular reference to restriction fragment length polymorphisms of apolipoprotein genes, are also discussed.

RÉSUMÉ

Les maladies coronariennes sont beaucoup moins courantes au Japon qu'en Amérique du Nord et en Europe. Etant donné que l'athérosclérose représente le principal facteur pathogénétique des maladies coronariennes, il est important de comparer les différences de facteurs athérogéniques, en particulier le métabolisme des lipides, entre le Japon et les pays de l'Ouest. Dans ce chapitre on examine quelques traits caractéristiques et quelques changements de l'athérosclérose survenus au Japon, en ce qui concerne le métabolisme des lipides, ces 35 dernières années. Une étude des taux de mortalité due à diverses maladies cardiaques au

Japon montre que le taux des maladies cardiaques ischémiques a augmenté ces 35 dernières années, mais il est encore beaucoup moins élevé que celui des pays occidentaux. Par contre, le taux global de mortalité due aux maladies cérébrovasculaires au Japon a considérablement diminué au cours de la même période, mais les chiffres sont toujours beaucoup plus élevés que ceux des pays occidentaux. Les changements dans le métabolisme des lipides ont largement contribué au développement de lésions athérosclérotiques, et de là aux taux de mortalités dues aux maladies coronariennes. Depuis 1960 il y a eu au Japon des accroissements des niveaux de cholestérol et de triglycérides et les niveaux de cholestérol atteignent aujourd'hui presque ceux des Etats-Unis. On pense que cet accroissement du taux de cholestérol chez les Japonais est principalement dû à un changement dans les habitudes alimentaires. La consommation de graisses, et en particulier de graisses animales saturées, a plus que doublé ces 20 dernières années au Japon. Les niveaux de cholestérol étant maintenant presque semblables à ceux des Etats-Unis on examine pourquoi les incidences de maladies coronariennes sont moins fréquentes au Japon qu'aux Etats-Unis. D'autres facteurs de risque, tels le mode de vie, l'hypertension et le tabac peuvent jouer un rôle important. On examine aussi les différences génétiques surtout en ce qui concerne les polymorphismes de la longueur des fragments de restriction.

ZUSAMMENFASSUNG

Koronare Herzkrankheit (CHD) ist in Japan viel weniger häufig als in Nordamerika oder in den europäischen Ländern. Da Atherosklerose der pathogenetische Hauptfaktor bei koronarer Herzkrankheit ist, ist es von Wert, die Unterschiede der atherogenen Faktoren, insbesondere den Lipidstoffwechsel, zwischen Japan und den westlichen Ländern zu vergleichen. Dieses Kapitel gibt einen Überblick über einige der charakteristischen Merkmale und der Veränderungen der Atherosklerose in Japan über den Zeitraum der letzten 35 Jahren in Bezug auf Lipidstoffwechsel. Eine Studie der Sterblichkeitsraten verursacht durch verschiedene Herzkrankheiten in Japan zeigt, daß die Rate von ischämischen Herzkrankheiten während der letzen 35 Jahre gestiegen ist, aber sie ist trotzdem wesentlich niedriger als in westlichen Ländern. Im Vergleich dazu ist die totale Todesrate durch zerebrovaskulare Krankheiten über dieselbe Zeitperiode in Japan erheblich gesunken, aber die Anzahl ist immer noch höher als die in westlichen Ländern. Veränderter Lipidstoffwechsel hat wesentlich zur Entstehung von atherosklerotischen Läsionen, und somit zu den Sterblichkeitsraten durch CHD beigetragen. Seit 1960 hat man in Japan Erhöhungen der Gesamtserum-Cholesterin- und Triglyzerid-Spiegel vorgefunden, und Serum-Cholesterin Spiegel nähern sich jetzt denen der Vereinigten Staaten. Ein Wechsel in der Diät unter den Japanern scheint ein Hauptfaktor zu sein, der zur Erhöhung des Serum-Cholesterins beiträgt. Ihr Konsum von Fett hat sich über die letzten 20 Jahre mehr als verdopplelt, mit besonders auffälliger Zunahme der gesättigten Tierfette. Gründe, die erklären können, warum das Vorkommen des CHD in Japan immer noch beachtlich niedriger ist als in den Vereinigten Staaten, sind geprüft, obwohl die Serum-Cholesterin-Spiegel jetzt ziemlich ähnlich scheinen. Andere Risikofaktoren, wie z.B. Lebenstil, Hypertension und das Rauchen von Zigaretten könnten von Bedeutung sein. Genetische Unterschiede mit besonderem Bezug auf Polymorphismen der Länge der Einschränkungsfragmente sind ebenfalls erörtert.

SOMMARIO

La malattia coronaria del cuore (MCC) è molto meno comune in Giappone che nell'America del Nord e nelle nazioni europee. Siccome l'aterosclerosi è il principale fattore patogenico nella malattia coronaria, è importante paragonare le differenze dei fattori aterogenici, particolarmente del metabolismo lipide fra il Giappone e le nazione dell'Ovest. Questo capitolo riassume alcune caratteristiche e alcuni cambiamenti dell'aterosclerosi nel Giappone, durante gli scorsi 35 anni, in relazione al metabolismo lipido. Uno studio sulle varie malattie del cuore nel Giappone dimostra che la percentuale sulla malattia ischemica del cuore è aumentata negli ultimi 35 anni, ma è ancora molto meno che nei paesi dell'Ovest. In contrasto, in Giappone, la percentuale dei morti per cerebro-vascolopatia è diminiuta durante lo stesso periodo di tempo, mentre nei paesi dell'ovest la percentuale è molto piú alta. Un cambiamento al metabolismo lipido ha contribuito immensamente allo sviluppo di lesioni ateroscolerotiche e quindi all'alta mortalità per MCC. In Giappone, dal 1960, c'è stato un'aumento nei livelli del colesterolo totale del siero e della trigliceride, adesso i livelli del colesterolo del siero si stanno avvicinando a quelli degli Stati Uniti. Si pensa che un cambiamento nella dieta fra il popolo giapponese abbia contribuito all'aumento del colesterolo del siero. Il consumo di grassi è piú che raddoppiato negli ultimi 20 anni, con un'aumento specifico nei grassi saturati d'animali. Vengono esaminate le ragioni per cui nel Giappone la MCC è tuttavia meno che negli Stati Uniti, sebbene i livelli del colesterolo del siero ne siano ormai quasi uguali. Si pensa che altri rischi, come il tipo di vita, l'ipertensione o il fumare potrebbero essere rilevanti. Vengono discusse le differenze genetiche, con un particolare accenno ai polimorfismi della lunghezza dei frammenti di restrizione.

SUMÁRIO

A cardiopátia coronária (CHD) é muito menos comum no Japão do que na América do Norte e nos países da Europa. Desde que a aterosclerose é o maior fator patogênico em cardiopátia coronária, vale a pena comparar as diferenças nos fatores aterogênicos, especialmente o metabolismo de lípidos, entre o Japão e os países do Ocidente. Este capítulo revista algumas das feições características e mudanças de aterosclerose no Japão durante os últimos 35 anos em relaçao ao metabolismo de lípidos. Um estudo das taxas de mortalidade de varias doenças do coração no Japão mostra que a taxa de doenças do coração isquémicas tem aumentado durante os últimos 35 anos, mas é ainda muito menos do que nos países do Ocidente. Em contraste, a taxa total de mortalidade de doença cerebrovascular no Japão tem diminuido significativamente durante o mesmo tempo, mas a cifra é ainda mais alta do que nos países do Ocidente. O metabolismo de lípidos alterado tem contribuido significativamente ao desenvolvimento de lesões ateroscleróticas, e assim às taxas de mortalidáde de CHD. Desde 1960 no Japão, têm havido aumentos nos níveis totais de colesterol no soro e de triglicéridos, e os níveis de colesterol no soro estão agora aproximando aquêles vistos nos Estados Unidos. Uma mudança de regime alimentar entre os Japonêses é considerado ser um fator importante contribuindo para o aumento em níveis de colesterol no soro. O consumo dêles des gordura tem mais do que dobrado durante os últimos 20 anos, com um aumento singularmente marcado nas gorduras saturadas animais. As razões porquê a incidência de CHD é ainda considerávelmente mais baixa no Japão do que nos Estados Unidos, mesmo que os níveis de colesterol no soro são agora muito semelhantes, são examinadas. Outros fatores de risco, tais como o estilo de vida, a hipertensão, e o fumar de cígaros, podem ser pertinentes. As diferenças genéticas, com uma referência especial a polimorfismos do comprimento dos fragmentos de restrição são também examinadas.

RESUMEN

La cardiopatía coronaria (CHD) es mucho menos frecuente en el Japón que en Norteamérica y en Europa. Ya que la aterosclerosis es el principal factor patogénico en la CHD, resulta valioso comparar las diferencias en los factores aterogénicos—en particular el metabolismo de los lípidos—que existen entre el Japón y los países occidentales. Se examinan algunas de las características y cambios en la aterosclerosis en el Japón durante los últimos 35 años, en relación con el metabolismo de los lípidos. Un estudio de los índices de mortalidad de distintas enfermedades del corazón en el Japón muestra que el índice de cardiopatía coronaria isquémica ha aumentado durante los últimos 35 años, pero todavía es mucho menor que en los países occidentales. En contraste, el índice total de muertes causadas por enfermedades cerebrovasculares en el Japón ha disminuido significativamente en el mismo período, pero la cifra es todavía más alta que en los países occidentales. Las alteraciones en el metabolismo de los lípidos han contribuido significativamente al desarrollo de lesiones ateroscleróticas, y consecuentemente a los índices de mortalidad causados por la CHD. A partir de 1960, en el Japón ha habido incrementos en los niveles séricos totales de colesterol y triglicéridos, y los niveles séricos de colesterol se están ahora aproximando a aquéllos vistos en los Estados Unidos. Se piensa que el cambio en la dieta de la población japonesa es un factor principal que ha contribuído al incremento en el nivel de colesterol sérico; su consumo de grasas ha aumentado a más del doble en los últimos 20 años, con un incremento particularmente notable en el consumo de grasas animales saturadas. Se examinan las razones por las que la incidencia de CHD todavía considerablemente reducida en el Japón en comparación con los Estados Unidos, incluso cuando se considera que los niveles séricos de colesterol son ahora bastante similares. Podrían haber otros factores de riesgo que juegan cierto papel, como por ejemplo el estilo de vida, hipertensión y tabaquismo. También se discuten diferencias genéticas, prestando particular atención a polimorfismos de restricción de longitud fragmentaria.

The Role of Cholesterol in Atherosclerosis:
New Therapeutic Opportunities, edited by S. M. Grundy
and A. G. Bearn, Hanley & Belfus, Inc., Philadelphia.

Discussion

JULIAN: Can you comment on Japanese who migrate to America?

IMURA: There are some comparative studies between Japanese in Japan and the Japanese in Hawaii. The incidence of coronary heart disease is higher in the Japanese in Hawaii, but it is still lower than in the Caucasians in Hawaii.

JULIAN: Could you explain the high incidence of other cardiac disease referred to in your presentation?

IMURA: It is possible that some coronary heart diseases are included in ''other types of heart diseases'' if there is no autopsy. The autopsy rate is high in major hospitals but low in small hospitals.

NORTH: Could you comment on the overall change in stroke incidence? Your slide showed that the incidence of cerebral infarction was going up while that of hemorrhage was coming down. In Western countries infarction is more common than hemorrhage as a cause of stroke. What is the overall change in stroke mortality in Japan over the past 20 years?

IMURA: Overall, mortality has been considerably decreased, the major reason being the decrease in the number of patients with hypertension. Hypertension is a major risk factor in cerebral hemorrhage, and now we can control hypertensive patients with drugs and diet; the daily sodium intake in Japanese has been decreased tremendously over the past 10 to 15 years through a government campaign. However, over the same period there has been an increase in cerebral infarction and this is partly caused by an altered lipid metabolism.

The Role of Cholesterol in Atherosclerosis:
New Therapeutic Opportunities, edited by S. M. Grundy
and A. G. Bearn, Hanley & Belfus, Inc., Philadelphia.

Roundtable 1: *Worldwide Prevalence of Atherosclerosis: Differences and Similarities*

Chairman: Michael J. S. Langman
Panelists: Detlev Ganten, Hiroo Imura, Barry Lewis, Kalevi Pyörälä, and Thomas W. Smith

Is there sufficient evidence of a direct correlation between serum cholesterol levels and coronary heart disease (CHD) to justify making a reduction in serum cholesterol the main objective of physicians, when clearly so many other factors are involved? Professor Langman, in opening the roundtable discussion on the prevalence of atherosclerosis, felt this central point should not be overlooked. "Are we satisfied that in all places and situations the reduction of serum cholesterol levels should be our prime objective when other strategies are available?" "This question," he said, "is underlined by the variation observed in international studies where coronary heart disease mortality rates are compared with national estimates of prevailing serum cholesterol levels. The correlation observed is not exact, even in men, and deviation is presumably, in part, telling us about the importance of other factors. In women the correlation is very poor indeed and underlines this point."

THE IMPORTANCE OF OTHER RISK FACTORS

The other factors alluded to by Professor Langman also concerned Dr. Ganten. He pointed out that there is a number of very important risk factors other than an elevated serum cholesterol that should be considered. Dr. Ganten referred to data from the PROCAM study carried out by Dr. Assman in Munster (Prospective Cardiovascular Munster Trial). "Looking at the risk factors in this study population derived from screening at the work site, the risk factor most prevalent was smoking (about 40% in males and females), followed by overweight (35% in both sexes), and next comes hypertension with a prevalence of about 15-20%, followed by low HDL cholesterol." Dr. Ganten agreed that decisions to treat a raised serum cholesterol should be based on absolute cut-points, but felt, in view of the low cut-points of the European recommendations (and the importance of these other risk factors), more emphasis should be placed on the nonpharmacologic therapy during this discussion.

"In the planning of a population-directed educational stategy," continued Dr. Ganten, "these extremely important risk factors must be taken into consideration. We have a National Hypertension Program in Germany, and a cholesterol program is at the present time being established, and there are anti-smoking and anti-alcohol groups. There is a danger that these groups are competing for the importance of one of 'their' risk factors. In different groups different emphasis is placed on different types of treatment. What is required is a coordinated program that incorporates all these risk factors, and with one set of recommendations, without necessarily giving up the identity of these groups."

Professor Lewis also felt that populated-directed education strategies were required. "If we say that the cut-off point which should trigger some level of therapy is 200 mg/dl (5.2 mmol/L), we are defining about 65% of the population of Britain into the 'require therapy' group. Clearly this is a problem which in the main must be dealt with by the population strategy of education in terms of optimal eating and optimal levels of physical exercise. However, when we come across such individuals in clinical practice it is important that we know how to counsel them."

THE INDIVIDUAL'S RESPONSE TO RISK FACTORS

Dr. Ganten pointed out that in addition to there being a number of different risk factors to consider, the individual's response to those risk factors also varies. "We all know of cases of smokers who live to 90 years of age. Everybody has his 'Churchill' in mind to excuse or justify his risky behavior. Some people are affected by risk factors; other are not. I think the genetic classification of the individual patient as a basis for individual counseling in general practice may be extremely important, and at the present time the restriction fragment length polymorphism appears to be the most important methodology to achieve this goal."

HETEROGENEITY IN POPULATIONS

Dr. Smith commented that when it comes to treating patients, heterogeneity within given populations can present problems. He pointed out that this is particularly a problem in the United States, where the level of heterogeneity of the population would be expected to be greater than in Japan or Scandinavia, for example. "This raises the question of subsets of populations," he said. "There are probably few medical therapies that are good for everyone or for no-one, and progress will depend to some extent on identifying subsets of patients that have a suitable risk:benefit ratio for any given therapeutic approach." He noted that the statistical power of many studies was a problem, and added "If one wants to stratify a U.S. population for all of the important variables, monumental n values are required for most important outcome endpoints."

Professor Lewis also felt that it was very important to be able to identify patients who are suitable for a given therapeutic approach. "About 1–2% of people in the population have major mutant genes conferring gross hyperlipidemia. One of the strong arguments for risk factor assessment as a population-wide activity is to identify these people, who, almost by definition, will not respond to the sort of educational measures that we are recommending to the population as a whole. Of the 120,000–140,000 people in the United Kingdom who probably have familial hypercholesterolemia in the heterozygous state, virtually none would respond to the changes in diet that are advocated for the population as a whole. There are other rarer diseases which similarly require recognition and individual therapy in a clinical setting if any progress is to be made. Untreated, such diseases confer very high risk of cardiovascular disease."

Professor Lewis continued: "We have to accept that there are few doctors in most Western European countries who are educated to handle such patients. There is, as of one year ago, a British Hyperlipidemia Association of which the membership started at 70 and has almost doubled since. That is the number of people who have classified themselves as having the expertise to handle this sort of clinical problem in district hospitals in Britain. I wouldn't imagine the prevalence is very different in most of Western Europe. So the magnitude of the problem is very great. Even if we were only going to deal by individual strategy with the 1% or so of the population at very high risk, we are still going to need to increase the number of trained physicians. If we are going to include in individual care, and I believe we should, the much larger number of people who have moderate hyperlipidemia and moderate increase in risk, but are vastly more important because of the high prevalence of that range, we are going to have to educate a second echelon of the medical population in Europe to handle simple hyperlipidemia as well. That is going to include drug therapy, although dietary therapy is the ideal approach for the great majority of patients," he concluded.

RELATIONSHIP BETWEEN SERUM CHOLESTEROL AND CHD

It has been well documented, as Professor Langman reminded the panel, that the correlation between serum cholesterol and CHD was particularly weak in women. Dr. Pyörälä was able to shed some light on this finding. "The apparent weakness of this correlation in women could be due to the lack of data from prospective studies on women compared to men. Although there appears to be no correlation between mean serum cholesterol and coronary heart disease (CHD) mortality in women under the age of 64 years (this was shown in the retrospective study by Dr. Simons (Simons: *Am J Cardiol* 1986; **57**:5G–10G), it has to be remembered that it is based on a small number of countries. Such data as are available from prospective population studies on women show that there is a correlation between cholesterol levels and CHD risk. Women, of course, have a reduced risk of developing CHD compared with men, probably due to hormonal factors. In Western populations, the first atherosclerotic lesions start to develop in men below 20 years of age, whereas in women it is about 10 years later, and women continue to lag about 10 years behind men in the occurrence of clinical events. In most populations, particularly middle-aged populations, mean serum cholesterol levels in women are a little higher than in men. In any event, I would caution against interpreting the data as suggesting that there is little relationship between cholesterol and coronary heart disease in women. There is a relationship, but it is difficult to show this because the data on women are more scarce than data on men''.

RELATIONSHIP BETWEEN OBESITY AND CHD

According to the data from the PROCAM study cited earlier by Dr. Ganten, obesity was the second major risk factor associated with CHD. There was some support for the view that such a relationship exists. The studies quoted (in particular the Framingham study and the Finnish Population Studies) suggested that the relationship between obesity and CHD might be stronger in the younger segments of the population.

Professor Julian pointed out that Professor Shaper's study (which showed no relationship) was confined to men over the age of 40 years. Dr. Grundy, referring to the Framingham data, said that although a relationship had not been seen initially and for many years, over an extended period of time the relationship became apparent.

Dr. Pyörälä commented that there had been confusion in the interpretation of data from population studies in which obesity was reported *not* to be a risk factor once the relationship has been adjusted for other major risk factors such as blood lipids and blood pressure. Dr. Pyörälä continued, ''It has to be taken into account that obesity is an important risk factor for hypertension, and is closely related to serum lipids, and so the finding of no independent effect of obesity in multivariate analysis does not mean that obesity is unimportant. Rather, it could be that because obesity is so strongly related to blood pressure and abnormal lipids it is really very important.''

Professor Lasagna added that a further factor that should be taken into account is the type of obesity. ''It has been suggested that the type of distribution of obesity has something to do with prognosis, and that one must distinguish between truncal and other kinds of obesity.''

RELATIONSHIP BETWEEN TOTAL MORTALITY AND CHD

Dr. Poole-Wilson felt that it was crucial to be able to demonstrate that intervention in people between the ages of 45 and 65 years affects total mortality and not just the incidence of CHD. ''If you look at the MRFIT data,'' he said, ''at least the version put out in the *American Journal of Cardiology* and the ERICA data of a couple of years ago, they showed a very weak relationship between total mortality and cholesterol.'' Dr. Poole-Wilson felt that it was reasonable for a patient to ask his doctor ''Is a high cholesterol associated with an increased mortality?'' The MRFIT data would seem to offer no such confirmation. ''Perhaps there are subgroups within these overall groups that are affected, but it is disappointing that there isn't a more obvious relationship,'' he concluded.

RELATIONSHIP BETWEEN RACE AND CHD

While it is not disputed that there is considerable variation in the incidence of coronary heart disease between races, whether these variations are due to genetic or environmental factors, or to both, is not clear. Professor Imura pointed out that at any given serum cholesterol level, there are also great racial differences in the incidence of CHD—a factor that should be borne in mind when deciding at which level of serum cholesterol treatment should start.

Professor Imura cited Japan and Thailand as an example. ''Dr. Murai has done some comparative studies between Japan and Thailand. The results showed that total cholesterol was about 10 mg/dl higher in Thailand than in Japan. Further, HDL cholesterol was about 10 mg/dl lower in Thailand than in Japan. However, CHD is quite uncommon in Thailand.'' (The exact incidence is not known, but there is no evidence that it is high in Thailand.)

When asked about the other risk factors in Thailand such as smoking, overweight, and hypertension, Professor Imura replied that these had not been studied, and added, ''Other risk factors may be very important. Perhaps the incidence of obesity is lower in Thailand?''

Professor Lewis pointed out that there is a very important problem of sampling in Thailand. ''The urban serum cholesterol level in Bangkok is almost the same as that in London. The rural serum cholesterol is little more than half as great.'' (Dr. Murai's study had been carried out in Chang Mai—a city, but not as large as Bangkok.)

CHD IN JAPAN

An interesting observation with regard to the incidence of CHD in the Japanese was made by Dr. Pyörälä. It was one, he said, which had been very important for the understanding of many of the aspects of atherosclerosis and CHD. ''Japanese living in their home islands have a high frequency of hypertension and they also have a relatively high frequency of smoking. Yet these two risk factors have relatively little impact on atherosclerosis and coronary heart disease in that population. But when the Japanese move to Hawaii or the United States their mean serum cholesterol values start to rise, and there will be a larger proportion of those Japanese who are above the threshold where there is enough substrate for atheroma to form. Then hypertension and smoking start to relate strongly to the occurrence of atherosclerosis and coronary heart disease as in Western populations. There are other examples of such migrant populations showing a similar development. There must be some kind of threshold above which LDL cholesterol levels have to be to produce mass occurrence of the disease in the population. As to the Japanese living in their home islands, a large part of the population so far has been living below that threshold. On the other hand, the Japanese example shows that CHD is not necessarily an accompaniment of industrialized society.''

Turning to the differences in the incidence and prevalence of CHD in Japan and England (Japan has a much lower incidence of CHD than the U.K.), Sir Richard Bayliss commented that he understood that the Japanese smoke very heavily. Professor Imura replied that the ratio of smokers to non-smokers in adult males in Japan is almost the same as in European countries. The lung cancer rate is much lower in Japan, but it has increased in the past 10 to 20 years.

Other changes that have been taking place in Japan were outlined by Professor Yoshitoshi. ''About 45 years ago, the first time that cholesterol was measured by the Japanese Circulation Society, serum cholesterol was found to be much lower than in the Western populations. These studies have been repeated many times, and the results show that Japanese cholesterol levels have gradually come closer to Western levels, such that it is anticipated that within 10 or 15 years there will be no difference at all.''

Professor Yoshitoshi reported another interesting observation that has recently been made in Japan. ''There are two types of senile dementia: Alzheimer's disease and an atherosclerotic type. In Japan, the atherosclerotic type occurs much more frequently than the Alzheimer type. Most psychiatrists in Japan believe that this is a very unusual type of senile dementia. Autopsy on these patients showed that atherosclerosis occurred mostly in the small arteries of the brain, as distinct from cerebral infarction.''

CHD IN DEVELOPING COUNTRIES

Speaking on behalf of a developing country, Brazil, Dr. Rocha commented that very few data are so far available. Recently there have been several reports showing that CHD is increasing in the larger cities, but there have been very few attempts to correlate serum lipid levels and death from CHD. In one such study, Giannini *et al.* looked at the incidence of myocardial infarction (MI) in people of lower socioeconomic class, and showed that patients who had a myocardial infarction had a higher total cholesterol, higher VLDL and LDL, and lower HDL. Dr. Rocha continued, ''We are aware of the NIH guidelines on serum lipids, but we do not know whether those levels are applicable in Brazil. There may be heterogeneity in populations of the United States, but in Brazil it is probably even greater.''

Dr. Rocha went on to comment on the Indian populations in Brazil who are thought to have a low incidence of CHD and related problems. For instance, a study by Franco (1981) showed that Indians from the high Xingu area had a total average cholesterol in males of 144 mg/dl (3.7 mmol/L) and in females 154 mg/dl (4.0 mmol/L). Perhaps surprisingly, in Giannini's study of people of lower socioeconomic classes in Sao Paulo (Brazil's largest city), the total serum cholesterol was 168 mg/dl (4.4 mmol/L) in males and 186 mg/dl (4.8 mmol/L) in females. "Not so different from the Indian population," said Dr. Rocha.

In concluding this roundtable discussion Professor Langman said that the heterogeneity of the available epidemiologic data indicated that the contribution of the individual factors that affect the incidence of CHD will naturally vary. Hypercholesterolemia is plainly an important factor everywhere.

The Role of Cholesterol in Atherosclerosis:
New Therapeutic Opportunities, edited by S. M. Grundy
and A. G. Bearn, Hanley & Belfus, Inc., Philadelphia.

Roundtable 2: *Attitudes Toward Cholesterol Reduction*

Chairman: Sir Colin Dollery
Panelists: Pierre Corvol, Scott M. Grundy, Colin I. Johnston, Philip A. Poole-Wilson, and Yawara Yoshitoshi

In Roundtable 1 Professor Langman opened the discussion by asking whether there was sufficient evidence of a correlation between serum cholesterol levels and coronary heart disease (CHD) to justify attempts to reduce cholesterol levels. The answer to this question, or at least the physician's perception of it, must inevitably affect his attitude toward cholesterol reduction.

If indeed, there, is a link between serum cholesterol and CHD, can elevated serum cholesterol levels be reduced by diet or by lipid-lowering drugs? Are other risk factors involved?—the discussion in Roundtable 1 suggested strongly that they are—and if so, are these other risk factors reversible?

RISK FACTORS AND REVERSIBILITY

It was with the subject of risk factors and their reversibility that Professor Sir Colin Dollery opened the second roundtable discussion. "Factors such as smoking," said Professor Dollery, "are powerful predictors of risk, and diabetes, obesity and certain dietary factors are also important. But to what extent does controlling these risk predictors reduce risk? How realistic is it to expect that correction of a risk factor such as a raised serum cholesterol will result in a proportionate reduction in risk?" This was a difficult question to answer. The desired or predicted results do not always occur. Professor Dollery cited as an example the University Group Diabetes Project (UGDP), a randomized controlled trial in which diabetes was treated with oral hypoglycemics, insulin and diet. The data have suggested that treatment with certain oral hypoglycemics had increased the risk of coronary disease. Altering a physiological variable (i.e., reducing blood sugar levels) should have resulted in a reduced risk, but this was not found to be the case. The MRC and ANBPS trial on mild hypertension showed a halving in the incidence of stroke but only a small reduction in myocardial infarction, whereas one might have expected a 20–25% reduction in CHD from the reduction in blood pressure. With regard to cholesterol,

Professor Dollery believes that it is a more powerful predictor in younger people than in older people (over 50 years of age). This suggests, he said, that a degree of irreversibility may occur with increasing age. But clinical coronary disease occurs mainly in the age range where cholesterol is a less powerful discriminant of risk.

Benefit and Cholesterol Reduction: A Linear Relationship?

There was some disagreement about whether a linear relationship can be assumed between benefit and cholesterol reduction, i.e., whether benefit will be obtained across a range of serum cholesterol levels, or indeed over varying degrees of development of atheromatous lesions. This question must inevitably affect at which serum cholesterol level doctors should intervene with treatment.

Professor Johnston suggested that although epidemiologists appear to assume that such linear benefit exists, it has not been proven. He pointed out that although there is a relationship between the risk of cerebrovascular disease and blood pressure, the effect of reducing blood pressure is not linear.

Professor Lewis's figures (p. 163) show that in order to make an impact on the incidence of coronary disease, it is necessary to lower the cholesterol levels of the general population, most of which are in the range of 5–6 mmol/L (193–232 mg/dl). "The majority of people who will suffer a heart attack," he said, "have cholesterol levels in the range of 5–7 mmol/L (193–270 mg/dl). If surveillance is focused on those at the high end of this range, the bulk of people at risk will go undetected. Because they are numerous, and the abnormality is mild, they are largely a public health problem."

Pointing out that Dr. Richard Peto's data on improved outcome through reduced risk factors were based on the highest cholesterol levels, Dr. Ledingham said that "Professor Lewis was making a significant assumption in suggesting that if you start at much lower levels, for example 6 mmol/L and come down to 5 mmol/L, that you will also be better off." "That is a question of faith," he said.

Dr. Corvol believes that risk factors may be significant at both high and low serum cholesterol levels. He referred to a study conducted by Ducimetiere and coworkers in Paris. They looked at the annual incidence of coronary disease in 7434 men between 42 and 53 years of age, and followed them for 6.6 years. They compared their risk factors with other prospective studies, in particular the risk associated with an increase in plasma cholesterol of 50 mg/dl (1.2 mmol/L). In the European Seven Countries studies, the mean cholesterol level at the start of the trial was 210 mg/dl (5.4 mmol/L), whereas in the Lipid Research Clinical Trial the mean plasma cholesterol was 290 mg/dl (7.5 mmol/L). In all these studies, the risk factor varied between 1.7 and 1.4 for each increase of 50 mg/dl of plasma cholesterol; i.e., it was the same in every study, whatever the starting level of cholesterol. This suggests that even at low plasma cholesterol levels, the risk factor is significant, and for every 50 mg/dl (1.2 mmol/L) increase, the risk of developing CHD increases by 40–70%. This does not imply, however, that there will be a 45% reduction in CHD mortality.

Are Atheromatous Lesions Reversible?

Professor Dollery felt that it was dangerous to equate a regression line with reversibility, pointing out that atheroma may not be reversible at all, and even if it is, it is not known to what degree or over what time scale. Dr. Poole-Wilson said that it was inconceivable that the treatment of hypertension would alter some atheromatous lesions, nor would any drug. "In America cholesterol predicts coronary events much better than in the U.K.—that may be related to differences in the nature of the lesions," he said. Professor Dollery asked about the thrombotic tendency of the blood. "We have been impressed by data from Lars Wilhelmsen and Tom Meade concerning coagulation proteins and their power as risk predictors for coronary disease." Dr. Poole-Wilson replied that the situation was even more complex. "Cholesterol may be affecting smooth muscle contraction and platelet activation. There is no theoretical reason for reversibility of the incidence of coronary events. We have to demonstrate that it does occur."

Professor Lasagna commented, "It is unreasonable to suppose that lowering the blood cholesterol by a given amount in someone who has vessels that are almost completely occluded will have the same impact as in a young person with a few fatty streaks." Dr. Grundy and Professor Lewis disagreed. "These people may be helped the most by lipid lowering," said Dr. Grundy. Dr. Moncloa added, "Of the vessels that are already occluded, 50–60% progress rapidly, and they are in the initial part of the curve that correlates occlusion with flow. These lesions may kill the patient, and this progression may be retarded by lowering cholesterol." Referring again to Dr. Peto's work, Professor Lewis said, "Peto has set up a series of regression lines relating the change in serum cholesterol to the change in coronary incidence in the published trial. The slope is parallel to the predictive relationship, which is one of the indications that treatment of hyperlipidemia reverses risk. The slope for the secondary prevention trials is the same as that for the primary prevention trials in which there has been no overt coronary heart disease."

DIET AND SMOKING IN CHOLESTEROL REDUCTION

While attitudes toward cholesterol reduction will clearly be affected by whether such a measure is effective in reducing CHD, attitudes toward the different methods of lowering serum cholesterol must also depend on their safety.

Professor Dollery drew attention to the dichotomy between measures that might be harmful (drugs) and those unlikely to cause harm (diet and stopping smoking). He said that advising patients to change their diets and to stop smoking may do good, and yet doctors have a very poor record of encouraging patients in this respect. Professor Lewis was concerned whether there were sufficient facilities to counsel all individuals with mild hypercholesterolemia. "The European recommendation for persons with mild hypercholesterolemia is that they should be strongly counseled to adopt the recommendations of the populations strategy on diet, smoking and other health habits.'' ''But,'' he continued, ''there are several times more people with cholesterol levels above 5 mmol/L (193mg/dl) than there are diabetics, yet we have difficulty providing adequate facilities for diabetic care.''

Professor Dollery suggested that in view of the fact that 70% of the population consults a doctor every year (this figure is even higher in older people) and 90% within three years, there was an opportunity to give advice about modifying the diet and stopping smoking when the patient consults about something else. ''Perhaps we should call them back and reinforce the advice. Fifteen to 20% of patients will stop smoking with such advice,'' he said.

Dr. Hay was doubtful whether sufficient benefit could be derived through dietary intervention. He said that while for some people who have moderately elevated serum cholesterol levels, diet is fairly effective, most studies showed that ''except in those people who are put on zucchini squash for the rest of their lives,'' a 10% reduction in serum cholesterol was the most that could be achieved. Dr. Hay pointed out that Taylor and Law, in the MRFIT population, were only able to achieve a 6.7% reduction in cholesterol through diet. He continued, ''I think there are a lot of people who would be very reluctant to give up hamburgers and ice cream to achieve the three week additional life expectancy.'' ''I don't know if lovastatin is an ideal drug, but I think we need to do better than what diet is capable of achieving.''

In France, attitudes toward diet seem to be somewhat different from those in the U.S. ''Food is extremely important in France,'' explained Dr. Corvol, ''yet we have contributed quite remarkably to the decrease in heavy and fatty food by the introduction of nouvelle cuisine. I think this example could be followed with advantage elsewhere.'' Dr. Corvol pointed out that the polyunsaturated:saturated (P:S) fat ratio of the food eaten in France is 0.35, and the cardiovascular mortality 2.5 times less than in the United States. He felt, therefore, that there was not the same urgency in France to treat mild to moderate hyperlipidemia with drugs, although familial homo-zygous and heterozygous hyperlipoproteinemia would be treated.

Dr. Ganten reminded the conference that hyperlipidemia was a chronic disease, and that there was plenty of time to decide on the correct form of treatment. ''It is probably impossible to decide at the first patient/doctor contact whether the patient will benefit from drug treatment or a diet. We have plenty of time and should use this time to discuss the disease process with the patient, and to try to help with diet alone.'' He continued, ''If the disease is progressing and the diet is clearly not sufficient, then it is time to consider drug treatment. Observation and counseling are an important part of the decision to use the drug or not, and the time available should be used unless the clinical situation mandates immediate action.''

IS A PUBLIC EDUCATION PROGRAM THE WAY FORWARD?

Professor Lewis's earlier remarks about population strategies raised again the question of whether treatment of the individual or wider public education is the best way forward in dealing with raised serum cholesterol levels. Dr. North suggested that "if two-thirds of the population need treatment, you don't waste time measuring cholesterol, you educate everybody to change their diet." "Doctors need to accept the importance of public education," he said. Dr. Lenfant, who has considerable experience of the effects of mass education through the U.S. National Cholesterol Education Program (p. 213), said that their surveys had shown a significant gain on all fronts. "However," he added, "the physicians are far behind the public in their awareness about cholesterol matters."

Dr. Norrby asked whether it would be feasible to screen everyone in the U.K. over the age of 35 years and to intervene in all those with values above a certain level. Professor Dollery commented that it would mean that if you wanted to modify the diet of a patient, you would modify the diet of the whole family. "It might be more sensible to modify the diet of the whole population." "The Americans have been more successful in this than we have," he said.

Hypercholesterolemia is not, of course, confined to adults. Dr. Mezey commented on some sobering data presented by Dr. Wynder at the American Health Foundation in New York about the incidence of hypercholesterolemia in the children of non-hypercholesterolemic parents. Dr. Lenfant explained that the American Health Foundation has a school-based program of intervention through which they provide information to school children. "The response has been quite good;" said Dr. Lenfant, "in fact Dr. Wynder has reported some very striking data to the effect that you can intervene in a school and produce a significant lowering of cholesterol over a period of time." Dr. Lenfant continued, "We do believe, in our program, that school intervention is a very nice way to tackle the problem. By and large, in the American family, the children get what they want, and therefore if you can educate the children there is a very strong possibility that the rest of the family will follow suit." But Dr. Lenfant cautioned that much more work needs to be done before final conclusions can be drawn with regard to children.

ATTITUDES TOWARD LIPID-LOWERING DRUGS

Lipid-Lowering Drugs—An Easy Option?

While efficacy and safety, discussed below, may be the main factors governing the physician's attitude toward lipid-lowering drugs, the possibility that many doctors may resort to drug therapy simply because it is easier than persuading a patient to stop smoking or keep to a strict diet concerned a number of the panelists. Professor Peters anticipated that the majority of those advised to give up smoking and to diet will fail, and will soon be consuming lipid-lowering drugs. Professor Lenfant also viewed this as a very real problem. "Doctors may soon be finding it easier to prescribe a drug than to impress upon their patients that they should follow a strict dietary regimen," he said. "'High risk' patients, quantified today by Dr. Grundy as those with serum cholesterol levels above 300 mg/dl (7.8 mmol/L), could tomorrow be those above 280 or 260 mg/dl or less." "In the United States," continued Dr. Lenfant, "we have 25–30 million people who are at risk, according to the Consensus Development Conference. It would be a sad thing to see so many people taking lovastatin in the morning and then going out for eggs and bacon for breakfast and a big fat steak in the evening."

Efficacy and Safety

Directing the discussion toward the important considerations of efficacy and safety of lipid-lowering drugs, Professor Dollery asked, "What should our attitude be toward these drugs? Should we go ahead and use them or should we insist that evidence must first be obtained that they are efficacious? Efficacy could be judged on various levels. It could be judged from angiographic studies or from studies in patients with angina. If angina could be improved dramatically, it would be powerful evidence that stenoses of coronary arteries were reversible. Or ought we to insist on there being outcome evidence, that is, evidence of reduction of myocardial infarction? The drugs, although effective, are not free of toxicity; for example, an elevation in creatine phosphokinase (CPK) in 9% of patients and a 0.5% incidence of myositis severe enough to cause the drug to be stopped have been reported. That is not entirely a trivial degree of toxicity. There is also still a tiny question mark about cataracts which no doubt can be answered by further studies."

Addressing Dr. Grundy, Professor Dollery asked whether he felt that lipid-lowering drugs should be limited to, for example, people with heterozygous familial hypercholesterolemia (FH). Dr. Grundy felt that the drug should be restricted to people with quite high serum cholesterol levels. The exact level of intervention would depend on the individual and the physician would have to judge accordingly. Dr. Grundy suggested that you might use the drugs more readily in younger people than in older. When pressed by Professor Dollery to give exact levels at which he would intervene, Dr. Grundy said at 350 mg/dl (9.1 mmol/L) he would almost certainly use drugs, at 300 mg/dl (7.8 mmol/L) probably, and at 280 mg/dl (7.3 mmol/L) perhaps not.

Dr. Grundy stressed that he was advocating that the use of drug treatment should develop slowly, starting with the worst cases—those at highest risk. "I think the patient should be labeled 'high risk' before getting the drug and not just 'moderate risk.' For example, a smoker should get the drug before a non-smoker, because smoking cigarettes is equivalent in risk to raising your serum cholesterol by around 100 mg/dl (2.6 mmol/L)."

Professor Dollery sounded a word of caution about the incremental policy that Dr. Grundy had described, fearing that it might become a policy of incremental drift. "We did that in hypertension, gradually treating people with milder and milder hypertension and forgetting to develop the evidence that we were doing any good until very late in the day."

Requirements Before Licensing

Professor Dollery asked the panel, "If you were drug regulators, would you insist on evidence of efficacy before you licensed the drug for general sale?" Dr. Grundy felt that this would depend on how much the drug was regulated after licensing, something that Professor Dollery suggested would be impracticable. Dr. Grundy was satisfied by the fact that the FDA in the United States was about to license lovastatin and accepted the argument that until the drug has been used in sufficiently large numbers of patients, comprehensive toxicity data will not be available. "I think we know about as much as we are going to know about its toxicity for the next 4 to 5 years," said Dr. Grundy. "There are many high-risk patients who would possibly benefit from the drug, so I am in favor of the approval, but I can certainly see the other side of the argument." Professor Dollery agreed that if one waited for data from large outcome trials prior to marketing, licensing could be delayed by five or ten years.

The Need for Trials

Although it seemed clear that trials should be conducted to provide hard data on drug safety and efficacy, there were some suggestions that there would be both ethical and practical problems in conducting such trials.

Professor Lewis said there was one situation in which trials would never be done. "I think that it will not be ethical to randomize patients with heterozygous familial hypercholesterolemia into the treatment versus no treatment trial. We have to decide whether to treat such patients on the basis of what we know about their risk without such a trial." Professor Dollery countered that these kinds of arguments had been employed in the past for not doing trials in serious conditions. "We have now realized years later that things are not so clear cut," he said. "If I were a regulator I might consider licensing lovastatin if I were convinced that large outcome trials were in progress, but without that assurance I would license it only for heterozygous FH."

Professor Langman was unsure how, once a drug was licensed, large outcome trials could be conducted. He felt that a definite outcome was unlikely to be reached for a long time. Professor Dollery said that this had been achieved in hypertension, even though many people were already on treatment. He continued, "The MRC elderly trial is a good illustration—70–75% of patients screened were already on treatment so we had a great deal of difficulty in recruiting patients for the study, but we did eventually succeed."

Dr. Moncloa, Group Director of Clinical Research at Merck, said that several trials were in progress. "We continue to follow up these patients from the Phase III studies in order to obtain long-term experience. We also have a large-scale trial in about 7500 patients, which will provide valuable information in terms of safety. We have two angiography studies to document efficacy regarding the progression and/or regression of atheroma.'' Merck also plans to start a third trial in patients with a history of coronary heart disease or peripheral vascular disease, and they are also committed to do an outcome study.

Professor Dollery suggested that Merck should also consider a trial of primary prevention in high-risk patients. ''I would also find it more impressive if you could relieve patients with the fixed stenosis type of angina rather than just show an improvement in atheroma in the angiography studies,'' he said. Professor Dollery's request for primary prevention studies was supported by Dr. Corvol.

Dr. Grundy concluded: ''We are lucky to have a drug that will lower cholesterol effectively. But it can be misused and we need to educate physicians to use it rationally.''

The final admonition came from Professor Dollery: ''The Merck scientists and also the Sankyo scientists in Japan have given us powerful weapons to reduce cholesterol; we have a great opportunity. Those of you in the lipid field should not repeat the mistakes we have made in the hypertension field and you should go after the hard outcome evidence early rather than late. If you do that, you will reap great rewards.''

The Role of Cholesterol in Atherosclerosis:
New Therapeutic Opportunities, edited by S. M. Grundy
and A. G. Bearn, Hanley & Belfus, Inc., Philadelphia.

The U.S. National Cholesterol Education Program: Raising Health Professional and Public Awareness About the Importance of Lowering High Blood Cholesterol

James I. Cleeman and Claude Lenfant

In November 1985, the National Heart, Lung, and Blood Institute (NHLBI) of the National Institutes of Health (NIH) launched the National Cholesterol Education Program (NCEP), a cooperative undertaking by major health and medically oriented organizations in the United States. The goal of the program is to reduce the prevalence of elevated blood cholesterol in this country and thereby contribute to reducing the morbidity and mortality that results from coronary heart disease (CHD). The NCEP seeks to achieve this goal through educational initiatives to encourage health professionals and the public to pay more attention to the need to control elevated blood cholesterol levels, and to increase their awareness that lowering high blood cholesterol is important in preventing CHD.

THE SCIENCE BASE OF THE NCEP

Like all "risk factor reduction programs" of NHLBI, the NCEP rests on a firm base of biomedical research findings. For some time this science base has built on results from basic studies of the atherosclerotic plaque as well as the use of animal models and genetic and epidemiologic approaches. The data have linked high levels of blood cholesterol to increased rates of CHD. What had been missing, however, was conclusive experimental evidence that lowering high blood cholesterol in humans actually reduces the risk of heart attack. When, in 1984, the NHLBI announced the results of a landmark study, the Coronary Primary Prevention Trial (CPPT), it provided the long-awaited definitive evidence.[1,2] In the CPPT, 3806 middle-aged men with high blood cholesterol levels were divided into two groups: one group was treated with diet and cholestyramine (a bile acid sequestrant), the other with diet and a placebo. The cholestyramine-treated group had an average 9% greater reduction in blood levels of total cholesterol than the placebo group, and this was associated with a 19% reduction in the risk of fatal and non-fatal heart attacks (Fig. 1).

In December 1984, the NIH convened a Consensus Development Conference to consider the findings of the CPPT as well as all other evidence linking serum cholesterol to CHD.[3] The Consensus Panel concluded that: (1) elevated blood cholesterol level is a major cause of CHD, and (2) lowering elevated blood cholesterol level will reduce the risk of heart attacks due to CHD. The Panel made two major recommendations:

1. Individuals with blood cholesterol levels above the 75th percentile (i.e., the upper 25%, or 1 in 4 Americans) should be treated, under medical supervision, to lower their levels and hence reduce their risk of CHD. For middle-aged Americans (40 and older), this translates into cholesterol levels above 240 mg/dl (6.2 mmol/L). The primary approach to treatment is a diet that reduces fat to less than 30% of total calories, saturated fat to less than 10% of calories, and dietary cholesterol to less than 300 mg a day. For people with significantly elevated blood cholesterol levels (generally above the 90th percentile) after an adequate trial of diet therapy, the addition of cholesterol-lowering drugs should be considered (Fig. 2).

2. All Americans (except children under 2 years of age) are advised to adopt a low saturated fat and low cholesterol diet.

The first of these recommendations, which is a patient-based or high-risk approach, entails the identification and treatment of individuals with cholesterol levels high enough to warrant medical intervention. It is this approach that has been emphasized in the early activities of the NCEP. The second recommendation, which is a population-based or public health approach, will be the focus of a new NCEP

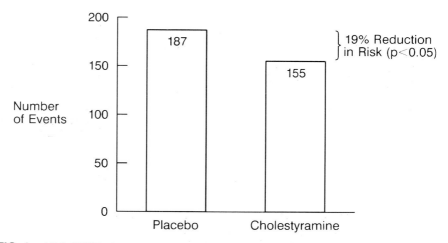

FIG. 1. LRC-CPPT primary endpoint (definite coronary heart disease death and/or non-fatal myocardial infarction).

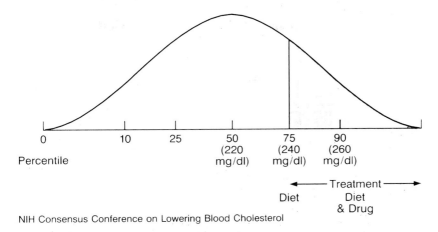

FIG. 2.   Consensus Panel recommendations applied to the U.S. cholesterol distribution.

panel currently being constituted. The two strategies are intended to be complementary.

NCEP CHOLESTEROL AWARENESS SURVEYS

Achieving better control of high blood cholesterol requires heightened awareness as a first step. Surveys conducted by NHLBI in 1983 and again in 1986 show that the cholesterol-related knowledge, attitudes, and practices of physicians and the public are improving but not yet adequate.[4,5] Both groups were asked a key attitudinal question: Would reducing elevated blood cholesterol have little or no effect, a moderate effect, or a large effect in preventing heart disease? Figure 3 shows that from 1983 to 1986, the percentage of physicians who thought that reducing elevated cholesterol levels would have a large preventive effect increased from 39% to 64%. The proportion of the public that expressed this view also increased from 64% to 72%. Attitudes of physicians and the public are changing in the desired direction, but work remains to be done to reach the still substantial percentage of individuals who are not yet fully convinced.

PHYSICIAN SURVEYS

Physicians were asked at what level of blood cholesterol they usually initiated diet and drug therapy for middle-aged, asymptomatic males. Table I shows the median response. In 1986, the reported median range for diet therapy was 240–259 mg/dl (6.2–6.7 mmol/L), down from 260–279 mg/dl (6.8–7.3 mmol/L) in 1983. The median range for drug therapy in 1986 was 300–319 mg/dl (7.8–8.3 mmol/L),

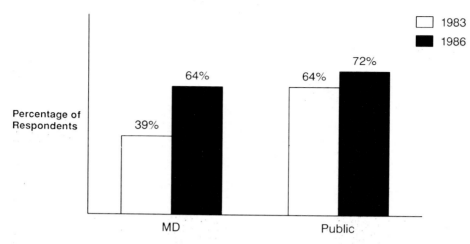

FIG. 3. Belief that reducing elevated blood cholesterol will have a large effect on heart disease.

down from 340–359 mg/dl (8.8–9.3 mmol/L). Thus, physicians were treating at lower levels of blood cholesterol in 1986 than in 1983, levels closer to the Consensus recommendations. Nevertheless, as shown in Table II, in 1986 50% of physicians were still starting diet therapy at levels above the recommended 240 mg/dl (6.2 mmol/L) level, and a total of 24% of all physicians were using diet treatment only for people with levels of 260 mg/dl (6.8 mmol/L) or higher. This means that some patients who should have been on diet therapy were not receiving it.

The cholesterol level at which physicians used drug therapy in addition to diet, where the effect of diet alone was insufficient, showed a modest downward shift toward the recommended level. Still, in 1986 a sizeable proportion of those at significantly increased risk were not receiving appropriate drug therapy. As shown in Table III, a total of 36% of all physicians were never or virtually never prescribing cholesterol-lowering drugs.

Physicians were asked which drugs they prescribed for middle-aged males with elevated low density lipoprotein (LDL) cholesterol and normal triglycerides. Table IV shows that both in 1983 and in 1986, physicians were prescribing a number of drugs; most frequently cited in 1986 were the bile-acid-binding resins, cholestyramine and colestipol. Moreover, three times as many physicians reported using resins in 1986 as in 1983. This was undoubtedly influenced by the results of the CPPT, in which cholestyramine was shown to be effective in reducing the risk of CHD.

TABLE I. *Median range of cholesterol level, mg/dl (mmol/L) for initiating therapy*

	1983		1986	
Diet Therapy	260–279	(6.8–7.3)	240–259	(6.2–6.7)
Drug Therapy	340–359	(8.8–9.3)	300–319	(7.8–8.3)

TABLE II. *Level of blood cholesterol for initiating diet therapy*

Cholesterol Level		Percent of Physicians	
mg/dl	(mmol/L)	1983	1986
≤240	(6.2)	—	50
<260	(6.8)	40	76
260–299	(6.8–7.7)	15	12
≥300	(7.8)	41	10
Never		4	2

TABLE III. *Level of blood cholesterol for initiating drug therapy*

Cholesterol Level		Percent of Physicians	
mg/dl	(mmol/L)	1983	1986
≤260	(6.8)	—	24
<280	(7.3)	9	28
280–339	(7.3–8.8)	24	36
≥340	(8.8)	39	23
Never		28	13

TABLE IV. *Drugs prescribed to lower blood cholesterol**

Drug		Prescription Frequency (%)	
		1983	1986
Cholestyramine	} Resins	13	44
Colestipol		4	7
Clofibrate		26	15
Gemfibrozil		19	25
Probucol		12	17
Nicotinic Acid		10	22

* Physicians could name more than one drug.

In 1986, the NCEP was particularly interested in assessing physician acceptance of the Consensus Conference recommendations. Respondents were told the treatment goal set forth by the Consensus Conference: to use medical intervention to achieve cholesterol lowering for people in the top 25% of the cholesterol distribution. It was explained that this would entail the treatment of 1 in 4 adults (in the middle-aged, those with cholesterol levels above 240 mg/dl [6.2 mmol/L]). Eighty-seven percent of the physicians surveyed thought this goal was warranted by scientific evidence, and 59% thought the goal was feasible in routine practice (Fig. 4). Other data from the surveys suggest that the 41% who thought it was not feasible may well have been reflecting a lack of proper educational tools and materials for carrying out diet treatment, as well as a lack of time and staff for diet counseling.

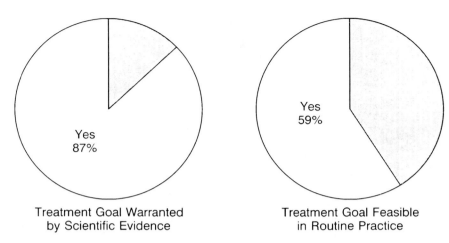

Treatment Goal Warranted
by Scientific Evidence

Treatment Goal Feasible
in Routine Practice

FIG. 4. Physician endorsement of Consensus Conference recommendation that the one in four adults with cholesterol levels above 240 mg/dl be treated (1986).

PUBLIC SURVEYS

The public surveys revealed that awareness of the condition called "high blood cholesterol" increased modestly from 1983 to 1986, from 77% to 81%, and appeared to be at a relatively high level (Fig. 5). In 1983 and 1986, in response to an open-ended question, over 60% of respondents were aware that high blood cholesterol is caused by dietary factors. In a prompted question, 70% and more recognized that high blood cholesterol could lead to heart attacks or hardening of the arteries (Table V).

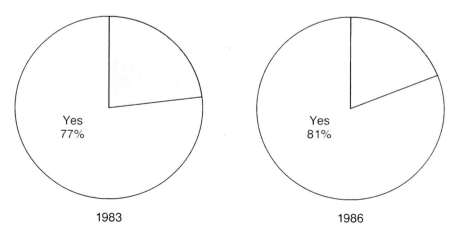

1983

1986

FIG. 5. Public response to the question: "Have you ever heard of high blood cholesterol, sometimes just called high cholesterol?"

TABLE V.   *Public awareness of causes and consequences of high blood cholesterol (percent)*

	1983	1986
High blood cholesterol is caused by dietary factors	61	65
High blood cholesterol leads to heart attacks	70	75
High blood cholesterol leads to hardening of the arteries	70	75

The surveys revealed an interesting pattern concerning public awareness of dietary actions to lower blood cholesterol. On the one hand, when a list of dietary actions was read to respondents, substantial percentages of them displayed an awareness of the basic dietary principles. Thus, in 1986, over 70% of the public knew that eating less fat and less dietary cholesterol would lower blood cholesterol levels. Moreover, the majority recognized that reducing the consumption of certain specific foods could be beneficial (see Fig. 6). It is not surprising that only modest increases in awareness were seen from 1983 to 1986, since the public appeared to be quite aware in these areas to begin with. However, as shown in Figure 7, a sizeable proportion of the public lacked specific knowledge about the effects and characteristics of saturated fat and polyunsaturated fat and where they are found, information that is necessary for translating dietary principles into practical eating patterns. Encouragingly, the percentage of people who reported they had attempted to make diet changes specifically to lower their blood cholesterol level, either on their own initiative or on a doctor's advice, increased from 14% in 1983 to 23% in 1986. Most of these changes were self-initiated.

The Consensus Panel and others have emphasized the importance of knowing one's own cholesterol level. In 1986, 46% of people reported having had their blood cholesterol checked, compared with 35% reported previously (Fig. 8). This increase may reflect better communication about cholesterol measurement between physician and patient, as well as increased attention to obtaining a cholesterol determination. Nevertheless, over half of the public said they had not had their cholesterol checked; fewer than 10% could recall their own blood cholesterol level; and the percentage of adults who reported being told that their blood cholesterol is high was only 8% in 1986, virtually unchanged from 7% in 1983. Ideally, if the Consensus Panel's recommendation to treat above 240 mg/dl (6.2 mmol/L) were being followed, about 25% of adults would have been told that their cholesterol is high.

IMPLICATIONS OF THE SURVEYS

In summary, the results of the physician and public cholesterol awareness surveys show that, between 1983 and 1986, there has been a significant change in the cholesterol-related attitudes and practices of physicians and a strengthening of positive attitudes and practices among the public. These gratifying developments hold

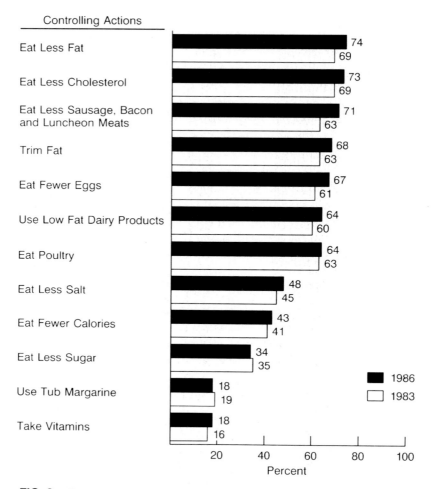

FIG. 6. Percent of public saying dietary actions would lower blood cholesterol.

promise for continued progress in the future. At the same time, the surveys clearly point to the existence of educational challenges that the NCEP will have to meet. The program will have to:

- Continue to provide the latest scientific information about the importance of lowering high blood cholesterol in preventing CHD;

- Reach physicians with messages to encourage appropriate use of diet and drugs to lower high blood cholesterol levels; and

- Recommend practical approaches to the successful management of high blood cholesterol.

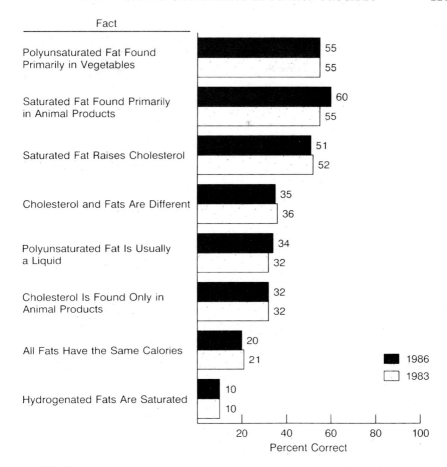

FIG. 7.   Public response to questions about knowledge of nutritional facts.

To address these needs, the program established an Expert Panel on Detection, Evaluation, and Treatment of High Blood Cholesterol in Adults (known as the Adult Treatment Panel) to develop detailed guidelines for physicians and other health professionals on the management of high blood cholesterol. This Panel issued its report in October 1987. It is anticipated that the guidelines will be of substantial practical help to physicians in managing the care of patients with high blood cholesterol.

The survey findings also have important implications for the public education activities of the NCEP. The program will have to:

● Continue the media campaign to convey the message: "Know your cholesterol—and do something about an elevated level"; and

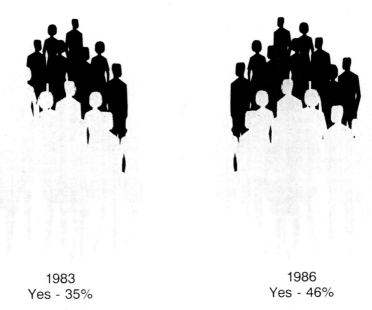

1983
Yes - 35%

1986
Yes - 46%

FIG. 8. Public response to the question: "Have you ever had your blood cholesterol checked?"

- Distribute information that translates basic dietary principles for lowering high blood cholesterol into practical advice about eating patterns that can be sustained over a lifetime.

PARTNERSHIP IN THE NCEP

In carrying out its activities, the NCEP uses a partnership approach, building cooperative relationships with a variety of "intermediary" organizations (Fig. 9) to control elevated blood cholesterol through education of professionals, patients, and the public. These cooperating organizations are called "intermediaries" because they have constituencies they can reach, and thus expand the scope of the NCEP. Working with a wide range of organizations and associations—including professional associations, community groups, industry and business, voluntary organizations, and government agencies at the federal, state, and local levels—enables the NCEP to bring a powerful array of resources to bear in a concerted fashion on cholesterol reduction and to extend the reach of NHLBI efforts.

A salient example of partnership in action is the NCEP Coordinating Committee. It comprises representatives of over 20 national organizations that are involved in health and medical affairs and concerned with cholesterol education (Table VI). Federal agencies with cholesterol-related interests have liaison representatives on the Coordinating Committee, and representatives of industry and members of the

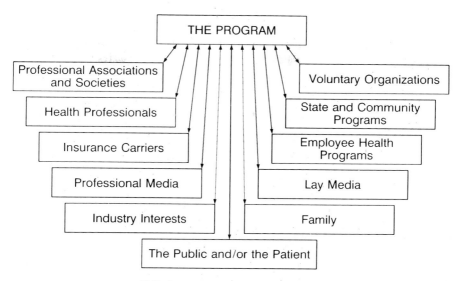

FIG. 9. The intermediary approach.

public attend the meetings and participate during the open forum portion of the agenda. The Coordinating Committee is the central body responsible for charting the course of the program. Its members address issues and suggest policies and strategies for the NCEP, and support the objectives of the program by carrying out activities through their organizations' own constituencies. With member organizations representing a spectrum of interests, the Coordinating Committee makes the NCEP a truly national effort and not just a federal program. If the NCEP is to succeed, it must be a broad-based endeavor that can generate enthusiasm and commitment at community, state, and national levels. The Coordinating Committee plays a crucial role in mobilizing the widest possible constituency for the NCEP.

TABLE VI. *NCEP Coordinating Committee: Member Organizations*

American Academy of Family Physicians	American Osteopathic Association
American Academy of Pediatrics	American Pharmaceutical Association
American Association of Occupational Health Nurses	American Public Health Association
American College of Cardiology	American Red Cross
American College of Physicians	Association of Black Cardiologists
American College of Preventive Medicine	Association of Life Insurance Medical Directors of America
American Dietetic Association	Association of State and Territorial Health Officials
American Heart Association	
American Hospital Association	Citizens for Public Action on Cholesterol
American Medical Association	National Black Nurses Association
American Nurses Association	National Heart, Lung, and Blood Institute
American Occupational Medical Association	National Medical Association
	Society for Nutrition Education

An important aspect of the NCEP's cooperative approach is the effort to build relationships with industry. The NHLBI staff met with representatives of the food, pharmaceutical, and medical devices industries before the NCEP was launched to obtain input about the directions of the program and to identify opportunities for collaboration. Such efforts are continuing and the Institute is gratified to see the extent of industry support for the educational thrusts of the NCEP.

NCEP ACTIVITIES

The initial activities of the NCEP are designed to establish the scientific base for the program and to deliver educational messages to health professionals and the American public. Surveys have repeatedly shown that the most frequently cited source of health information is the physician. Hence, a primary emphasis of the NCEP at this stage is on professional education. Some of the program's early initiatives are highlighted below:

1. Panels on treatment guidelines will inform physicians and other health professionals about the management of high blood cholesterol. The Expert Panel on Detection, Evaluation, and Treatment of High Blood Cholesterol in Adults (Adult Treatment Panel) issued guidelines in October 1987 dealing with detection and evaluation, diet therapy, and drug treatment. A second panel will be convened in 1988 to formulate recommendations on the management of high blood cholesterol in children. Yet a third panel is being formed to develop recommendations for reducing cholesterol levels in the general population.

2. A panel on laboratory standardization comprises representatives of the laboratory professions, government, and industry, and is developing recommendations to improve the accuracy and precision of laboratory cholesterol measurements. This effort is particularly important in light of the recommendation to treat all adults above a particular cutpoint, which requires that all laboratories produce comparable values for cholesterol measurements. The Laboratory Standardization Panel will also recommend standardized reporting of cholesterol values.

3. "Physician First" campaigns are being used to reach physicians with educational messages. The NCEP is cooperating and coordinating its efforts with two "Physician First" projects that are targeting physicians as one of the first audiences for cholesterol education. One, being conducted out of New York by the Science and Medicine group, is an extensive education project that will use a variety of media over a three-year period. A second project, being conducted at Johns Hopkins, is concentrated within a shorter time period and has offered physicians an opportunity to have their own cholesterol levels measured. Physician interest in these campaigns appears quite high. Officials of NHLBI sit on the advisory boards of these two projects.

4. "Cholesterol Counts" and a Continuing Medical Eduction (CME) module is another educational initiative. This effort centers on a booklet entitled "Cholesterol Counts," which distilled the experience of three physicians and two dietitians who participated in the CPPT. It provided interim guidance to professionals on the management of high blood cholesterol until the definitive guidelines from the Adult Treatment Panel became available. A CME module has been built around "Cholesterol Counts." The module has a loose-leaf format and is intended to be used in a self-study mode. It provides some of the classic articles in the literature and offers an overview of what is known today about cholesterol. "Cholesterol Counts" has been distributed to primary care physicians. The CME module is being distributed through the major physician organizations in the United States and will be updated to reflect the new guidelines for treatment of adults.

5. Public education is an early priority of the NCEP. Surveys have shown that, after the physician, the mass media are the most frequently cited source of health information. To educate the public about cholesterol, the NCEP media campaign is using television, radio, and print messages that are distributed nationwide. These public service announcements have a central theme: "Know your blood cholesterol number." The NCEP is encouraging the public to ask about blood cholesterol the next time they see their doctor; to have their level checked if this has not already been done; to know what their number or level is; and to learn whether this level is too high and needs to be reduced. The public (as well as health professionals) can also obtain information from the NCEP Information Center. One of the publications available is "Facts About Blood Cholesterol," which gives an introduction to the subject of cholesterol and answers some common questions. The program is currently developing nutrition-related brochures and a cookbook to provide advice about how to eat to lower elevated blood cholesterol levels.

6. Surveys of cholesterol awareness among physicians and the public will be repeated periodically by the NCEP as one means of monitoring the progress of the program. In addition, planning for a survey of nurses and dietitians is under way. If diet, the first line of treatment for high blood cholesterol, is to be successful, the expertise of nurses and dietitians will have to be applied in education and counseling. At present, however, we know too little about their cholesterol-related knowledge, attitudes, and practices. The planned survey will form an essential part of the information base for fully involving nurses and dietitians in cholesterol education and reduction.

CONCLUSIONS

Raising health professional and public awareness is a critically important element of the NCEP strategy for controlling elevated blood cholesterol. The program will succeed only if a wide range of organizations and individuals contribute their efforts to the national endeavor.

REFERENCES

1. Lipid Research Clinics Program. The Lipid Research Clinics Coronary Primary Prevention Trial Results. I. Reduction in incidence of coronary heart disease. *JAMA* 1984; **251**:351–364.
2. Lipid Research Clinics Program. The Lipid Research Clinics Coronary Primary Prevention Trial Results. II. The relationship of reduction in incidence of coronary heart disease to cholesterol lowering. *JAMA* 1984; **251**:365–374.
3. U.S. Department of Health and Human Services, Public Health Service. National Institutes of Health Consensus Development Conference Statement: Lowering Blood Cholesterol to Prevent Heart Disease. 1985; Vol. 5, Number 7.
4. Schucker B, Wittes JT, Cutler JA, *et al*. Change in physician perspective on cholesterol and heart disease: results from two national surveys. Submitted for publication February 1987.
5. Schucker B, Bailey K, Heimbach JT, *et al*. Change in public perspective on cholesterol and heart disease: results from two national surveys. Submitted for publication February 1987.

SUMMARY

If elevated blood cholesterol levels are to be controlled it is essential that health professionals and the public be fully aware of the importance of lowering raised serum cholesterol to reduce the risk of coronary heart disease. The National Cholesterol Education Program (NCEP) was launched in November 1985 by the National Heart, Lung, and Blood Institute in partnership with other major health and medical organizations with the goal of reducing the prevalence of elevated blood cholesterol in the United States. During 1986, the NCEP carried out cholesterol awareness surveys among physicians and the public. The results showed that between 1983 and 1986 there had been a significant change in cholesterol-related attitudes and practices among physicians and a strengthening of positive attitudes and practices among the public. At the same time, the study indicated that further improvements are necessary. It also highlighted a public lack of awareness about its own cholesterol levels and a lack of information as to how to translate basic dietary principles for lowering high blood cholesterol into practical advice about eating patterns that can be sustained over a lifetime. Some of the ongoing NCEP activities are described. These include developing and distributing detailed treatment guidelines for physicians and other health professionals, improving laboratory standardization of cholesterol measurement and several public and physician education initiatives.

RÉSUMÉ

Si l'on doit contrôler les niveaux élevés de cholestérol dans le sang il est essentiel que les médecins, les professionnels de la santé et le public soient pleinement conscients de l'importance qu'il y a à faire tomber les niveaux de cholestérol afin de diminuer les risques de maladies coronariennes. En novembre 1985, l'Institut Nationaux du Coeur, des Poumons et du Sang, en coopération avec d'autres organismes médicaux, ont lancé un programme d'enseignement et de formation: le "National Cholesterol Education Program," qui a pour objectif de réduire la prédominance des taux élevés de cholestérol dans le sang aux Etats-

Unis. Au cours de l'année 1986, le "National Cholesterol Education Program" a fait des sondages de prise de conscience des niveaux de cholestérol auprès des médecins et du public. Les résultats ont montré qu'entre 1983 et 1986 les médecins ont changé radicalement d'attitudes et de méthodes en ce qui concerne le cholestérol et que le public a également adopté une attitude plus positive et une mise en pratique. Mais en même temps, cette étude a montré qu'il était encore nécessaire d'améliorer ces résultats. Elle a aussi souligné l'ignorance générale des gens en ce qui concerne leurs propres niveaux de cholestérol ainsi qu'une absence de notions de diététique. Les gens ne savent pas comment modifier leur régime alimentaire afin de faire baisser leur niveau de cholestérol et adopter des principes de sélection alimentaire à observer toute leur vie. On décrit ici quelques-unes des activités actuelles du programme du "National Cholesterol Education Program." Celles-ci comprennent le développement et la distribution de conseils et indications détaillés de traitement auprès des médecins et d'autres professionnels de la santé, l'amélioration des processus de laboratoire pour mesurer les niveaux de cholestérol et plusieurs activités de formation et d'enseignement de notions auprès du public et des médecins.

ZUSAMMENFASSUNG

Wenn man erhöhte Blut-Cholesterin-Spiegel unter Kontrolle bringen will, ist es unbedingt nötig, daß Fachkräfte im Gesundheitsdienst und die Öffentlichkeit sich über die Wichtigkeit der Senkung von erhöhtem Serum-Cholesterin zur Verminderung des Risikos der koronaren Herzkrankheit bewußt werden. Das "Nationale Cholesterin-Schulungsprogramm" (NCEP) wurde im November 1985 durch die "Nationale Herz-, Lungen- und Blut-Institute" in Partnerschaft mit anderen wichtigen Gesundheits- und ärztlichen Organisationen ins Leben gerufen, mit dem Ziel der Reduzierung des Überhandnehmens des erhöhten Blut-Cholesterins in den Vereinigten Staaten. Im Laufe vom 1986 führte die NCEP Cholesterin-Kenntnis-Umfragen unter Ärzten und in der Öffentlichkeit durch. Die Resultate zeigten, daß zwischen 1983 und 1986 ein wichtiger Wechsel in der Haltung und in der Praxis gegenüber Cholesterin unter den Ärzten und eine Verstärkung von positiven Einstellungen und Praktiken unter der Öffentlichkeit eintrat. Gleichzeitig deutete die Studie darauf hin, daß weitere Verbesserungen nötig sind. Die Studie betonte außerdem, daß die Öffentlichkeit sich nicht über ihren eigenen Cholesterin-Spiegel bewußt ist und ein Mangel an Informationen betreffend die Frage wie man grundlegende Diätprinzipien zur Erniedrigung von hohem Blut-Cholesterin in praktische Ratschläge über Eßgewohnheiten, die lebenslang beibehalten werden kónnen, übersetzt. Einige der fortlaufenden NCEP-Tätigkeiten sind beschrieben. Diese schließen die Entwicklung und Verteilung ausführlicher Behandlungsrichtlinien für Ärzte und andere Fachkräfte des Gesundheitsystems und Verbesserung der Labormaßstabe für das Messen von Cholesterin und einige öffentliche und Arztschulungsinitiativen ein.

SOMMARIO

Se bisogna controllare gli alti livelli del colesterolo nel sangue allora è essenziale che professionisti e pubblico siano assolutamente al corrente dell'importanza di abbassare l' elevato colesterolo nel siero per ridurre il rischio della malattia coronaria del cuore. Il Programma Nazionale d'Istruzione sul Colesterolo (PNIC) è stato lanciato dagli Istituti Nazionali del Cuore, Polmoni e Sangue insieme con altre maggiori organizzazzioni mediche, sperando di ridurre l'alto livello del colesterolo nel sangue prevalente negli Stati Uniti. Durante il 1986, il PNIC ha condotto uno studio per medici e pubblico sulla consapevolezza del colesterolo. I risultati dimostrarono che fra l'83 e l'86 era avvenuto un cambiamento significativo in quanto agli atteggiamenti e alle pratiche del colesterolo fra i medici e un'rafforzamento di abitudini e atteggiamenti positivi fra il pubblico. Allo stesso tempo, lo studio indico la necessità di ulteriori miglioramenti. [Lo studio] dimostrò inoltre una certa mancanza, da parte del pubblico, verso il proprio livello di colesterolo e una mancanza d'informazione su come tradurre principi basilari dietari, far ridurre l'alto colesterolo nel sangue, tramite una dieta che puo' essere eseguita per tutta la vita. Alcune delle attività del PNIC sono descritte. Alcune di queste sono lo sviluppo e la distribuzione di dettagliate direzioni di cura per medici e altri professionisti, il miglioramento per misurare il livello del colesterolo nel laboratorio e alcune iniziative per l'educazione del pubblico e del medico.

SUMÁRIO

Se os níveis elevados de colesterol no sangue deviam ser controlados, é essencial que os profissionais da saúde e o público estejam completamente conscientes da importância de baixar os níveis elevados de colesterol no soro para reduzir o risco de cardiopátia coronária. O "National Cholesterol Education Program" (NCEP) (O Programa Nacional de Intrução sobre Colesterol) foi iniciado em Novembro de 1985 pelos Instituto Nacionais de Coração, Pulmoes e Sangue em associação com outras organizações médicas importantes com a meta de reduzir a prevalência de níveis elevados de colesterol no sangue nos Estados Unidos. Durante 1986, o NCEP realizou estudos sobre o conhecimento de colesterol entre os médicos e o público. Os resultados mostraram que entre 1983 e 1986 tinha havido uma mudança significativa nas atitudes e na prática em relação ao colesterol entre médicos, e um fortalecimento de atitudes positivas e hábitos entre o público. Ao mesmo tempo, o estudo indicou que mais progresso é preciso. Também realçou uma falta pública de conhecimento sobre os seus próprios níveis de colesterol e uma falta de informação como transferir os princípios básicos de regime alimentar para baixar níveis elevados de colesterol no sangue em informação prática sobre hábitos de alimentação que podem ser mantidos durante a vida tôda. Algumas das atividades atuais do NCEP são narradas. Estas contêm o desenvolvimento e a distribuição de normas detalhadas sobre o tratamento para os médicos e outros profissionais de saude, como melhorar a estandardização no laboratório da medição de colesterol, e algumas iniciativas públicas e de instrução para os médicos.

RESUMEN

Si vamos a controlar los niveles elevados de colesterol sérico es esencial que los profesionales de la salud y el público estén totalmente al tanto de la importancia de reducir el colesterol sérico para lograr una disminución en el riesgo de cardiopatía coronaria. En noviembre de

1985 se dio inicio al National Cholesterol Education Program—NCEP—(Programa nacional de educación sobre el colesterol) por parte del National Heart, Lung, and Blood Institute (Instituto Nacional del Corazón, Pulmones y Sangre) en colaboración con otras importantes organizaciones médicas y sanitarias, con el propósito de reducir la prevalencia de elevados niveles de colesterol sérico en los Estados Unidos. Durante 1986 el NCEP llevó a cabo encuestas para determinar el nivel de conocimientos sobre el colesterol entre los médicos y el público. Los resultados demonstraron que entre 1983 y 1986 había habido un cambio significativo en las actitudes y prácticas de los médicos con respecto al colesterol y un reforzamiento de las actitudes y prácticas positivas entre el público. Al mismo tiempo, el estudio indicó que se necesitaba mejorar aun más. También se subraya la falta de conocimiento del público en cuanto a los niveles personales de colesterol y falta de información con respecto a cómo transformar principios dietéticos básicos para reducir los niveles elevados de colesterol sérico en consejos prácticos que puedan mantenerse durante toda la vida. Se describen algunas de las actividades que actualmente lleva a cabo el NCEP. Entre éstas se incluyen el desarrollo y distribución de guías terapéuticas detalladas para médicos y otros profesionales de la salud, mejoría en la estandarización de los métodos de medición del colesterol en el laboratorio, así como varias iniciativas para educar al público y a los médicos.

The Role of Cholesterol in Atherosclerosis:
New Therapeutic Opportunities, edited by S. M. Grundy
and A. G. Bearn, Hanley & Belfus, Inc., Philadelphia.

Discussion

JULIAN: As far as the public and the medical profession are concerned the situation in Britain is very different from that in the United States. In the United Kingdom physicians are being driven by the public for more information about cholesterol and diet. There is a lack of conviction among physicians about the level of serum and cholesterol at which one should intervene and only about 5% of the population in the United Kingdom have had their serum cholesterol levels measured. Britain is often castigated for its high level of coronary disease and its failure to change, but in younger age groups (i.e., between 35 and 55 years of age) the mortality has fallen by about 25%, and is now lower than in the United States. But I think the fall in mortality requires further analysis—the situation is not as simple as it appears.

LASAGNA: The results of a Louis Harris survey, which asks if Americans avoid eating too much fat and high cholesterol foods such as eggs, dairy products, and fatty meats, show that the numbers have not changed much between 1983 and 1986.

LENFANT: These surveys are difficult to conduct. Sometimes the questions can be misleading and do not call for precise enough answers. If you look at the consumption of meat and eggs in the United States, it does not seem to have changed much in the last few years. However, the quality of the meat has changed from fatter to leaner meat; the Cattleman's Association in the United States is now producing meat containing much less fat than five years ago. The number of eggs consumed remains the same but there is evidence that only the white is eaten and not the yolks.

LASAGNA: I would agree about the change in beef. Now you can buy different grades of leanness of hamburger meat in local American supermarkets.

LENFANT: Meat must have at least 7% fat to be palatable and acceptable to the consumer. The fat content used to be as much as 20–25% but now you can buy meat with only 10–12% fat. The Department of Agriculture in the United States has changed the criteria for "prime beef" so there is a shift toward leaner meat. A program such as our National Cholesterol Education Program must have wide support from both the public and the food producer. Dietary educational changes must be presented not as a "punishment" but are intended to shift the emphasis from one food to another while still enjoying eating. It is also important not to cause political problems by dealing with the food producers in an adversarial fashion.

GRUNDY: There is a great interest in the United States now about altering beef and pork to a more favorable ratio of fat to protein and to improving the composition of fat by reducing saturated fatty acids.

JOHNSTON: In Australia some years ago a method was developed for making beef fat polyunsaturated. However, it was more expensive and after a market survey it was abandoned because the public was not prepared to bear the extra cost.

GRUNDY: I have served on a Committee of the National Academy of Sciences where we have looked at the different options for meat and animal products, and there will be a report available soon which was compiled by interviewing many different representatives of the beef and pork industries. The public wants a change in the quality of their meat and this will be the driving force in making it come about.

230

NORTH: Could we hear about sequential changes in mean serum cholesterol observed in the United States over the past 10 years?

LENFANT: We have some data from previous national surveys such as the Health and Nutrition Examination Survey. Blood cholesterol seems to have decreased in the American population, although these measurements may not have been performed with the rigor which we now think necessary. We are now committed to making further measurements of blood cholesterol in a National Survey of a cross section of about 60,000 people throughout the United States. These surveys will be repeated every three years—the next will be in 1989.

BAYLISS: What was the male/female ratio in the public surveys? I believe women in the United Kingdom are more aware than men, most likely due to the influence of women's magazines which are very potent in educating women, probably more effective than education pamphlets put out by the DHSS.

LENFANT: What you say is correct. Last year we put out a heart quiz that allowed people to assess their own knowledge about heart disease and what to do to prevent it. It was distributed to the media and was picked up mostly by women's magazines. The quiz was answered by about 42 million people in the United States, mostly women.

LANGMAN: I wonder why women respond to advice about diet but do not seem to modify their smoking habits in the same way, whereas men do respond to smoking advice.

DOLLERY: What is the legal and administrative framework for giving dietary advice in the United States? The dairy industry in Britain has been quite successful in preventing manufacturers of polyunsaturated fats such as margarines from making any kind of health claims in support of their products. Therefore it has been difficult to bring home to people through advertising that they should switch from butter or cream to polyunsaturated fats. Are there similar constraints in the United States?

LENFANT: Yes, but we can work with them. Any dietary information or recommendation coming from the Government has to be made or approved by the Department of Agriculture. However, the legislation regulating this advocates that there should be a combined effort between the Departments of Agriculture and Health. Our National Cholesterol Education Program is governed by a coordinating committee made up of representatives from 30–35 professional organizations. The Department of Agriculture participates in all the discussions. We also have representatives from the food industry and their trade unions. They understand what is going on and cooperate in implementing our recommendations. Next year we intend to have a National Cholesterol Conference for all the health professionals to review the current state of knowledge. To our surprise the representative of the Egg Producers of America offered to help finance this conference. Once or twice I have had to explain to Congress what we are doing but so far there have been no problems for us.

DOLLERY: You surprise me.

CORVOL: I am not surprised to find that physicians are involved in diet regulation because they are extremely motivated to undertake this job. What is your future strategy? Do you want to bypass the physicians and go direct to the public or do you wish to increase the involvement of the physicians in helping the patients in management of their lives?

LENFANT: We want to work with the physicians and hope to get them to see that dietary intervention is part of the therapeutic strategy. It takes more time than writing a prescription for drugs but we hope to succeed in persuading them to give dietary advice.

PYORALA: In Finland we have been able to follow changes in habitual diet and to some extent mean cholesterol levels since the 1960s. Finnish diet started to change before any organized public health education campaign, probably following the publicity that followed the Seven Countries Study results. Improved diet was reflected in the population's mean serum cholesterol levels from the beginning of the 1970s; since then coronary heart disease rates have been falling. Awareness of the problem and health education, however, are not enough and the agricultural, political and marketing policies should be developed in a better direction. I agree with Dr. Lenfant's point that it is important to work with the food producing and marketing circles if further achievements are to be made.

BEARN: Could we have some discussion about fish oils? Alex Leaf in Boston has some interesting data on fish oil, particularly that from fish in colder waters—the omega-3 fatty acids.

SMITH: There is great interest in this and now one sees Eskimos in television advertisements touting the benefits of omega-3 fatty acids! The NIH is making available a source of standardized fish oil high in eicosapentaenoic acid (EPA) and other essential polyunsaturated fatty acids to facilitate clinical trials. Trials are in progress to study the effects of fish oil capsules in patients post-PTCA, in whom there is a 20–30% probability of early occlusive disease in the region of the angioplasty.

LEWIS: It is important to distinguish between the epidemiology of fish consumption, which is quite consistently inversely related to coronary mortality, and the attribution of this relationship to omega-3 fatty acid intake, which I think is unproven and could even be a red herring! Omega-3 fatty acids are potent at lowering plasma triglyceride when consumed in large quantities. Except in very high intake, the majority of studies suggest that they neither lower LDL cholesterol nor increase HDL. Hence they may not fully explain the typical lipoprotein pattern of the Eskimos. So if they are important in preventing the complications of atherosclerosis, it is much more likely that the mechanism is related to changes in prostaglandin production.

LENFANT: In the United States a group at Vanderbilt University has undertaken to disprove the attribution to fish oil on the basis that the mechanism is not known.

LASAGNA: In some populations with a high consumption of fish the incidence of gastric cancer is higher.

LANGMAN: I do not think the evidence connecting gastric cancer with fish consumption is very good. The best correlations are with factors such as carbohydrate intake, and perhaps with smoked foods in some areas (but not in the United States). It tends to be impoverished populations such as Eastern Europeans with high carbohydrate diets who are at high risk.

GRUNDY: I think it is right to be cautious about recommending fish oils for the general public but we also have to recognize from the pharmacologic point of view that these oils contain very potent materials and that they do have many interesting metabolic effects. They need to be studied extensively because they may have more potential than we realize for affecting systems such as the immune system.

The Role of Cholesterol in Atherosclerosis:
New Therapeutic Opportunities, edited by S. M. Grundy
and A. G. Bearn, Hanley & Belfus, Inc., Philadelphia.

Roundtable 3: *Medical and Economic Implications of Lovastatin*

Chairman: Louis Lasagna
Panelists: C. Boyd Clarke, Pierre Corvol, Joel W. Hay, Michael J. S. Langman, John G. G. Ledingham, and Derek K. North.
Other Discussants: Alexander G. Bearn, Kalman C. Mezey, Claude Lenfant, Scott M. Grundy, and Barry Lewis.

This third roundtable discussion examined the medical and economic implications of the introduction of the new lipid-lowering drug, lovastatin. What is likely to be the physician's response to lovastatin? In whom will it be used and under what circumstances? What benefits will be derived? And, very importantly, does the reduction in serum cholesterol produced by the drug translate into a reduction in coronary events and coronary mortality?

WHEN SHOULD LOVASTATIN BE USED?

Physicians' attitudes toward cholesterol reduction were discussed in Roundtable 2. Dr. Ledingham continued the theme by considering what the attitude of the general physician in the U.K. might be toward lovastatin and when the drug might be used. Like Dr. Grundy, Dr. Ledingham felt that the age of the patient was important and that physicians would be more inclined to tackle hyperlipidemia seriously in younger patients. "Most clinicians in the United Kingdom are not inclined to intervene with regard to serum lipid levels in patients much over the age of 65 years, whereas they are beginning to intervene for patients in their 20s and early 30s," he said. "I am sure, despite Sir Richard's comments earlier (p. 231), that although women may be more aware of the importance of cholesterol, it is the men who require the attention by physicians, and so one would be more inclined to tackle the male sex at a given level of risk factor."

The question of diet versus drug was addressed in Roundtable 2. The general view was that dietary therapy and persuading patients to stop smoking were the first steps to take, but that these would not be sufficient in all patients, and indeed there might be considerable numbers of patients requiring drug therapy. Dr. Ledingham's comments supported this view. He continued: "I am sure we should be

233

trying to implement diet therapy in these patients first, but there will be a hard core of patients in whom diet cannot be applied or in whom it fails. Many patients will have heterozygous FH or familial combined hyperlipidemia, with a prevalence in the United Kingdom of about 1 in 500 and 1 in 300, respectively. So there may be about 1 in 200 patients in the younger age groups on lipid-lowering diets who will have serum lipid levels that may require drug intervention. If you look at the males only, it may be 1 in 400, but it could be a larger number." In practice, the actual numbers who may be given drug therapy will be much lower than that, since it cannot be assumed that all the affected individuals will be identified.

Professor Lasagna asked if Dr. Ledingham would consider whether a patient had already had a stroke, heart attack, or coronary bypass surgery in deciding whether to use drug therapy. Dr. Ledingham felt that, in such circumstances, it was likely— and not necessarily for very scientific reasons—that drug therapy would be offered. After such an event, said Dr. Ledingham, "the patient is very likely to ask his physician what he should do, and I think we should offer some sort of life-line."

Professor North said that in terms of primary prevention, he would, at present, choose to intervene with drug therapy at serum cholesterol levels of 300 mg/dl (7.8 mmol/L), coming down as he became more confident with its wider general use. Professor North continued, "It appeared from the economic data that if you had a serum cholesterol of 260 mg/dl (6.7 mmol/L), according to the Framingham data of low-risk patients, you would buy, on average, 9 months of life at the age of 37 years, or 2 months at ages in the 50s. This rises to 2 to 5 years in the high-risk group. So clearly significant gains could be made by using this drug if it proves to be safe."

MULTIPLE RISK FACTORS

In deciding which patients to treat, Dr. Ledingham stressed again the point first raised by Dr. Ganten in Roundtable 1; namely, the importance of multiple risk factors. "Their importance should not be ignored, but commonly is," said Dr. Ledingham. "The Framingham data showed that if there is only one risk factor the risk is minute in absolute and relative terms compared with if you have more than one. I think this cannot be overemphasized. Risk factors such as smoking, diabetes, hypertension, and male sex must all be taken into account more than they are at present. Obesity is probably less important."

IMPORTANCE OF SHOWING BENEFIT FROM DRUG THERAPY

The importance of showing benefit from lovastatin therapy has both medical and economic implications. From a medical standpoint, as Professor North and Professor Langman pointed out, the drug must be shown to be both safe and effective if physicians are to be persuaded to use it. From the economic standpoint, unless it can be shown that the reduction in serum cholesterol is accompanied by a concomitant decrease in CHD morbidity and mortality, it is impossible to make an economic assessment of the benefits. This last point was stressed forcefully by Professor Lasagna; he felt that many of the assumptions about benefit of lovastatin were yet to be proved.

The importance of conducting trials to establish the efficacy and safety of lovastatin was raised by Professor Dollery in Roundtable 2, something that both Professor Lasagna and Professor North supported. "I think it is important that Merck go ahead and conduct the studies to show that there is direct benefit from lovastatin therapy," said Professor North. "At present the only information that is available comes from Blankenhorn *et al.* and was published recently in *JAMA*.[1] They showed a reduction in serum LDL cholesterol of 41% and an increase in HDL cholesterol of 37%. They were able to show that 16% of patients who took the drugs (colestipol and nicotinic acid) had an improvement in the narrowing of their coronary arteries. This was a group that had already undergone coronary bypass surgery. More studies of this type would give the direct assurance that lovastatin is doing good, as well as just reducing the serum cholesterol. Once these data are available the commitment by physicians to the use of lovastatin will be greater." Dr. Bearn commented that a European double-blind placebo-controlled trial involving some 300 patients was planned. "It will examine atherosclerosis regression using central laboratory angiography," said Dr. Bearn. "Although this will take some time, such a trial should provide some very useful evidence on this point."

Professor Lasagna continued his argument that a more scientific basis needed to be adopted when trying to estimate benefit. He felt that it was reasonable to question whether a 1% drop in cholesterol actually produces a 2% fall in coronary events, a point that was raised earlier in the meeting (p. 175). "To begin with, there is no consistency about what is counted as a coronary artery event. Furthermore, I don't think that ratio follows just by dividing one number into another. For example, in blood pressure trials we don't divide the average drop in blood pressure into the average benefit and say that 1 mm Hg drop in blood pressure gives a certain benefit."

Dr. Grundy countered Professor Lasagna's criticism of the 1%–2% relationship by commenting on four clinical trials: the Lipid Research Clinics Coronary Primary Prevention Trial using cholestyramine; the WHO trial using clofibrate; the Coronary Drug Project using nicotinic acid; and the Oslo trial using polyunsaturated fat and a low fat diet. "In all of these trials the 1–2% relationship held good," said Dr. Grundy. "Starting out with hypercholesterolemic men, when cholesterol was lowered by, on average, 1%, it resulted in a 2% reduction in coronary events. So the data support that relationship: you might not believe it intuitively, and certainly there is a lot of individual variation, but if you take the data that exist and analyze them, that is what the results show." Professor Lasagna disagreed, saying that other data did not support this view.

Professor Lewis, however, felt that the predictive relationship between serum cholesterol, or any other continuous variable, and coronary heart disease may be underestimated. "There is reason to think that, in fact, the reported epidemiology attenuates the relationship," said Professor Lewis. "There is no basis for suggesting that it is exaggerated. That is because most longitudinal studies have been based on a single measurement, be it blood pressure, cholesterol or HDL. That single measurement has an error, and the error in the extremes of the distribution would tend to exaggerate the distribution, whereas the true distribution would have been narrower because of regression to the mean. Therefore, the slope of the predictive relationship would end up steeper than 2:1. This doesn't answer the problem of what happens during therapy, but at least the predictive relationship may be more powerful than we have been led to expect in the past."

Dr. Hay said that, interestingly, the Framingham risk estimates do not suggest a 1–2% rule. In fact smokers, who also have raised systolic blood pressures, can achieve 5–10 times as much benefit from cholesterol lowering as the 1–2% rule suggests over the cross-section. "Unfortunately," he continued, "the LRC study is the only prospective study that looks at that, and it was that study that came up with the 1–2% rule. If you use the Framingham data, it tends to be more conservative than the 1–2% rule for the typical average male member of the population, and yet it still suggests that there are substantial benefits from lowering cholesterol."

Professor Lasagna concluded this part of the discussion by saying that all the data support cholesterol as *a* factor in coronary artery disease, not *the* factor. "I would submit that making statements such as 'a 1% drop gives a 2% decrease in coronary disease' are oversimplified and quantitatively indefensible statements to make."

POST-MARKETING PROBLEMS

However rigorously a drug is tested during its clinical development, the drug and its manufacturers will face a number of problems in the post-marketing phase.

The question of side effects was introduced by Professor North. If the side effects of a drug are rare and nonspecific, then it is unlikely that sufficient numbers of patients will have been tested with that drug for the side-effect profile to develop prior to marketing. Such a situation seems likely to be the case with lovastatin. Professor North felt that it may take 4–5 years for lovastatin's side-effect profile to be fully developed. He agreed with Dr. Grundy's earlier comments that there will be progressive relaxation of attitudes as more people are treated for longer periods of time without evidence of serious adverse effects. "I am not concerned about the side effects observed so far," said Professor North. "I feel that liver changes are an acceptable risk since they are reversible and only appear to occur in about 2% of treated individuals."

Professor North continued, "To date, less than 1000 patients have received the drug for 1 year, so as yet there is no large data-base, and physicians will need to be cautious at first. When it comes to selecting on medical grounds the patients to treat, I think we should broadly be following the policy described by Dr. Ledingham in relation to multiple risk factors for CHD. I think the drive will come from the patients who have had a heart attack or known narrowing of the arteries for secondary prevention, and this demand will come at serum cholesterol levels that are considerably lower than those recommended for primary prevention.''

Another, unavoidable, problem was highlighted by Professor Langman, based on his own post-marketing experience with the H2-receptor antagonist, cimetidine. This problem stems from the fact that new drugs are more likely to be given to high-risk patients in the first instance, which can result in an excess mortality among treated patients during the early years. It may be difficult to convince people that this increased death rate is not caused by the drug itself.

Professor Langman described some parallels between lovastatin and cimetidine. ''First, the group who will receive the drug will be smokers and probably heavy drinkers, which was true of cimetidine. Second, it will be used fairly widely in practice, which was certainly true of cimetidine. In 1977 we started to collect data on 10,000 people treated with cimetidine. In the first year there were some 360 deaths, whereas the expectation in the population was half of that. So first we had to rebut the suggestion that this drug was actually killing people. This was relatively easy except in the area of cancer of the stomach and also cancer of the lung. It has taken 4 years for mortality to fall to population expectation, and we still do not believe that the drug was responsible for any of this mortality; it was all due to confounding factors.''

Professor Langman continued, ''If we transpose this situation to lovastatin, there will almost certainly be an excess mortality in the first year from CHD, because we will be selecting people who are at high risk. There will also be an excessive risk for cancer and an excess all-cases risk, which will be about a doubling. So in a 10,000 sample there may be 180 excess deaths, with at least 25 excess deaths from coronary heart disease (with, perhaps, an expectation of 50 and an observed of 75), and a 50% excess or more for cancer (with, say, 25 to 30 deaths when the expected figure is half that number). In the following year, however, instead of 180 excess deaths, the figure might be 100. In the third year that figure will perhaps fall to about 50 deaths, but it is only in the fourth year that it will drop to population expectation. At no point will we be able to see from post-marketing surveillance an apparent benefit. I don't believe this proves that the drug is a disaster. I think in a post-Opren world it means that it will be important to have some evidence of drug efficacy to set against these figures and to be able to say that we have reason to believe that the drug works and that we will not be put off by post-marketing surveillance. The effects we are seeing are those of confounding: they raise questions about the effectiveness of post-marketing surveillance, because against a background of commonly detected ordinary disease it will be difficult to detect drug-induced disease. Any pattern of increased morbidity or mortality which is detected during post-marketing surveillance will inevitably, and wrongly, be used to cast doubts on drug efficacy. It will, therefore, be all the more important to provide proper evidence of efficacy apart from indicating cholesterol-lowering effects.''

HOW RELIABLE ARE THE CHOLESTEROL MEASUREMENTS?

Professor Lasagna felt strongly that focusing excessively on serum cholesterol levels, while ignoring all sorts of other risk factors and other therapeutic modifications, was a mistake. He also questioned the accuracy of those cholesterol measurements. He quoted from a recent issue of the *Medical Letter*[2] which described a study conducted in 1985 by the College of American Pathologists. They sent out samples of blood, for which, according to the Centers for Disease Control (CDC), the correct value was 262 mg/dl (6.8 mmol/L). Samples were sent to over 100 laboratories. Laboratories using the DuPont machine reported values ranging from 222–270 mg/dl (5.8–7.0 mmol/L), whereas those using the Technicon ranged from 250–294 mg/dl (6.5–7.6 mmol/L). For all instruments and all laboratories using enzymatic methods the range of concentrations reported for a single specimen was 197–379 mg/dl (5.1–9.8 mmol/L). "Clearly," said Professor Lasagna, "the precision of measuring cholesterol leaves a lot to be desired and makes it difficult to detect correlations, even when they exist. I would use that fact as one argument against picking an arbitrary level of cholesterol as the cutoff point above which the drug should be used and below which the drug should not be used." Professor Lasagna was also concerned that a fixed cutoff level leads us to try to make some statement not only about what is abnormal but what is normal. "It is hard to agree on what is an abnormal serum cholesterol: it is even harder to agree on what is normal and on what might happen if you lower the level in someone who already has a 'normal' serum cholesterol," he concluded.

Dr. Lenfant said that Professor Lasagna was right to be concerned about the lack of reliability of measurements and equipment but felt that the problem applied only to certain population-based strategies that are being considered now in several countries. "This is particularly true in the United States," continued Dr. Lenfant, "where many organizations want to go out and do some population-based mass screening. However, it does not apply to the conclusions that have been discussed here for the last two days, because the studies that have been reported here have been based on measurements that were exceedingly carefully controlled against a standard. Therefore, I don't think there is any reason to question the reliability which has led to the conclusions that have been discussed here."

Dr. Lenfant continued, "At the National Heart, Lung and Blood Institute we are greatly concerned about the question of quality control of measurements, so much so, that at the present time we have deferred making any statement in favor of population-based strategy. For that we have taken a lot of flak from groups that are much more pressing and active than we are with regard to population-based strategies."

ECONOMIC IMPLICATIONS

What are the economic implications of an effective lipid-lowering drug that in turn decreases morbidity and mortality from CHD? Dr. Hay's presentation suggested that there could be considerable economic savings from reducing mortality in this way. As Professor Lasagna pointed out earlier, it must first be shown that there is a reduction in mortality. Dr. Ledingham felt that the economic implications were intangible, and referring to Dr. Hay's presentation commented that not enough attention was being paid to what hyperlipidemic patients were going to die of if they were no longer going to die of coronary disease. "The costs of long-term care of patients with Alzheimer's disease and other chronic diseases of old age must be far greater than those of, for example, coronary bypass surgery," he said.

Dr. Hay argued that in the young and middle-aged hyperlipidemic patients there was evidence from Framingham and elsewhere that this was not the case. These individuals, with primary manifestations of CHD, either fatal or non-fatal, do not have a very good prognosis. Within 5–8 years the cumulative survival is very low. Dr. Hay continued, "Both the economic model and the underlying Framingham risk models suggest that those are the people for whom intervention would be the most advantageous. Those people probably have relatively low risks of death from other types of disease, and so, again, everything suggests that intervention in the young to middle-aged adult male may be very effective."

Professor Lasagna pointed out that the most recent Framingham study also showed that after the age of 50, there is no increased overall mortality with either high or low serum cholesterol levels, and this risk factor is confounded by other factors. Dr. Hay responded that more recently, they had just started to include the HDL components into the risk assessments of people over the age of 50. "When this adjustment is made you see benefits of lowering cholesterol," he concluded.

In concluding this roundtable discussion, Professor Lasagna quoted from a letter to the _Lancet_[3] from Ancel Keys, a long-time proponent of the importance of serum cholesterol. "Most readers in the general public certainly will fail to note that over most of the range of serum cholesterol (in the MRFIT study), there was little or no relation between serum cholesterol and total mortality. I would be the last to argue against the importance of serum cholesterol; . . . but the MRFIT study . . . leaves unanswered most of the questions about the way to attack the coronary problem, and what can be expected from efforts to control the level of serum cholesterol in middle-age and later years."

Professor Lasagna warned the meeting against losing sight of the fact that risk factors other than a raised serum cholesterol contribute to the incidence and severity of coronary heart disease, and that other therapeutic modifications must also be employed in the management of these patients. Fortunately, the discussions that have taken place during this two-day meeting suggest that a much broader awareness of the problem prevails.

REFERENCES

1. Blankenhorn DH, Nessim SA, Johnson RL, _et al_. Beneficial effects of combined colestipol-niacin therapy on coronary atherosclerosis and coronary venous bypass grafts. _JAMA_ 1987; **257**:3233–3240.
2. Serum cholesterol determinations. _Med Lett_ 1987; **29**:41–42.
3. Keys A. Combined risk factors and coronary heart disease (letter). _Lancet_ 1987; **1**:812–813.

The Role of Cholesterol in Atherosclerosis:
New Therapeutic Opportunities, edited by S. M. Grundy
and A. G. Bearn, Hanley & Belfus, Inc., Philadelphia.

Future Approaches to Therapy for Dyslipidemia

Scott M. Grundy

A relation between abnormalities in plasma lipids and lipoproteins (dyslipidemia) and coronary heart disease (CHD) is well established. Clinical trials have shown that drug therapy of hypercholesterolemia will both prevent the progression of coronary atherosclerosis and decrease the risk for CHD. However, while we now have a solid rationale for cholesterol lowering, the application of this approach in clinical medicine remains to be developed. There are several areas in which opportunities exist for the development of new forms of therapy in dyslipidemia, and these are reviewed here.

SEVERE HYPERCHOLESTEROLEMIA

For patients with heterozygous familial hypercholesterolemia (FH) and other forms of severe primary hypercholesterolemia—serum cholesterol levels persistently at 300 mg/dl (7.8 mmol/L) and over with a corresponding elevation of LDL-cholesterol—the advent of HMG-CoA reductase inhibitors provides great promise for a major reduction in coronary risk. If these drugs prove to be safe, they can be used in most patients with severe forms of primary and familial hypercholesterolemia. Data so far available, however, indicate that treatment with reductase inhibitors does not completely normalize cholesterol levels for most patients in this category. There is, therefore, a need to use a combination of drugs for the more resistant patients. Nicotinic acid, for example, is effective and may be used with an HMG-CoA reductase inhibitor; but because of its many side effects, it is not a practical drug for many patients and other medications may be needed.

PRIMARY MODERATE HYPERCHOLESTEROLEMIA

Up to 20% of the adult population has primary moderate hypercholesterolemia, and the risk of developing CHD is increased 2–3 fold. Many investigators are skeptical that the powerful lipid-lowering drugs, such as HMG-CoA reductase inhibitors, will be appropriate for most patients in this group. The long-range side effects of these drugs have not yet been determined and therefore it is difficult to assess the risk/benefit ratio at this time: much more research is needed in this area. Clearly, diet therapy is indicated for patients with moderately elevated serum cholesterol levels (250–300 mg/dl; 6.5–7.8 mmol/L), but for those patients who remain hypercholesterolemic in spite of diet therapy, drug treatment should be considered.

241

Reductase inhibitors will normalize cholesterol levels in most patients of this type, and if these agents prove to be safe, their use in patients with primary moderate hypercholesterolemia who are unresponsive to diet can be given consideration.

An alternative approach would be to develop highly efficient drugs that act entirely within the intestinal tract to inhibit the absorption of either bile acids or cholesterol. Such drugs should not be absorbed and should therefore have a minimal toxicity. If such drugs can be developed, they could have widespread use in the treatment of primary moderate hypercholesterolemia.

HYPOALPHALIPOPROTEINEMIA

There is a firm association between low levels of high density lipoprotein (HDL) cholesterol and risk for CHD. The mechanism for this association is unknown. One of the most common causes of a low HDL cholesterol, however, appears to be a disturbance in the metabolism of triglycerides. Most patients with hypertriglyceridemia have low HDL cholesterol levels. It has yet to be proven that raising the HDL cholesterol level will prevent the development of atherosclerosis, although it is highly probable that this would occur. A fruitful area for future research, therefore, could be to develop new drugs that raise the HDL cholesterol concentration.

Diabetic Dyslipidemia

Diabetes mellitus, particularly non-insulin-dependent diabetes mellitus (NIDDM), is a strong risk factor for CHD. The mechanisms for the increased risk are not well understood, but abnormalities in plasma lipoproteins—very low density lipoproteins (VLDL), LDL, and HDL—probably contribute substantially to the acceleration of atherosclerosis in patients with NIDDM. To a moderate extent, control of hyperglycemia in patients with NIDDM will improve dyslipidemia. However, for most patients, perfect glycemic control is impossible to obtain, and consequently some degree of dyslipidemia will persist. If, however, the dyslipidemia could be eliminated by independent pharmacologic means, the coronary risk of diabetics should be substantially reduced. Studies in our laboratory suggest that HMG-CoA reductase inhibitors are one approach to controlling elevated cholesterol levels in diabetics. They are especially effective in reducing elevated levels of LDL. On the other hand, these drugs do not correct elevations of VLDL or reductions of HDL-cholesterol that are common in diabetic patients, and new pharmacological approaches are needed.

High-Risk Patients with Dyslipidemia

Patients with various forms of dyslipidemia who have other risk factors, for example, cigarettte smoking, hypertension, and established atherosclerotic disease, deserve special consideration. These patients are at high risk for primary or secondary coronary events, and any degrees of dyslipidemia only enhances their risk. They may be candidates for potent drugs, such as reductase inhibitors. Clinical trials of drug therapy in such patients could be especially valuable. There is a great opportunity to use pharmacologic therapy in high-risk patients because of the great size of this population and because of the danger associated with further progression of atherosclerosis.

SUMMARY

When the relationship between abnormalities in plasma lipids and lipoproteins and coronary heart disease was established, it became clear that opportunities existed for the development of new forms of therapy for dyslipidemia. The type of therapy required varies according to the severity and type of dyslipidemia. In severe hypercholesterolemia, the potent HMG-CoA reductase inhibitors are likely to prove the most appropriate form of therapy, and a combination of drugs may be needed. Such drugs may also be appropriate in moderate hypercholesterolemia, but diet therapy should be tried first. The possibility of developing alternative forms of therapy—highly efficient drugs that absorb bile acids or cholesterol—for the treatment of patients with moderate hypercholesterolemia is considered. The value of treating hypoalphalipoproteinemia (lowered HDL), diabetic dyslipidemia and other high risk patients with dyslipidemia is discussed.

RÉSUMÉ

Quand les rapports entre les anormalités dans les lipides plasmatiques et les lipoprotéines et les maladies coronariennes ont été établis, il est apparu évident que le moment était venu de se lancer dans le développement de nouvelles formes thérapeutiques pour le traitement de la dyslipidémie. La thérapie recommandée varie selon la gravité des types de dyslipidémie. Dand les cas d'hypercholestérolémie grave il est probable que les inhibiteurs puissants de réductase HGM-CoA seront à adopter, et dans ce cas il sera peu-être nécessaire de prescrire une association de plusieurs médicaments. De tels médicaments peuvent également convenir dans le traitement d'hypercholestérolémie modérée, mais la première chose à essayer est la modification du régime alimentaire. On examine ici la possibilité de développer d'autres formes thérapeutiques pour le traitement des malades atteints d'hypercholestérolémie modérée: à savoir le développement de médicaments très efficaces qui permettent l'absorption des acides biliaires ou du cholestérol. On discute de l'importance de traiter l'hypoalphalipoprotéinémie (lipoprotéines de forte densité en baisse), la dyslipidémie diabétique et les autres patients ̧a hauts risques atteints de dyslipidémie.

ZUSAMMENFASSUNG

Als das Verhältnis zwischen Abnormalitäten der Lipide und Lipoproteine im Plasma und koronarer Herzkrankheit festgestellt wurde, wurde es klar, daß Möglichkeiten für die Entwicklung von neuen Formen der Therapie für Dyslipämie existierten. Der Typ der benötigten Therapie variiert in Überstimmung mit der Schwere der Krankheit und dem Typ der Dyslipämie. Bei schweren Fäullen von Hypercholesterinämie sind die starken HMG-CoA Reduktase-Hemmer wahrscheinlich die geeignete Form der Therapie, und eine Kombination von Medikamenten kann angemessen sein. Diese Medikamente mögen ebenfalls im Falle von mittelmäßiger Hypercholesterinämie zuerst versucht werden. Die Möglichkeit der Entwicklung von alternativen Arten der Therapie—Behandlung mit sehr wirksamen Gallensäure-

oder Cholesterin-absorbierenden Medikamenten—für die Behandlung von Patienten mit mittelmäßiger Hypercholesterinämie ist berücksichtigt. Der Wert einer Behandlung von Patienten mit Hypoalphalipoproteinämie (erniedrigtem HDL) und anderen Patienten mit Dyslipämie, die sich in hohen Gefahr befinden, ist diskutiert.

SOMMARIO

Quando fu stabilita la relazione fra le anormalità dei lipidi del plasma, delle lipoproteine e delle malattie coronarie del cuore, si evidenziò un'opportunità per lo sviluppo di nuove forme di terapia per la dislipidemia. Il tipo di terapia necessaria varia assecondo della gravità e del tipo di dislipidemia. In caso di severa ipercolesterolemia, i potenti inibitori di riduttasi HMG-CoA sarebbero probabilmente la terapia piú appropriata, e potrebbe anche servire una combinazione di medicine. Tali medicine potrebbero essere appropriate anche nel caso di un'ipercolesterolemia moderata, anche se in questo caso si dovrebbe inizialmente povare con una terapia dietetica. Viene considerata la possibilità di sviluppare forme alternative di terapia—efficacissime medicine che assorbino gli acidi della bile o del colesterolo—per la cura di quei pazienti con ipercolesterolemia moderata. Viene inoltre discussa l'importanza di curare l'ipoalfalipoproteinemia (minore LAD), la dislipidemia diabetica e altri pazienti di maggior rischio con dislipidemia.

SUMÁRIO

Quando a relação entre anormalidades nos lípidos no plasma e nas lipoproteínas e a cardiopátia coronária foi estabelecida, ficou claro que oportunidades existiam para o desenvolvimento de novas formas de terapia para dislipidemia. O tipo de terapia exigida varia conforme a severidade e o tipo de dislipidemia. Em hipercolesterolemia severa, os inibidores potentes da HMG-CoA-reductasa são capazes de ser a forma de terapia mais apropriada, e uma combinação de remédios pode ser necessária. Tais remédios podem ser apropriados em hipercolesterolemia moderada mas uma terapia de regime alimentar deve ser tentada primeiro. A possibilidade de desenvolver formas alternativas de terapia—remédios altamente eficientes que absorvem ácidos biliares ou colesterol—para o tratamento de pacientes com hipercolesterolemia moderada é considerada. O valor de tratar hiperalfalipoproteinemia (HDL baixada), dislipidemia diabética e outros pacientes de alto risco com dislipidemia é examinado.

RESUMEN

El descubrimiento de la relación existente entre las anormalidades en los lípidos plasmáticos y las lipoproteínas y la cardiopatía coronaria, creó una oportunidad para desarrollar nuevas formas de tratamiento de la dislipidemia. El tipo de tratamiento requerido varía de acuerdo a la severidad y tipo de dislipidemia. En los casos de hipercolesterolemia severa, los potentes inhibidores de la HMG-CoA-reductasa probablemente van a demostrar que son la forma más apropiada de tratamiento, y podría ser necesaria una combinación de fármacos. Tales fármacos también podrían ser apropiados en los casos de hipercolesterolemia moderada, pero primero se debe probar un tratamiento dietético. Se considera la posibilidad de desarrollar formas alternativas de tratamiento—fármacos muy eficaces que absorban los ácidos biliares o el colesterol—para el tratamiento de pacientes con hipercolesterolemia moderada. Se discute el valor del tratamiento de la hipoalfalipoproteinemia (reducido nivel de HDL), dislipidemia diabética y de pacientes con riesgo elevado de dislipidemia.

The Role of Cholesterol in Atherosclerosis:
New Therapeutic Opportunities, edited by S. M. Grundy
and A. G. Bearn, Hanley & Belfus, Inc., Philadelphia.

Roundtable 4: *Future Areas of Clinical and Scientific Opportunity: Genetic Predisposition/DNA Probes*

Chairman: D. Keith Peters
Panelists: Detlev Ganten, Scott M. Grundy, Barry Lewis, Kalevi Pyörälä, Eve E. Slater, and Thomas W. Smith.
Other Discussants: Hiroo Imura, Colin T. Dollery, Robert W. Mahley, and Alexander G. Bearn.

By the opening of the final roundtable discussions, an impressive body of information had already been presented on the role of cholesterol in atherosclerosis and on ways of treating hyperlipidemia, with particular emphasis on pharmacologic intervention using new lipid-lowering drugs such as lovastatin. But it became clear from the discussions in this roundtable that scientific and clinical research in the field of molecular pathology and genetics is really only just beginning, and some very exciting prospects lie ahead. A number of general comments made by some of the panelists are worth emphasizing at this stage, since they tie in with many of the questions raised throughout this meeting—in Professor Lewis's words, "who to treat, when to treat and how to treat."

Dr. Pyörälä pointed out that the effective reduction of cholesterol levels through diet would mean that the influence of genetic abnormalities would become more obvious and by implication more important.

Dr. Ganten emphasized that the future for more appropriate treatment of atherosclerosis must be based on a better understanding of the underlying genetics and molecular pathophysiology. By defining patients who will respond to diet and different sorts of treatment, indiscriminate therapy could be avoided.

Many questions remain unanswered. Dr. Smith said that over the past 20 years, our views about cholesterol levels have chiefly been in terms of the inexorable accumulation of atheromatous material in vessels, leading to gradual occlusion. What influences the transition from a stable, atheromatous plaque to an unstable lesion that will produce thrombosis? Work currently under way in Dr. Smith's and also in Dr. Cotran's laboratory may, in the future, provide the answers. Dr. Grundy pointed out that although considerable advances have been made in our understanding of the causes of severe hypercholesterolemia, for example heterozygous FH, almost nothing is known about the causes of moderate hypercholesterolemia, which

245

affects the bulk of the hypercholesterolemic population. "We think it might have something to do with LDL receptors, but we don't know what is wrong with the receptors, why they are down-regulated, or whether there are post-translational modifications in the receptor. We don't know what is wrong with the apolipoproteins, or their regulation or production rates. There is a vast area for research," Dr. Grundy concluded.

Some of the inroads, in molecular pathological terms, that have been made into this area were outlined in short presentations by Dr. Mahley and Professor Lewis. First, the scene for this discussion was set by the Chairman, Professor Keith Peters: "We are dealing with a group of diseases whose genetic basis is varied. There is a multiplicity of defects affecting the LDL receptor, affecting the lipoproteins, and affecting enzymes involved in lipid metabolism; and we have heard of the influence of a variety of environmental factors. The consequences are abnormalities of blood lipids, mostly crudely indicated by elevation of blood cholesterol. We have heard that such hyperlipidemia creates predisposition to the development of a complicated disease process in which changes occur in the blood vessel wall characterized by lipid deposition and thrombosis. And we have heard from Dr. Smith that there is a non-linear relation between blood vessel disease of this kind and critical stenosis of the lumen. There are, therefore, many factors that potentially influence the relationships between genetic predisposition and clinically important organ dysfunction presenting much later in life. To a practicing clinician, concerned with disease, there are three questions—who to treat, when to treat, and how to treat. In this connection we should ask whether the spectacular advances in the molecular genetics of these disorders are proving to be clinically useful and we need to turn to the epidemiologists to inquire whether what might be termed "molecular epidemiology" can help us define better the relationship between genetic changes and the diseases they subtend."

THE MOLECULAR PATHOLOGY OF PREMATURE CORONARY ARTERY ATHEROSCLEROSIS

Dr. Mahley outlined the extent of our understanding of the structure and function of the apolipoproteins and of LDL receptor activity in terms of amino acid sequence and gene structure. Mutations have been observed in both apolipoprotein (apo-) B and apo-E and the LDL receptor. Dr. Mahley discussed how these might be responsible for elevations in plasma cholesterol. He pointed out that we are now rapidly moving beyond the simple measurement of blood total cholesterol and HDL-cholesterol toward an understanding of the effects of a limited number of genes on the development of premature heart disease.

"The LDL receptor regulates the plasma cholesterol level by mediating the uptake of specific lipoproteins (for review, see Brown and Goldstein, *Science* 1986; **232**:34). Apolipoprotein E is the mediator protein for the uptake of remnant lipoproteins, including chylomicrons of intestinal origin and very low density lipoproteins (VLDL) of hepatic origin. Apolipoprotein B mediates LDL uptake. The LDL receptor has a short cytoplasmic tail in which specific mutations can alter the way the receptor functions. A single substitution impairs the internalization of the receptor. There is a membrane-spanning region and then an extracellular region that show remarkable amino acid sequence homology with the epidermal growth factor precursor, which, according to Goldstein and Brown, is an important "spacer" region. There is also a ligand binding domain responsible for interacting with apo-B and apo-E. This region contains numerous cysteine residues and seven repeated sequences that appear to be important in binding the ligands. There are about a dozen different mutations that Russell, Goldstein, Brown, and their associates have identified, with varying effects on function. One result is the production of no protein at all—a receptor-negative phenotype. Another type of mutation deletes an entire repeated ligand binding domain, and the LDL will not bind, whereas apo-E-containing lipoproteins do bind. Several other specific mutations are being identified, and they continue to shed light on the function of specific regions of the LDL receptor. As we learn more about the structure of the LDL receptor and the regulation of its gene, I think we will find some patients with moderate or mild hypercholesterolemia who have more subtle changes in the LDL receptor which allow an elevation in plasma cholesterol and have a predisposition for premature heart disease.

"A considerable amount is known about apo-E and its structure and function (for review, see Mahley and Innerarity, *Biochim Biophys Acta* 1983; **737**:197, and Mahley *et al.*, *J Lipid Res* 1984; **25**:1277). Apolipoprotein E3 is the parent form, and there are two major variant forms, E4 and E2, that have different impacts on plasma cholesterol levels. Apolipoprotein E is secreted as a 299-amino acid protein (Fig. 1). The gene structure is known, and the promoter elements are being mapped.

"We know that the region of apo-E responsible for binding to the LDL receptor residues is in the vicinity of amino acid residues 140 to 160. There are four variants that occur in the human population that affect receptor binding activity. They include single amino acid substitutions occurring at residues 142, 145, 146, and 158 and involve neutral amino acids being substituted for either arginine or lysine residues (Fig. 2). It is now possible to use site-directed mutagenesis to map further the key residues important in mediating apo-E binding to the lipoprotein receptors. Figure 3 shows the region of apo-E that is important in binding apo-E-containing lipoproteins to the receptor.

"The structure of apo-B has been determined in the last few months (Fig. 4) (Knott *et al.*, *Nature* 1986; **323**:734). Apolipoprotein B is a very large protein composed of 4563 amino acids with a molecular weight of 550,000, and there is one molecule of apo-B per LDL particle. The gene has been mapped in our laboratory, and is 43 kilobases in length (Blackhart *et al.*, *J Biol Chem* 1986; **261**:15364). The promoter is presently being studied.

"As a natural extension of our studies designed to map the receptor binding domain of apo-E, we have been trying to define the receptor binding domain of apo-B. Most of the data indicate that there are two relatively small regions, each composed of a dozen amino acids or so, that may be responsible for mediating

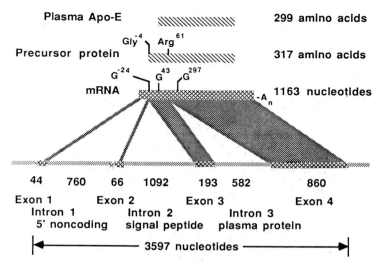

FIG. 1.   Structure of human apolipoprotein E gene, mRNA, and mature protein.

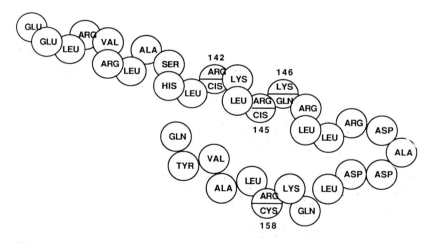

FIG. 2.   Region of apo-E involved in mediating its binding to the LDL receptor.

Apo-E
(residues 140-150)   -His-Leu-Arg-Lys-Leu-Arg-Lys-Arg-Leu-Leu-Arg-

Apo-B,E (LDL)   Cys-**Asp**-X-X-X-**Asp**-Cys-X-**Asp**-Gly-Ser-**Asp**-**Glu**-
receptor

FIG. 3.   Receptor binding domain of apo-E and the postulated ligand binding domain of the
LDL receptor.

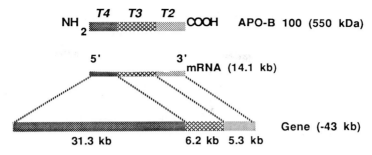

FIG. 4.   Apolipoprotein B100 gene, mRNA, and mature protein.

apo-B binding to the LDL receptor (Fig. 5). The sequence of these two regions is shown in Figure 6. There is a striking homology with the receptor binding domain of apo-E.

"It is certainly possible that there are numerous mutations of apo-B that could be responsible for elevated plasma cholesterol levels. At present we are studying a family that we believe to be the first such individuals with a recognized mutation of apo-E (Innerarity *et al.*, *Proc Natl Acad Sci USA* 1987; **84**:6919), possibly a mutation within one of these two regions (Fig. 6). The LDL from the affected individuals does have abnormal receptor binding activity, and, in fact, it may have zero ability to bind to the LDL receptor. We believe there are many more patients to be discovered with abnormal apo-B structure."

Professor Peters asked whether there was any relationship between the molecular configuration of either the apoproteins or the receptors and the capacity of macrophages to clear up cholesterol from sites of deposition.

Dr. Mahley responded: "Yes. We are beginning to appreciate that the structure and function of the LDL receptor could be modulated differently in different cells, to alter the way cells handle lipoprotein cholesterol delivered via the different ligands (either apo-B or apo-E). In the macrophage, the uptake of diet-induced lipoproteins (so-called β-VLDL) is mediated by apo-E. The β-VLDL cause a marked cholesterol accumulation in macrophages. On the other hand, LDL (uptake mediated by apo-B) do not have that effect. Thus, there may be discrimination at the level of the

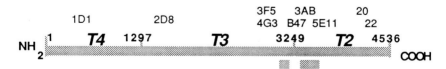

FIG. 5.   Epitopes of apo-B monoclonal antibodies that inhibit LDL binding to the receptor. The location of the two putative binding sites is indicated by the bars. As can be seen, these regions are located near the carboxyl terminus of the apo-B molecule. (See Knott *et al.*, *Nature* 1986; **323**:734, for a more complete discussion of the data.)

Apo-E	-His- X -Arg-Lys- X -Arg-Lys-Arg- X - X -Arg-
Apo-B	- X - X -Arg- X - X -Arg-Lys-Arg- X - X -Lys-
Apo-B	-His-Arg -His-Lys- X -Lys-Lys- X - X - X -Lys-
Apo-B,E (LDL) receptor	-**Asp**- X - X - X -**Asp**-Cys- X -**Asp**-Gly-Ser-**Asp**-**Glu**-

FIG. 6. Comparison of the possible receptor binding domains of apo-B and apo-E. An ionic interaction of the ligands with the binding domain of the LDL receptor has been postulated.

receptor, at the level of the ligand mediating the uptake of the lipoproteins, or at the level of regulation of intracellular cholesterol metabolism.''

Dr. Slater expressed her hope that investigators would be able to refine hyper-cholesterolemia therapies based upon genetic classifications. Sudhof et al.[1] have identified a short segment, 42 base pairs, of the 5'-flanking region of the human LDL receptor gene, which appears to mediate its expression by sterols. Perhaps one could find a drug molecule that interacts at the segment, which would up-regulate the receptor. So far, however, there is no precedent for small molecules acting at the level of gene expression with the specificity that would be required for such a drug.

EPIDEMIOLOGY OF GENETIC POLYMORPHISMS

Professor Peters asked whether we can address epidemiological questions with such genetic tools as those described by Dr. Mahley.

Professor Lewis replied: ''There have been reports in the last year of studies of polymorphisms of Apo-B and their association with coronary heart disease. There seems to be a geographical variation in these associations which is not entirely consistent in different reports. On the other hand, the more familiar polymorphism of Apo-E has an association with coronary heart disease and with LDL-cholesterol. There are two forms of variation of serum cholestrol among normal subjects. First, there is a considerable variation in mean levels between different populations. Much of this is due to diet, and the role of the environment is underlined by rapid changes among population groups during migration to a country with a contrasting life-style. But there is also evidence that the prevalence of polymorphic forms of apolipoproteins differs in different countries, and this may explain a small part of the interpopulation variation. Within populations there is also a wide variation between individuals. This is explained only to a small extent by dietary differences, but genetic factors are likely to play a much larger role. These two forms of variation and their determinants are important since they underlie a wide variation in the risk of coronary heart disease.''

Professor Lewis continued, ''We have studied the role of a particular poly-morphism of Apo-B, described by the Xba1 restriction enzyme, in subjects randomly recruited from a general practice list in Sheffield. The fractional catabolic rate of

LDL, the production of LDL, and the degradation *in vitro* of LDL by blood lymphocytes were examined in relation to this polymorphism. It looks as though the mechanism for the variation in serum cholesterol described by this restriction fragment length polymorphism in Apo-B is mediated by differences in the fractional catabolic rate of LDL, which is highest in those subjects with the lowest levels of LDL-cholesterol. If we know the Xba1 typing of Apo-B, we can explain about 40% of the variance of LDL fractional catabolism in this population. This may, however, prove to be only a small component of within-population variation. There may be differences in amino acid sequence in Apo-B that influence the ligand binding by the LDL receptor and ultimately influence plasma cholesterol level. We were intrigued because Dr. Grundy has described a minority of patients with moderate hypercholesterolemia in whom normal LDL showed normal fractional catabolism but the patients' own LDL showed impaired fractional catabolism. In some of these families a polymorphism of Apo-B such as we have identified may account for the impaired metabolism. This disorder may, therefore, be one kind of common moderate hypercholesterolemia.

"Variation within a population may also be due to variation in the responsiveness to a given dietary milieu. Individuals are consistent in their plasma cholesterol responsiveness to the challenge of a change in the intake of dietary cholesterol, as Katan and colleagues have found. We have observed, in collaboration with Katan, that hyper-responders to dietary cholesterol differ from hypo-responders in the extent to which LDL production is stimulated by this dietary change. While this has not, as yet, been shown to be genetically determined in man, there is no doubt that hyper-response is an inherited characteristic in laboratory animals."

Dr. Pyörälä commented: "With regard to the distribution differences of Apo-E polymorphisms in the population, we will apparently soon have data for calculations as to how far these differences could explain cholesterol distribution differences between populations. It looks as though they would not explain great differences in the mean values between populations, but they may affect the upper tail of the distributions.

"In populations in whom, due to changes in the habitual diet, cholesterol levels are shifting downward, the influence of genetic abnormalities on the shape of the upper end of the distribution may become more clearly evident. Those individuals who do not respond well to diet may be the subgroup in whom we have to look for those genetic markers."

GENETIC POLYMORPHISMS IN JAPAN

In his presentation, Professor Imura had commented on the fact that the incidence of coronary heart disease in Japan is still considerably lower than in the United States, even though there is now very little difference in their respective serum cholesterol levels. The significance of genetic polymorphism, within a population, and genetic differences between countries is, therefore, of particular interest.

Professor Dollery asked what is known about the prevalence of genetic polymorphisms in Japan. "Historically, the Japanese with their low serum cholesterol
level, have had a low incidence of coronary disease. You could argue that if they
have a similar distribution of lipoprotein/LDL receptor polymorphisms, such polymorphisms do not matter if you keep the serum cholesterol low enough."

Professor Imura replied that the studies in Japan showed some differences in
restriction fragment length polymorphisms in the Apo-AI-CIII gene. The phenotype
of Apo-E has also been studied. The differences are mainly that E3/3 is higher in
Japanese (more than 70%), and E2/E2, E3/E2 and E4/E2 are lower. "I think there
may be a difference in Apo-E and Apo-AI-CIII genes," said Professor Imura.

Professor Peters asked what contribution polymorphism of Apo-E makes to the
presence of hypercholesterolemia in the Western world from which the importance
of the Japanese information could be assessed.

The incidence of various alleles is presented in Dr. Mahley's chapter (pp. 175).
Dr. Mahley explained: "In Western populations, the apo-E4 allele occurs in about
20% of individuals. I do not know its level of occurrence in the Japanese. However,
the apo-E phenotypes of plasma samples sent to us from Japan have revealed some
abnormal forms of apo-E which we have not seen in any other population." He
continued, "Dr. Slater referred to a small molecule that might modulate gene
function directly. However, as the field continues to study the structure and function
of the promoter regions for the LDL receptor, apo-E, and apo-B genes, various
positive and negative regulatory elements will be defined. We may be able to study
not only small molecules that may interact directly, but also molecules that modulate
the different regulatory proteins to up-regulate and down-regulate these genes."

CELLULAR PATHOPHYSIOLOGY OF ATHEROSCLEROSIS

Dr. Smith commented on some of the recent advances in the understanding of
atherosclerosis at the cellular level. "We have thought, over the last couple of
decades, about cholesterol levels chiefly in terms of the inexorable accumulation
of atheromatous material in vessels, leading to gradual occlusion and eventually
some untoward outcome when the vessel reaches a critical degree of stenosis. The
work that is currently being performed in Dr. Cotran's department and also in ours
is representative of exciting cell biology regarding vascular smooth muscle cells
and their interaction with endothelial cells, the biology of the macrophage, and the
effects of agents such as interleukins that may influence the transition from a stable
atheromatous plaque to an unstable lesion that will produce thrombosis. We are
only just beginning to learn about the ways whereby a patient with stable angina
or even an asymptomatic patient makes the transition from such a stable to unstable
angina or acute myocardial infarction."

"Lipoproteins are likely to be important in this process as well as in their influence
on the accumulation of atheromatous plaques in vessels. We have shown, for
example, that cardiac myocytes cultured in the presence of lipoprotein-depleted

serum change their receptor properties. Lipoprotein-depleted serum has a pronounced effect on the expression of muscarinic cholinergic receptors and also fast sodium channels in cardiac myocytes.

"Returning to the clinical level, I think that the importance of stratification of patients deserves emphasis. Stratification for genotype will become increasingly important, along with LDL, HDL and LP(a) levels, gender, age, weight, smoking history, carbohydrate tolerance, blood pressure, family history, platelets and clotting factors, and perhaps fatty acid content of the diet—and this is only a partial list."

INDEX

Page numbers in **boldface type** indicate chapters or major discussions.